Pediatric Hematology

A Practical Guide

D1334241

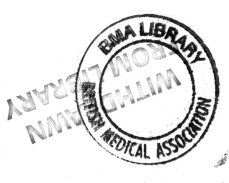

Pediatric Hematology

A Practical Guide

Edited by

Robert Wynn
University of Manchester and Royal Manchester Children's Hospital, Manchester,
United Kingdom

Rukhmi Bhat
Northwestern University's Feinberg School of Medicine and the Ann & Robert H. Lurie
Children's Hospital, Chicago, Illinois

Paul Monagle
University of Melbourne and Royal Children's Hospital, Melbourne, Australia

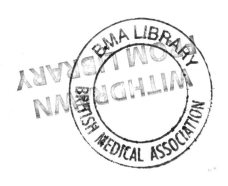

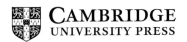

CAMBRIDGE
UNIVERSITY PRESS

CAMBRIDGE
UNIVERSITY PRESS

University Printing House, Cambridge CB2 8BS, United Kingdom

Cambridge University Press is part of the University of Cambridge.

It furthers the University's mission by disseminating knowledge
in the pursuit of education, learning and research at the highest
international levels of excellence.

www.cambridge.org
Information on this title: www.cambridge.org/9781107439368

First published 2017

Printed in the United Kingdom by Clays, St Ives plc

A catalog record for this publication is available from the British Library

Library of Congress Cataloging-in-Publication Data
Names: Wynn, Robert F. (Robert Francis), editor. | Monagle, Paul T.,
editor. | Bhat, Rukhmi, editor.
Title: Pediatric hematology : a practical guide / edited by Robert Wynn,
Paul Monagle, Rukhmi Bhat.
Other titles: Pediatric hematology (Wynn)
Description: Cambridge, United Kingdom : Cambridge University
Press, [2016]
Identifiers: LCCN 2016022434 | ISBN 9781107439368 (Paperback)
Subjects: | MESH: Hematologic Diseases | Child
Classification: LCC RJ411 | NLM WS 300 | DDC 618.92/15–dc23 LC
record available at https://lccn.loc.gov/2016022434

ISBN 978-1-107-43936-8 Paperback

Contents

Contents

Preface

This book is for all those who have contact with pediatric hematology – medical students, doctors-in-training, nurses, pharmacy staff, and patients and their families. We, as clinicians and here as authors, spend much of our time explaining the principles and practice of our subject, making it easy to understand. This book summarizes that teaching.

Each chapter covers a single area of our subject and follows a standard format, including a summary of the key disease-related points. Understanding the chapter will allow the student or practitioner to understand his or her patient, the family to understand better the illness affecting their child, and the exam candidate to deal with pediatric hematology to a postgraduate level (with the book chapters mirroring international exam syllabuses).

There are separate clinical scenarios that detail the practical management of several common hematologic situations, including newly diagnosed leukemia and its emergency situations, the child with pancytopenia, and the child with neutropenia and fever. These scenarios complement the didactic chapters, encouraging readers to manage effectively the more common problems in both a patient- and problem-oriented manner.

Normal Hematopoiesis and the Physiology of Blood

Key Messages

1. Cellular elements of blood are produced predominantly in the bone marrow during extrauterine life.

2. Blood cells are constantly renewed (in predictable time frames), so the bone marrow is very metabolically active.

3. The bone marrow environment is complex, and the release of blood cells from the bone marrow stroma is controlled by multiple adhesion molecules.

4. Pluripotent stem cells are capable of self-renewal and differentiation into all hemopoietic cell lines.

5. Hematopoietic growth factors drive the production and differentiation of all blood cell lineages.

6. Iron, vitamin B_{12}, and folate are essential hematinics required for blood cell production.

7. Hemoglobin is the essential component within red blood cells that carries oxygen.

8. The principal function of red blood cells is oxygen delivery. Tissue oxygen delivery is a function of cardiac output, hemoglobin concentration, and oxygen saturation levels.

9. White blood cells have multiple roles in inflammation, immunity, and wound repair.

10. Platelets are predominantly involved in primary hemostasis.

11. The vascular endothelium is a dynamic interactive surface that in combination with the blood vessel walls contributes significantly to many aspects of blood flow and function.

Introduction

Blood is the essential transport system that enables life in large multicellular, multiorgan animals. Without blood flow, there is no life, and arguably the most important element being transported is oxygen, which requires hemoglobin contained within red blood cells (RBCs). The ability to deal with infection and make an adequate inflammatory response to challenges depends on the white cell fraction of blood, which can transition rapidly into specific tissues as required. The requirement for blood to flow, and hence remain fluid, requires significant infrastructure and mechanisms to deal with inevitable breaches of the vascular endothelium. The function of the hemostatic system will be dealt with in Chapter 2. Diseases of almost every other organ can have an impact on blood, and conversely, diseases of blood can produce symptoms related to almost every other organ system. Understanding normal hematopoiesis and the physiology of normal blood is therefore essential to all healthcare professionals.

The Site of Blood Production

In the early weeks of embryonic life, blood cells are produced within the yolk sac. From approximately 6 weeks through 7 months of gestation, the predominant sites of blood production are the liver and spleen. The bone marrow becomes the main production site of blood from 7 months of gestation onward. Initially, in infants, the active bone marrow is located throughout most axial and long bones of the skeleton, but there is progressive fatty replacement of marrow throughout life, with constriction of the active bone marrow toward the axial skeleton. By early adult life, active bone marrow is mostly restricted to the skull, sternum, vertebrae, ribs, and pelvis. Even in sites of active hemopoiesis, the bone marrow consists of approximately 50 percent fat spaces. Active bone marrow has a relatively high blood flow and is functionally in continuity with blood.

Clinical Implications

1. The reticuloendothelial system (liver and spleen) can be re-recruited for hemopoiesis during childhood in cases of bone marrow replacement or clonal disease. Hence, hepatosplenomegaly is commonly a feature of diseases of the hemopoietic system.
2. Bone marrow examination is usually performed by accessing the marrow space in the pelvis via the posterosuperior iliac spine. However, in infants, the tibia can be used.
3. The use of intraosseous injection of fluids or drugs during acute resuscitation when intravenous access is not attainable results in an almost immediate impact of the fluid or drug on the central circulation.

Amount and Rate of Blood Production

Blood volumes vary with age, from 85 ml/kg in the neonate to 70 ml/kg in adults. Thus, the circulating volume of a 600-g premature infant is 50 ml compared to 250 ml in a 3-kg term baby, 850 ml in a 10-kg one-year-old, and approximately 5 liters in an average adult. The various cell counts and blood parameters also vary considerably with age. For further discussion of normal age-related values, see Chapter 3.

The total number of RBCs in circulation at any time for a healthy person is approximately 4 to 5 × 10^{12}/liter, and total RBC volume is replaced every 120 days. The total white blood cell (WBC) count varies from 2 to 8 × 10^9/liter and is replaced every 3 to 5 days. The total platelet count is 150 to 400 × 10^9/liter and is replaced every 10 days.

Clinical Implications

1. Iatrogenic blood loss (and resulting transfusion requirements) is a major problem in managing sick infants due to their small circulating blood volumes. Special techniques to analyze smaller-volume samples as well as judicious ordering of blood tests are critical elements of successful neonatal and pediatric centers.
2. RBCs predominate in peripheral blood examinations due to their relative abundance (three orders of magnitude more cells than WBCs or platelets), but for bone marrow examination, WBC precursors are dominant because their comparatively shortened life span requires higher production requirements (myeloid-to-erythroid ratio in bone marrow is usually 2:1 to 7:1, with granulocyte precursors making up 40 to 65 percent of counted cells).
3. The high production rates of large numbers of blood cells required to maintain normal blood demands considerable metabolic effort and a constant supply of hematinics and protein. Thus, the blood is often affected in systemic disease and is often the dose-limiting factor in the ability to give antimetabolic or chemotherapeutic agents.

The Bone Marrow Environment

The bone marrow stroma provides a specific microenvironment for hematopoiesis to occur. This involves many types of cells, including macrophages, fibroblasts, endothelial cells, fat cells, and reticulum cells. The extracellular matrix is equally important, and key components include fibronectin, hemonectin, laminin, collagen, and various proteoglycans. The progression of cells through the bone marrow stroma and their release into the circulation are usually highly regulated by complex interaction between adhesion molecules on the cells themselves and the bone marrow stroma. Thus, the presence of immature cells in the peripheral blood is highly significant and occurs as a physiologic response either to bone marrow stress or to bone marrow pathology. The pattern of cell surface markers on the cells can be used to ascertain their maturity and place within the cell lineages.

Clinical Implications

1. When bone marrow is transplanted, it is simply infused into the peripheral blood of the recipient, and the blood progenitors will 'home' to their preferred microenvironment within the bone marrow, as governed by respective adhesion molecules.
2. Immunophenotyping of WBCs is a critical part of the classification of leukemias, which is based on cell lineage and maturation.
3. Left shift or the presence of neutrophil precursors in the peripheral blood is a physiologic response to infection. The presence of nucleated RBCs in the peripheral blood is a physiologic response to hemolysis or blood loss but is also (to a small degree) common in normal neonates.

Understanding the Bone Marrow Compartment

The bone marrow compartment and its production of mature blood cells are best considered as three cell populations that are linked (Figure 1.1). Other tissues of the body are similarly organized, and malignant tissue – including leukemia – has similar cell hierarchies, but they are disordered:

- *The stem cell compartment.* Pluripotent hemopoietic stem cells (HSCs) have two key properties: they are capable of self-renewal and thus form a self-perpetuating pool, and they give rise to progeny that are capable – on demand – of multilineage differentiation into all cell lineages of the blood, including lymphocytes and osteoclasts. Their proliferative rate is low – they check and repair DNA rigorously – but their proliferative capacity is large because of this self-renewal ability. They cannot be identified visually on morphologic examination of the bone marrow but have been proven to exist in small numbers by their ability to initiate and sustain long-term *in vitro* hematopoiesis and their ability to repopulate hematopoiesis and rescue a lethally irradiated immunodeficient mouse model.

- *Hemopoietic progenitor cells.* These cells have a high replicative rate and are derived from HSCs. Their replicative potential is limited, and their differentiation potential is increasingly lineage restricted. Their survival and proliferation are supported by cytokines and growth factors, and they are recognizable in short-term *in vitro* clonogenic assays, where these growth factors are added to medium. Such cells will not rescue a lethally irradiated individual because their replicative and differentiation potential is limited.

- *Mature cells.* These are the cells of the blood. They are single-lineage only, for example, RBCs or neutrophils, and these cells have zero replicative potential. However, some cells can replicate; for example, antigen-specific T cells can expand in response to infection.

Clinical Implications

1. Clinical bone marrow transplant currently involves the transfer of many donor cells that will not contribute to the reconstitution of the recipient bone marrow, but we are limited by our inability to recognize and isolate pluripotent stem cells.

2. Our understanding of the pathophysiology of bone marrow failure syndromes is somewhat limited by our difficulty in identifying stem cells to enable specific study of functional relationships.

3. This cell hierarchy can be considered a mechanism for preventing malignancy. The longer-lived cells have a lower proliferative rate, and DNA mistakes and mutations are more likely to arise in those cells with a limited replicative

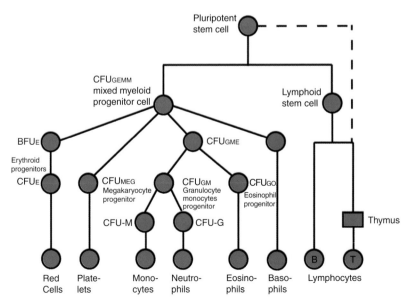

Figure 1.1 Cells produced in the bone marrow move sequentially through three cell 'compartments' that are functionally separate. The stem cells, hemopoietic progenitor cells, and mature blood cells constitute three distinct cell populations, although this is not obvious from visual examination of bone marrow aspirates or trephines.

potential (and so the mistake dies with the death of the cell).

4. Accumulating mistakes in the HSC pool will lead to cell-cycle exit and to aplastic anemia. This is more pronounced in disorders of DNA repair such as Fanconi anemia. Clonal escape and leukemia are also features of this disease.

5. In malignant disease, this hierarchy – albeit disorganized – is replicated. In chronic leukemia, there are more mature cells, whereas in acute leukemia, there is less differentiation and a higher proliferative rate. However, there are leukemia stem cells, and only these cells are capable of establishing the leukemia within an immunodeficient animal model.

Hematopoietic Growth Factors

Hemopoietic growth factors are predominantly glycoprotein hormones that have both local and circulating actions via specific surface receptors. There is considerable redundancy in the system, with multiple growth factors affecting different lineages, whereas others are quite specific, for example, erythropoietin (Figure 1.2).

The effects of the growth factors vary at different levels of maturation such that the same growth hormone might promote survival and replication in an immature progenitor and functional activation in a mature cell. Hemopoietic growth factors are produced by numerous cells involved in the inflammatory, immune, and wound-repair pathways and are integral to these pathways as well as normal blood cell production. Erythropoietin is produced predominantly (90 percent) in the kidneys, and tissue oxygenation is the most essential regulator of RBC production.

Clinical Implications

1. Strong clinical stimulus to produce a specific blood cell often may produce some collateral increase in other cell lineages due to the nonspecificity of some hematopoietic growth factors.

2. Erythropoietin has established clinical use in anemia of renal failure and may be of benefit in other clinical situations.

3. Granulocyte colony stimulating factor (G-CSF) has enabled significant intensification of chemotherapy regimes by providing the ability to restore neutrophil counts rapidly and hence reduce septic deaths.

4. Thrombopoietin has recently been introduced for the management of thrombocytopenia in specific circumstances, including idiopathic thrombocytopenic purpura (ITP).

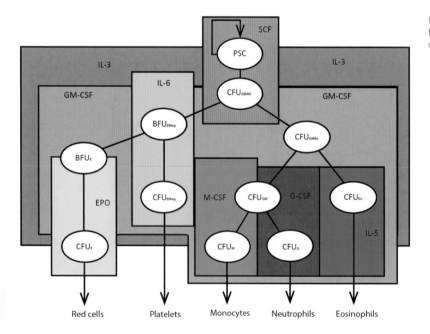

Figure 1.2 The hemopoietic growth factors exhibit redundancy and considerable overlap in their effects.

Specific Hematinics

While general nutritional status is important for adequate hematopoiesis because of the high rate of production, vitamin B_{12}, folate, and iron are specifically required in considerable amounts to adequately support hematopoiesis. Both vitamin B_{12} (found in animal products such as meat, fish, and dairy) and folate (found in green leafy vegetables) are essential for the synthesis of DNA. In this regard, they are crucial for all cellular growth and development, but given that the bone marrow is one of the most rapidly growing and reproducing tissues in the body, the effects of deficiencies of these two elements are frequently first seen in the blood. Further detail of the pathophysiology and clinical consequences of vitamin B_{12} or folate problems is given in Chapter 17.

Iron is crucial for the formation of hemoglobin and so is particularly relevant for RBC production. Approximately 65 percent of total-body iron is in hemoglobin, and a further 15 to 30 percent is stored in the form of ferritin. Iron stores are transferred from mother to fetus predominantly in the third trimester, so premature infants will readily become iron deficient if not appropriately supplemented. In contrast, term infants are almost never iron deficient during the first six months in the absence of blood loss (iatrogenic or pathologic). Most infant formulas are iron fortified, as are many early infant foods such as cereals. Further discussion of iron and iron deficiency is given in Chapter 18.

Hemoglobin

Hemoglobin is the core element of the RBCs and is responsible for carrying oxygen. Hemoglobin comprises four chains, predominantly two alpha (α) chains and two nonalpha (non-α) chains. The predominance of the hemoglobin chains varies with age (Figure 1.3). The two α genes are located on chromosome 16, as is the zeta (ζ) gene. The beta (β) gene is located on chromosome 11, as is the epsilon(ϵ), delta (δ), and two gamma (γ) genes. The embryonic hemoglobins consist of Gower-1 ($\zeta_2\epsilon_2$), Gower-2 ($\alpha_2\epsilon_2$), Portland-1 ($\zeta_2\gamma_2$), and Portland-2 ($\zeta_2\beta_2$). Fetal hemoglobin comprises $\alpha_2\gamma_2$, whereas the adult hemoglobins, hemoglobin A and A_2, are $\alpha_2\beta_2$ and $\alpha_2\delta_2$, respectively.

Clinical Implications

1. β-Chain switch does not occur until 6 months of life, so β-chain abnormalities such as sickle cell disease or β-thalassemia do not present before that time.
2. Microcytosis in the first months of life for term babies must represent alpha-thalassemia in the absence of blood loss.
3. Hemolysis in the newborn period rarely relates to abnormal fetal hemoglobin but will be

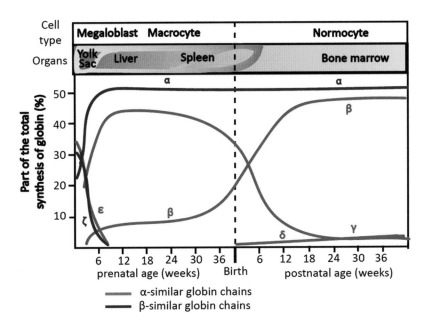

Figure 1.3 The globin chain changes with age.

self-limiting, and a conclusive diagnosis is usually difficult and not required.

RBCs and Oxygen Delivery

The physiology of oxygen delivery is important. The oxygen dissociation curve is frequently discussed, but actually just as important in terms of daily clinical practice is the tissue oxygen delivery equation:

$$\text{Tissue oxygen delivery}(ml/min) =$$
$$cardiac\ output(liters/min) \times \text{Hb}(g/liter) \times$$
$$\text{oxygen saturation}(\%) \times 1.34\ ml/g(constant:$$
$$amount\ of\ oxygen\ per\ gram\ of\ normal\ Hb)$$

Cardiac output is the product of heart rate and stroke volume, and given that stroke volume rarely changes acutely, the cardiac compensation for rapid loss of Hb is reflected in the heart rate.

Clinical Implications

1. Transfusion decisions (the decision to transfuse or not, as well as the urgency of transfusion) should never be based on the Hb concentration alone but rather on an understanding of the ability of the patient to deliver oxygen and the ability to cope with the additional demands being made on cardiac output.
2. The equation involves oxygen saturation and not PaO$_2$. Thus, oxygen therapy is of little use to a patient who has reduced Hb because the Hb the patient does have is usually 100 percent saturated in the absence of concurrent lung disease.
3. In the absence of fever (which will increase the heart rate), the heart rate is very effective for monitoring anemic patients' progress acutely because it will increase or decrease in an inverse linear relationship with the Hb. Thus, knowing the vital signs is a mandatory part of the clinical assessment of any patient suspected of anemia, especially acute blood loss or hemolysis.

Vascular Endothelium

The vascular system is not an inert series of tubes but an active, dynamic organ that is fundamentally different in different parts of the body. Overall, the vascular system can be described as three separate entities: the arterial system, the venous system, and the microvascular or capillary system. However, each of these components also differs in specific organ sites in terms of their ability to regulate blood flow, vascular resistance, and pressure. In addition, there may be variation in endothelial cell expression and secretion of adhesion molecules, coagulation-related factors, and soluble proteins, which fundamentally change the local response to blood cells. There is animal model data to confirm that there are age-related differences in the function of the vascular endothelium in both venous and arterial systems, although this remains a poorly studied organ in humans. Disturbances of the vascular endothelium appear to be critical in the development of atherosclerosis and vascular disease, both of which cause enormous morbidity and mortality in the adult population. The origins of these disturbances are identifiable during childhood, and perhaps even fetal life, and a better understanding of developmental changes in the vascular endothelium may provide the answers to enable prevention of cardiovascular disease in adults.

Clinical Implications

1. Disseminated intravascular coagulation (DIC) is a disease of the vascular endothelium that usually is measured by the impact on the coagulation system.
2. The pathophysiology of arterial thrombosis and venous thrombosis is usually different, and this needs to be considered when determining treatment, including the agents used and their intensity and duration of administration.
3. There are no clinically useful tests for measuring the integrity of the vascular endothelium or its function despite the obvious clinical importance.
4. A number of clinically relevant vasculitides have their primary presentations during infancy and childhood.

Conclusions

Understanding normal hematopoiesis and the physiology of blood is important, but in pediatric hematology it is crucial to understand the age-related differences in normal quantities and function. There are rapid changes in the hematologic system during childhood, but especially after birth and during early infancy. There remains lots to be learned about these developmental changes, and our current lack of knowledge impairs our ability to understand diseases of both childhood and adult life.

The Coagulation System

Key Messages

1. The hemostatic or coagulation system is a complex homeostatic system that is essential for maintaining healthy life.

2. Disturbances of the hemostatic system account for a large proportion of the noninfectious morbidity and mortality in westernized societies.

3. Rudolf Virchow, in the mid-1800s, described the critical components of hemostasis as being the blood vessel wall, blood composition, and blood flow (Virchow's triad), and clinically, this is still probably the most important way to think of the system.

4. The hemostatic system interacts with other physiologic systems such as wound repair, inflammation, immunity, and angiogenesis in a complex and as yet incompletely understood manner. The impact of hemostatic agents on these parallel systems, especially in children, remains largely unknown.

5. Hemostasis is a dynamic, evolving process that is age dependent and begins *in utero*. The evolution of the hemostatic system continues throughout life, as evidenced by studies of the coagulation system in centenarians. However, the changes are most marked during childhood and hence are of most clinical relevance during this time.

6. The term *developmental hemostasis* was coined in the late 1980s by Dr. Maureen Andrew to describe this phenomenon. Understanding developmental hemostasis is critical to the appropriate diagnosis and treatment of infants and children with hemostatic disorders.

7. No currently available test of the hemostatic system considers true physiology, that is, the combination of platelets and plasma proteins interacting with vascular endothelium under variable-flow conditions, and as such, all tests should be considered surrogate measures of various components of the system. Thus, studies providing clinical outcome data should be considered to validate the use of any test used in clinical practice. Sadly, such studies, especially in children, are often not yet done.

8. Our knowledge of the hemostatic system is rapidly expanding, especially in children, so the physiology that we describe today will likely be modified substantially even in a further five years.

9. While division of the plasma coagulation proteins into the extrinsic, intrinsic, and common pathways is helpful to understanding the meaning of routine coagulation tests such as the *activated partial thromboplastin time* (APTT) and the *prothrombin time* (PT), this division is totally nonphysiologic. The hemostatic system's response to vessel injury is best considered under the headings of primary hemostasis, secondary hemostasis, and fibrinolysis. The plasma coagulation proteins are best considered as having initiation, amplification, and propagation phases.

Introduction

The coagulation system is a fundamental biological system integral to survival for large multicellular organisms. The terminology is often confusing. Terms such as *coagulation system* and *hemostatic system* are often used interchangeably without clear definition. Conceptually, blood must stay in fluid form to function as a transport system, and hence, there must be a defense mechanism to deal with breaches of the vascular system at any level. Thus, in its broadest sense, the *hemostatic system* refers to the complex interplay of the vascular endothelium, blood cellular elements (especially platelets), and plasma proteins, all working together to promote an appropriate response to vascular injury, minimizing blood loss while maximizing ongoing flow throughout the vascular system. The term *coagulation system* is often used to describe the specific plasma proteins that are identified as being part of the plasma coagulation cascade, which results in the conversion of prothrombin into thrombin and the subsequent conversion of fibrinogen into fibrin, the basic framework of a blood clot. This terminology is further confused by the fact that the laboratory tests often referred to as *coagulation studies* are in fact tests of the plasma proteins in isolation from all other hemostatic components. Traditionally, this terminology has excluded the proteins that form the fibrinolytic system and that subsequently break down formed thrombus. However, with time, the interplay between the coagulation and fibrinolytic systems is becoming increasingly recognized. Global hemostatic tests are also now potentially available that consider the multiple components of the hemostatic system (e.g. thromboelastography or rotational thromboelastometry [ROTEM]) and are performed with whole blood.

However, the fundamental problem remains. All tests of the hemostatic system are surrogate measures that assess various components of the hemostatic system under artificial conditions. For example, the temperature is uniformly controlled, and there are no flow conditions, let alone the ability to account for arterial versus venous flow or flow conditions in sick patients versus healthy patients. The tests occur in the absence of interactions with the vascular endothelium. In this context, no hemostatic test should be considered a true reflection of physiology or pathophysiology but rather a surrogate measure, the value of which depends on the extent to which studies have demonstrated the ability of the test result to predict the behavior of the patient. For some tests, for example, the International Normalized Ratio (INR) in warfarinized patients, there are relatively good data that demonstrate a linear relationship between the INR and the risk of bleeding such that rational, clinical decisions can be made based on the level of the INR. Sadly for many other tests in a wide range of clinical situations (especially in children and neonates), such data relating laboratory tests to clinical outcomes are lacking. While there is some relationship between the

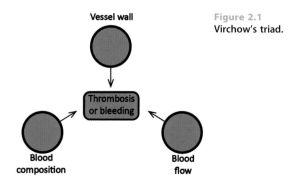

Figure 2.1
Virchow's triad.

test result and the behavior of the patient, accurate predictions of patient behavior remain impossible. Specific hemostatic tests and their interpretation will be discussed in Chapter 3.

Virchow's Triad

Virchow's triad (Figure 2.1) was originally used to describe the factors that lead to thrombosis, but in fact it is a useful paradigm for thinking about all disturbances of the hemostatic system. The presence of abnormal bleeding or clotting is the result of the interplay between the blood vessel wall, blood flow, and the blood constituents (cellular elements and plasma proteins). In fact, this interplay can often explain why patients, for example, with liver disease, can be bleeding and clotting in different vascular beds at the same time as blood flow and blood vessel wall damage exert their local effects. Indeed, it is often the impact of changes in flow or blood vessel wall damage that explain why a patient with an abnormal coagulation profile bleeds or clots at a particular point in time. This is important to remember because management of flow (by avoiding hypotension/dehydration, or controlling blood pressure) particularly at the time of vessel wall damage (e.g. central line insertion) is often underestimated in terms of usefulness in protecting against potential clotting or bleeding complications. The old adage that bleeding only occurs when there is a hole in the blood vessel wall remains true, and no amount of coagulopathy leads to bleeding without a vessel wall breach of some degree.

The Hemostatic System

Primary hemostasis describes the cellular interaction of platelets and the endothelium and the initiation of the platelet plug that is localized to the point of injury at the vessel wall. *Secondary hemostasis* describes the

INJURY

Primary Haemostasis
- Vasoconstriction (immediately)
- Platelet adhesion (seconds)
- Platelet aggregation (minutes)

Secondary Haemostasis
- Activation of coagulation factors (minutes)
- Formation of fibrin (minutes)

Tertiary Haemostasis
- Activation of fibrinolysis (minutes)
- Lysis of the clot (hours)

Figure 2.2 The hemostatic system response to injury.

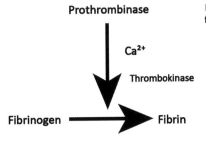

Figure 2.3 The four-factor theory.

activation of the coagulation system that is initiated, amplified, and prolonged in a sequence of activations of coagulation proteins and regulated by a series of positive- and negative-feedback mechanisms. *Tertiary hemostasis* is a description of the fibrinolytic system that regulates the breakdown of blood clots as healing vessels regain vascular integrity. In reality, none of these components acts in isolation. Nor do these processes act in perfectly sequential time frames, as their names would suggest. However, such terminology is useful in allowing an incredibly complex and interwoven system to be considered in a way that helps us to understand the pathophysiology of diseases, explain clinical presentations, and direct our currently available therapies (Figure 2.2).

The Coagulation System

In the plasma, a series of cascades involving coagulation proteins and enzymes, as well as cell surfaces (platelets and endothelial cells), work together to generate thrombin, the key enzyme in coagulation, subsequently leading to the formation of a fibrin clot. However, there also exist direct and indirect inhibitors of thrombin to ensure that clot formation does not go uncontrolled.

The initial descriptions of the coagulation cascade in the 1930s involved just four factors (Figure 2.3). Over the next 30 years, as more components of the system were discovered, the terminology of *intrinsic*, *extrinsic*, and *common pathways* came into vogue (Figure 2.4), and while this representation is very useful for interpreting a number of commonly used coagulation tests (e.g. APTT, PT, thrombin time [TT], ecarin time, dilute Russell viper venom time [DRVVT], and so on) it is not so useful in understanding the physiologic relationships of the *in vivo* coagulation system, nor the response of coagulation tests to a variety of

anticoagulant drugs. Recognition of the critical nature of cellular blood components as activating surfaces, recognition of positive- and negative-feedback loops, increased understanding of thrombin inhibitors, and recognition of crosstalk between the fibrinolytic and coagulation systems (e.g. via thrombin-activated fibrinolysis inhibitor [TAFI]) have only served to further illustrate the complexity of hemostasis in reality. A full exposition of the hemostatic pathway is beyond the scope of this book. However, a useful principle to remember is that the discovery of new components and new relationships within the hemostatic system continues. In particular, the relationships with other biological systems critical to survival – such as wound repair, inflammation, and angiogenesis, just to name a few – is expanding rapidly. Thus the likelihood that our understanding of the hemostatic system will continue to evolve and change over the coming years is high. Very little of our current teaching on the workings of the hemostatic system should be viewed as absolute truth, and as clinicians, we should continue to question our interpretation of mechanisms of diseases related to hemostasis and our interpretation of hemostatic tests.

In physiologic terms, the coagulation system is probably better considered in terms of phases rather than pathways. Blood vessel wall injury leads to contact between the blood and subendothelial components that activates tissue factor. Tissue factor binds to factor VII, converting it to factor VIIA, which subsequently activates factors IX and X to factors IXa and Xa, respectively. Factor Xa binds to factor Va on cellular surfaces. This phase is collectively described as the *initiation phase* (Figure 2.5).

During the *amplification phase*, the activated tenase complex (factors Xa and Va) converts small amounts of prothrombin (factor II) to thrombin (factor IIa). Positive-feedback loops activate factors XI, VIII, and V, which are then bound to activated - platelets (Figure 2.6).

9

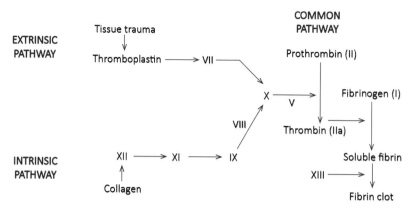

Figure 2.4 The coagulation cascade, divided into extrinsic, intrinsic, and common pathways. Many steps are calcium dependent and require a phospholipid surface. The diagram excludes all thrombin inhibitors and feedback loops.

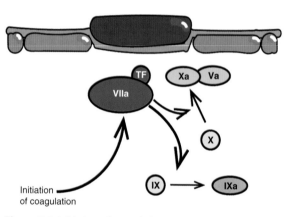

Figure 2.5 Initiation of coagulation.

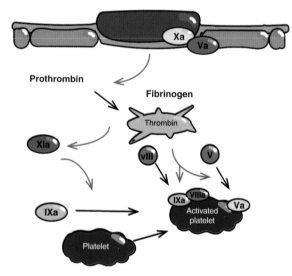

Figure 2.6 The amplification phase of coagulation.

Finally, in the *propagation phase*, The factor VIIIa/IXa complex activates factor X on the surfaces of activated platelets. Factor Xa in association with factor Va converts large amounts of prothrombin into thrombin, creating a *thrombin burst*. The thrombin burst leads to the formation of a stable *fibrin clot* (Figure 2.7).

In summary, the hemostatic system is a critical homeostatic system. Failure of the hemostatic system to be able to effectively plug holes in blood vessel walls leads to bleeding. Activation of the hemostatic system to create intravascular blood clots in the absence of blood vessel wall breaches leads to pathologic thrombosis. Collectively, abnormalities of bleeding and clotting constitute an enormous healthcare burden in Western society. For example, in the United States, bleeding accounts for approximately 40 percent of trauma mortality. On admission, approximately 35 percent of trauma patients present with coagulopathy, which is associated with a several-fold increase in morbidity and mortality. Bleeding-related complications are common in surgical hospitalization, where the associated incremental cost per hospitalization is between $2,805 and $17,279 per patient. At the other end of the spectrum, cardiovascular disease is the number one cause of death globally, accounting for 17.3 million deaths, or 34 percent of all deaths in 2008. The common final mechanism of almost all related diseases (i.e. ischemic heart disease, stroke, deep venous thrombosis, and pulmonary embolism) is blood vessel occlusion by thrombosis. Venous thromboembolism (VTE) is a common cause of morbidity and one of the most common preventable causes of in-hospital deaths. Outcomes for those affected by VTE include death (30 percent of individuals die within 30 days), recurrence (30 percent

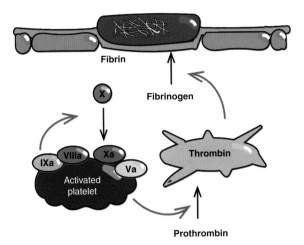

Figure 2.7 The propagation phase of coagulation resulting in a fibrin clot. Physiologically, the fibrin clot has red cells and other cells captured within the mesh to further enhance the impermeability of the repair.

within 10 years), and major bleeding due to treatment with anticoagulants. Understanding hemostasis is fundamental to the care of critically ill and hospitalized patients.

Developmental Hemostasis

The term *developmental hemostasis* was first introduced by Maureen Andrews in the 1980s to describe the age-related physiologic changes of the coagulation system (predominantly secondary hemostasis) observed progressively over time from fetal, neonatal, pediatric to adult life. Subsequently, the evolution of the hemostatic system was shown to continue throughout life, as evidenced by studies of the coagulation system in centenarians. However, the changes are most marked during childhood and hence are of most clinical relevance during this time. Our understanding of hemostatic physiology in neonates and infants remains poor compared with our knowledge of this subject in adults. The reasons for this are multiple: in neonates and infants, multiple reference ranges are required because these patients have rapidly changing systems, blood sampling in the young is technically difficult, only small blood volumes can be obtained, microtechniques are required, and greater interindividual variability in plasma concentrations of coagulation proteins makes interpretation of mechanistic studies difficult.

The fundamental principle underlying developmental hemostasis is that the functional levels of coagulation proteins change in a predictable way with changes in age. While the absolute values of these changes are reagent and analyzer dependent, the trends observed are consistent across a number of studies. These changes in functional protein levels lead to corresponding changes in global tests of coagulation such as the APTT. Other global measures of hemostasis may be more or less sensitive to age-related changes. For example, there is little difference in normal thromboelastography (TEG) with age. Studies to date have predominantly involved functional assays of the coagulation proteins due to the fact that these assays are commonly used in clinical practice. Whether these changes represent true changes in plasma protein concentrations, functional changes associated with posttranslational protein modifications, or the presence or absence of other as yet unidentified cofactors remains unknown. Initial studies also suggest that there are age-related changes in vascular endothelial function as well as platelet structure and function.

Despite the changes in individual protein levels and in global tests of coagulation, the hemostatic system in neonates and children does not seem disadvantageous compared with the 'normal' coagulation system as measured in adults. There are no data to support either an increased bleeding or thrombotic risk during infancy and childhood for any given stimulus, and on the contrary, one could argue that the hemostatic system in neonates and children is protective against bleeding and thrombotic complications compared with adults. This is despite the fact that when considering individual proteins, many proteins exist at levels during stages of infancy that would be associated with disease in adults. The absolute levels of hemostatic proteins as measured by the currently available functional assays are clearly not the key factor in determining clinical phenotype, and there remains much research to be performed to better understand the relationships between levels of hemostatic proteins and functional outcomes of the hemostatic system.

Developmental hemostasis has a number of specific implications for managing bleeding and clotting disorders in neonates and children. Arguably, the most important implication is the definition of normal age-related reference ranges. This will be discussed in detail in Chapter 4. The diagnosis of disease is even more complex. The level at which results define clinically relevant disease probably differs from the results that are outside the 95 percent confidence limits of the healthy population. To date, there have been no specific studies in children that address this issue. Correlation of phenotype and genotype, as well as longitudinal studies mapping the hemostatic protein changes in a cohort of patients in conjunction with their clinical outcomes, would be most helpful. One must always consider that a positive diagnosis of a hemostatic disorder should include the presence of a family history, a positive clinical phenotype, and reproducible abnormal laboratory results.

The introduction of all new assays into clinical use in children should be based on specific clinical studies in children that confirm the clinical predictive value of the assays or at the very least should be based on a thorough understanding of the developmental changes in the hemostatic system. Similar critical thinking must be applied to clinical decision-making algorithms. Risk stratification for treatment or prophylaxis often depends on clinical algorithms that involve the results of laboratory assays. Algorithms that use the D-dimer in determining the likelihood of pulmonary embolism have rarely been clinically tested in children, and the only studies addressing this issue have reported that the algorithms are not valid in children. The reasons for the lack of validity may include the age-related variation in the normal hemostatic system, uncertainties about the ability to truly diagnose asymptomatic hemostatic disease, and probably the pathophysiologic differences in bleeding and thrombosis development. However, the evidence to date would suggest that this and similar algorithms used in adults are unlikely to be valid in children without modifications that need to be specifically tested in the pediatric population. This poses a constant dilemma for clinicians, who in the absence of specific pediatric data often look to adult practice for guidance, and yet the basic principles on which the guidance is based are likely flawed.

Developmental hemostasis likely has an impact on anticoagulant therapy in numerous ways. This is discussed in more detail in Chapter 36. There have been no studies to determine target therapeutic ranges for any anticoagulant drug in children based on the 'gold standard' of clinical outcome. The only studies performed to date have reported the doses required in children to achieve the therapeutic ranges determined for given indications in adults. The likelihood that these therapeutic ranges are correct in children seems small. First, given that the reference ranges for coagulation assays in healthy children are different from those in healthy adults, then, for example, in the case of APTT monitoring of unfractionated heparin, the incremental increase in APTT to achieve the therapeutic range is clearly different. Second, the impact on thrombin generation for identical doses of anticoagulants in children versus adults has been shown to be different, suggesting that the target therapeutic ranges likewise will be different. Third, and perhaps most important, adult target therapeutic ranges for anticoagulation are based on clinical studies confirming that the target range provides the optimal therapeutic benefit for the least risk (of bleeding). The different biology of thrombosis (related in part to developmental hemostasis) and the different risk of bleeding (related to the clinical state of the children) make it unreasonable to assume that the target ranges will be identical for such vastly different patient populations. In addition, there are considerable data to show that there is a lack of correlation of related monitoring assays, for example, APTT versus anti-factor Xa assays for monitoring unfractionated heparin in children compared with adults, and that the ability to distinguish 'therapeutic' from 'nontherapeutic' is reduced.

Perhaps the most intriguing aspect of developmental hemostasis is understanding the rationale for such marked age-related changes. One can hypothesize that the hemostatic system is so dramatically different in neonates and children for reasons unrelated to hemostasis. There is increasing evidence that the proteins involved in the hemostatic system have multiple functions in multiple physiologic systems within the body, such as angiogenesis, inflammation, and wound repair. One theory is that it is these systems drive the developmental changes in the hemostatic system, which are therefore seen as necessary compensations to allow normal hemostatic function.

Given the limitations of our testing constructs and the difficulties of performing this research in children, much about the true nature of developmental hemostasis remains to be determined. Further research is required not only to improve our clinical understanding of hemostatic disorders in children but also to improve our understanding of the basic physiology of human growth and development. In the meantime, we must manage our patients clinically in the context of this lack of knowledge, and certainly carefully detailed outcome studies are going to be vital in improving clinical decision making.

Common Laboratory Tests Used in Hematology and How to Interpret Them

Key Messages

1. Patient identification errors cause more harm than lack of understanding about laboratory tests in children. All healthcare workers should be absolutely pedantic about patient identification for any laboratory test, not just transfusion-related tests, which tend to engender more care.

2. Sample integrity is a fundamental issue for all laboratory testing but is particularly relevant in pediatrics because of the difficulty in obtaining samples, the small volumes obtained, and the amount of distress collecting blood samples can cause for children, their parents, and healthcare professionals.

3. In general, it is better to make a clinical decision based on no laboratory data than to make a decision based on erroneous data. Hence, particular attention must be paid to Key Messages 1 and 2 at all times. Sources of preanalytical error (e.g. identification, sample integrity) and analytical error must always be considered when results do not match clinical expectations.

4. All laboratory tests have limitations. Frequent consultation with laboratory specialists is advised to assist in interpretation, especially in neonates and children.

5. All laboratory tests have optimal collection methodologies (e.g. venous versus capillary, type of anticoagulant in collection tube), collection volumes, optimal storage, and allowable times until processing. In general, cell counting is more robust than coagulation testing.

6. Interpretation of any laboratory tests is impossible without knowledge of normal values and the potential impact of disease.

Age-related reference ranges are discussed in Chapter 4.

7. Laboratory tests are reported in specific units, and these may vary from laboratory to laboratory despite the convention that diagnostic laboratories should use Système International (SI) units for all clinical tests. Clinicians must understand and not confuse the units for any parameter.

8. Laboratories must have active and well-maintained quality-assurance and quality-control systems to ensure that test results are accurate and reliable. Even automated tests that clinicians take for granted are subject to many causes of error, and constant monitoring of test performance is required.

9. Different methodologies can give entirely different results even for the same test. Careful consideration must be given whenever test results from different laboratories are being compared or results from different time frames. Appropriate calibration is an essential consideration whenever analyzers are changed or replaced.

10. The clinical relevance of any test result should be determined by studies showing a direct correlation between test results and clinical behavior of the patient. Unfortunately in pediatrics, such studies have often not been performed. Therefore, test interpretation must be guarded in a variety of clinical situations.

11. Understanding the principles of laboratory tests helps clinicians to interpret test results in settings of reduced clinical outcome data and also to anticipate patients in whom analytical and some causes of preanalytical sources of error might occur.

12. Full blood examination (FBE), full blood count (FBC), and complete blood count (CBC) are all names for a series of tests that count blood cells and determine useful parameters related to RBCs. Blood film morphology is a critical adjunct to interpretation of FBE results.

13. Common coagulation tests include the prothrombin time (PT), the activated partial thromboplastin time (APTT), the thrombin time (TT), and fibrinogen and D-dimers. The international normalized ratio (INR) is a mathematical manipulation of the PT that is useful for monitoring patients on warfarin therapy.

14. There are a wide range of general hemostatic tests used predominantly as near-patient tests that have variable clinical utility depending on the clinical situation, for example, thromboelastography (TEG) and rotational thromboelastometry (ROTEM).

15. There are many other tests of specific aspects of the coagulation system, including factor assays, inhibitor assays, and platelet function assays, to name a few. Functional assays are prone to error, so one should never label a patient with a hemostatic disease based on the results of one assay. Personal history, family history, and repeated consistently abnormal laboratory tests across at least 3 months are required for the diagnosis of most bleeding or clotting disorders.

Introduction

Modern medicine depends on laboratory testing to diagnose and exclude disease states, as well as to monitor response to and toxicity of therapy. For many clinicians, thinking about laboratory tests stops with completion of the request slip and recommences with reading of the test results without any consideration of the multitude of steps in between and the multiple sources of error. For effective clinical hematology practice, a deeper understanding of at least the common hematologic tests is essential.

Correct patient identification is the cornerstone of almost all laboratory quality systems. Simple administrative errors are responsible for too many lives lost in our current healthcare systems. Many laboratories now have a zero-tolerance policy for errors of labeling and patient identification, and while this often frustrates clinicians who can only think of the difficult conversations in explaining the need for rebleeding to parents or indeed the pragmatic difficulty in obtaining another sample, time and time again investigation of serious adverse events has justified the need for strict adherence to such policies.

The most common cause of error when collecting blood for hematologic tests in children is sample activation or clotting during the collection process. This may relate to prolonged attempts at drawing the blood, high suction pressures due to small-gauge needles, failure to mix the blood with the anticoagulant in the tube adequately on collection, or overfilling of the tubes such that there is inadequate anticoagulation of the blood. Similar processes may lead to cell hemolysis within the sample. Blood clots may or may not be visible to the naked eye on initial inspection. Blood clots will lead to erroneous cell counts, especially platelet counts, but all cell lines can be falsely reduced. In coagulation testing, clots commonly lead to prolongation of clotting times due to factor consumption, but occasionally times are shortened. Another frequent problem is contamination of the samples, most frequently with heparin, as samples are collected from previously inserted vascular access devices. This will invalidate all coagulation studies and, depending on the heparin concentration, may induce platelet and leukocyte clumping that affect cell counting. Finally, capillary collections are not pure blood and contain small amounts of interstitial and intracellular fluids. Excessive squeezing of the skin or poor peripheral blood flow can result in significantly wrong results through a variety of mechanisms. Capillary cell counts may be slightly different from venous collections even with optimal collection techniques, and from a coagulation perspective, most tests, with the exception of specific point-of-care PT/INR tests, cannot be reliably performed on capillary samples.

Hematologic tests are usually performed on whole blood (cell counting), for which ethylenediaminetetraacetic acid (EDTA) is the usual anticoagulant, or plasma (coagulation tests) separated from the cellular component by centrifugation of whole-blood samples, for which trisodium citrate is the usual anticoagulant. This is specifically platelet-poor plasma (requires more centrifugation, as distinct from platelet-rich plasma) as the ongoing presence of platelets will interfere not only with coagulation through phospholipid surfaces but also with a number of clot-detection methods. Serum, which is the supernatant after blood has clotted, lacks fibrinogen and some clotting factors and is usually collected in tubes without anticoagulant, can be used for antibody testing but mostly is useful for biochemical tests. Heparin is rarely used for hematologic tests but is the anticoagulant of choice for blood gas analysis.

EDTA irreversibly binds calcium and is usually a dry-powder coat on the inside of collection tubes. Hence, immediate inversion and mixing are critical to avoid blood clotting. In excess, it causes RBC and leukocyte shrinkage and degenerative changes, as well as platelet destruction. Blood counts are best performed within 2 to 4 h of collection if the sample is kept at room temperature, but at 4°C, accurate results can be maintained for up to 24 h. Freezing will destroy the cells. Occasional patients' platelets clump whenever they are exposed to EDTA, and in such patients, cell counting may need to be done on a citrate sample and then manually adjusted for the change in volume (citrate being a liquid).

Trisodium citrate at 32 g/liter (109 mmol/liter) is ideal for coagulation studies because the calcium chelation is reversible, so the coagulation system can regain activity (which is required for measurement) on recalcification. The ratio of plasma to citrate must be 9:1 for coagulation test results to be accurate. Thus, in patients with high or low hematocrit, an adjusted tube will need to be made manually by the laboratory with the correct amount of citrate. Coagulation tests are time and temperature critical, and optimal results are obtained with testing within 2 h for samples stores at room temperature, 4 h for those stores at 4°C, 2 weeks for those stores at –20°C, and 6 months for those stored at –70°C. Plasma must be separated from cells by centrifugation prior to freezing.

The volumes required for hematologic testing vary with the test, the analyzer, and the method being used. In general, the limiting factor for cell counting is the dead space of the analyzer and the volume required to actually perform the test, so <0.5 ml will often suffice, whatever the size of the collection tube. Small samples, however, may be not suitable for automated analysis and may require manual loading into the machine. Pediatric samples need to be dealt with differently in the laboratory. Smaller-volume samples increase the impact of the EDTA artifact and so reduce the time between sample collection and when adequate blood films for morphology can be made. In contrast, coagulation samples must be matched to the amount of citrate in the collection tube and hence must be within ±10 percent of the designated collection volume.

Full Blood Examination

Full blood examination (FBE) is arguably the most commonly performed hematologic test. The test is easily accessible from venous, arterial, or capillary blood with good reproducibility. The hemoglobin and RBC indices, white blood cell (WBC) and platelet count, and differential are useful in diagnosis, assessing severity, and monitoring of many diseases, not just those of the hematologic system. The automated analyzers of today provide an enormous amount of information, but one should never underestimate the value of blood film morphology as an integral component of the FBE.

The principles of how the various components of the FBE are determined are useful for the clinical hematologist to understand to the extent that they explain some of the potential sources of error that may occur in specific patient populations and disease situations. Table 3.1 lists the usual parameters obtained from an automated FBE, as well as the relevant SI units, relevant methodologic points, and some important situations that lead to abnormal results. Perhaps most important, adequate mixing of the sample immediately prior to processing is important to avoid settling of the cellular elements in the tube and hence erroneous sampling.

Hemostatic Testing

As explained in Chapter 2, there are multiple components to the hemostatic system, and yet our ability to test the system remains very limited, as indicated in Table 3.2.

Within the coagulation system, there has been a rapid increase in the number of tests available over recent years. The available tests can be divided into general tests that assess multiple parts of the system, but for the most part, these are only useful in predicting bleeding behavior. There are no tests that reliably predict overall thrombotic tendency; rather, only tests that measure specific abnormalities known to be associated with increased clotting risk, for example, antithrombin levels. Genetic tests remain of limited

15

Table 3.1 The Full Blood Examination

Parameter	SI units	Methodology	Key clinical utility	Sources of error
Hemoglobin (Hb)	g/liter*	Gold standard is the cyanmethemoglobin method. Key feature is that the RBCs are lysed, and the Hb is converted to HBcyanide before absorbance is recorded at 540 nm in very dilute sample via spectrophotometry or photoelectric colorimetry.	Major measure of oxygen-carrying capacity of blood, used to determine presence or absence of anemia of any cause	Multiple preanalytical errors can lead to falsely low result. Brisk intravascular hemolysis can lead to falsely high result because cells lysed in vivo still contribute to measured Hb despite not effectively carrying oxygen. Observation of sample for plasma discoloration and correlation with RBC count is helpful.
Hematocrit (Hct) or packed cell volume (PCV)	Ratio	Can be measured directly by microhematocrit method (centrifugation in standard microtube) and then direct measure of packed cells to plasma ratio. Most analyzers measure as a derived value utilizing the measured RBC count and mean corpuscular volume. Effective calibration of the analyzer is critical.	Has been used as a transfusion trigger in neonates. More useful than Hb in determining polycythemia. Used to determine other RBC indices. Used to assess suitability of blood samples for coagulation testing. An important input for some ventricular-assist device settings	By microtube method, plasma trapping may lead to falsely elevated results, as will as delays in reading the result. In analyzers where it is a derived value, severe microcytosis and spherocytosis may lead to false results, as may RBC agglutination, for example, secondary to cold agglutinins.
Red cell count (RCC)	$\times 10^{12}/$ liter	RBCs are measured by impedance counting or optical detection. The principles are similar: cells are passed in single file through the detector, and each electrical pulse (impedence) or interruption of light detection (optical) is counted as a cell. RBCs are discriminated from platelets based on size. Number of cells per volume is calculated.	Critical for calculation of MCV and MCH. Useful but not diagnostic in distinguishing iron-deficiency microcytosis (low RCC) from thalassemia (normal/high RCC).	Rarely affected by high platelet counts because of orders of magnitude difference in counts.
Mean corpuscular hemoglobin (MCH)	pg	MCH = Hb/RCC	Hypochromia seen in iron deficiency	Elevated in spherocytosis

Table 3.1 (cont.)

Parameter	SI units	Methodology	Key clinical utility	Sources of error
Mean corpuscular volume (MCV)	fl	Measured directly as mean of size of impedance or light impulses as RBCs are counted Can be derived by dividing Hct by RCC	Normochromic, microcytic, macrocytic are important in classification and diagnosis of anemia.	RBC agglutination will falsely elevate, as will severe rouleaux. Increased if significant reticulocytosis as new RBC are larger. Severe hyperglycemia may falsely elevate result.
Red cell distribution width (RDW)	% or fl	The coefficient of variation of the measured RBC volumes during cell counting. If expressed as standard deviation is in fl.	Useful in distinguishing iron deficiency (increased) from thalassemia (normal) As well as megaloblastosis (increased) from other causes macrocytosis (normal)	–
Platelets	× 10⁹/ liter	Similar to RBC counting but distinguished on size (2–20 fl)	Key hemostatic parameter	Falsely elevated if severe microcytosis Loss of accuracy at very low counts Normal West Indians and Africans may have lower counts than Caucasians. Large platelets may be counted as RBCs, falsely reducing the platelet count.
White cell count (WCC)	× 10⁹/ liter	Counting of WBCs by impedance or optical counting or both in sample that has RBCs lysed	White cell count for detection infection, hematologic malignancy, and monitoring response of bone marrow to chemotherapy etc.	Presence of nucleated RBCs will falsely elevate automated count. Can be corrected by manual counting on blood film.
Automated differential white cell count	× 10⁹/ liter	Five-part differential (segmented neutrophils, monocytes, lymphocytes, eosinophils, basophils) is performed by a variety of technologies that use either forward and side-scatter light characteristics of WBCs counted after RBC lysis or impedance with differing frequencies or, alternatively, direct flow-cytometry methods	Differential count critical for determining neutropenia or neutrophilia or lymphocytosis or lymphopenia etc with relevant clinical significance	Automated counts often struggle in infants, and manual differential counting on blood film is required. Beware of making decisions about recovery of neutrophil counts on interim (automated results) because final results (confirmed by blood film examination) often differ in low-count states. Automated counts cannot distinguish left shift and so determination of band (and earlier)

Table 3.1 (*cont.*)

Parameter	SI units	Methodology	Key clinical utility	Sources of error
				neutrophil forms, and hence determination of IT ratio requires manual blood film cell counting.
Manual differential WCC	$\times 10^9/$ liter	Consecutive counting of 100 to 200 nucleated cells on blood film and then multiply percents of each type of WBC counted by the total WCC to give the actual counts of the differential	Gold standard determination of white cell differential and separation of nucleated RBCs. Can also comment on toxic changes, left shift, and morphology of cells.	Operator dependent
Blood film	–	Manual microscopic examination of appropriately stained blood sample	RBC morphology. Confirmation of platelet number and morphology. May determine fibrin strands that could have caused errors in automated counting. WBC morphology	Delays in making slide can negatively affect morphology. Water artefact in hot ambient temperatures. Operator dependent.

* Hb should be reported in g/liter; however, some laboratories persist in reporting in g/dl. This is of real clinical relevance. Normal adult range of Hb is ~120–140 g/liter, which is 12–14 g/dl. For example, if the patient has a Hb of 10, in g/liter, this is a life-threatening severe anemia; however, in g/dl, this would be a mild anemia that may or may not cause symptoms. Multiple cases are reported where laboratories have rung clinicians to report a Hb of 10 g/liter, and the clinician has assumed the result was in g/dl and not acted appropriately. Clarification and understanding of the units being reported are essential, especially when results are being taken verbally or come from a different laboratory with which the clinician is not used to working.

Table 3.2 The Tests Available for Different Components of the Hemostatic System

Hemostatic component	Tests available
Blood vessel wall	Skin bleeding time no longer used: no effective tests
Platelets	Number Function (aggregometry) Appearance (electron microscopy)
Coagulation system (including fibrinolytic system)	Range of tests

Table 3.3 Types of Tests Available Depending on Purpose of Testing

Risk of bleeding	Risk of clotting	Monitor anticoagulant drugs
Global tests	No global tests	Global tests
Specific assays	Specific assays	Specific assays
Genotype for specific disorders	Genotype for specific disorders	Genotype to predict responsiveness

value. For bleeding disorders, functional tests remain more important, although genotype may be useful in predicting, for example, risk of developing inhibitors in hemophiliacs. Genetic tests are more specific for the risk of thrombosis, to the extent that the factor V Leiden mutation and prothrombin gene mutation are assessed by genetic tests rather than functional assays (Table 3.3).

Coagulation Testing

Coagulation assays also can be described in terms of the type of methodology involved. Immunologic assays measure the amount of protein actually present but make no comment about the functionality of the protein. They are used often in conjunction with functional assays to determine the subtype of a given abnormality. Functional assays may be chromogenic, in which a light-emitting substrate to a specific enzyme reaction is incubated with the patient's plasma, and then the emitted light is measured using a luminometer. True coagulation (clot)–based functional assays measure the potential for clot formation within the plasma under a variety of conditions. The results from immunologic, chromogenic, and coagulation-based assays are not directly comparable (Table 3.4).

Coagulation (clot)–based assays all work on a similar principle. The coagulation system in the patient sample is in limbo owing to the chelation of calcium. Recalcification of the sample occurs at the same time as an activator (variable depending on the test being performed) is added, and the time to clot formation is measured. The assays are all performed at 37°C, and all require a calibrator, which usually needs to be made from a pool of at least 20 donors to minimize the impact of individual differences in protein levels. This usually needs to be validated against a reference standard material. In addition, control samples are usually run with each batch of assays, and many assays are run in duplicate. Intralaboratory variation will still exist, likely related to dilution

and pipeting variability. Acceptable coefficients of variation can be as high as 10 percent for some functional assays. Interlaboratory variation is large and reflects differences in methods, analyzers, and reagents. This is particularly important if laboratories are interchanging point-of-care methods (e.g. for INR testing) with laboratory assays, and correlation studies must be performed regularly.

Coagulation assays themselves do not take much time to perform, but sample preparation does. Adequate centrifugation to properly separate platelet-poor plasma from the cellular elements takes at least 15 minutes, and combined with specimen reception, sample identification, sample warming and assay performance, verification, and control checking, turnaround times on laboratory coagulation tests remain approximately 20 to 30 minutes, even with the best of good will.

Coagulation assays depend on clot detection, and there are three main methods for detecting clot. While manual visual clot detection (operator observing the reaction in duplicate test tubes in a water bath) is still used in World Health Organization (WHO) calibration schemes, it is rarely used in routine diagnostic laboratories except for verification of results where automated technology results are questioned. Automated analyzers detect clot by either electromechanical or optical methods. In electromechanical detection, a steel ball is dropped into the cuvette containing the patient sample, which is within a strong magnetic field. Once the coagulation assay is begun, the formation of fibrin either causes or stops movement of the ball, which is then detected by motion sensor or change in the magnetic field, and the time to clot formation is recorded. In optical methods, as the clot forms, the transmission of light (usually 660 nm) through the sample will be changed, and clot is detected when a preset calibrated endpoint of light detection is reached. There are a variety of methods for

Table 3.4 Types of Assays Used to Assess the Coagulation System

Assay Type	Advantage	Disadvantage
Functional clot-based assays	Reflect physiology better	Technically difficult
Chromogenic assays	More reproducible Technically easier	Physiologic relevance Limited scope
Immunologic assays	Measure amount of protein	Do not tell you functional capacity

determining the endpoint. The key clinical implication of these methods relates to possible causes of interference. Jaundice and lipemia will both interfere with optical detection and hence many pediatric hospitals, with large neonatal populations prefer electromechanical detection methods which are not influenced by these variables.

The most commonly used coagulation tests are the prothrombin time (PT), the activated partial thromboplastin time (APTT), the thrombin time (TT), and the fibrinogen assay. All these tests combined are often referred to as a *coagulation* or *clotting screen* and, in conjunction with the platelet count, are used to assess the risk of bleeding. Clinicians should order the individual tests rather than a clotting screen to avoid interlaboratory variation in what actually constitutes a clotting screen. Individual assays also may be used specifically to monitor anticoagulant therapy (APTT for heparin therapy, PT converted to INR for warfarin therapy). The fact that other anticoagulants, with target proteins within the scope of these tests, cannot be monitored reliably by them is a constant reminder that the tests are artificial constructs that generate a number that has little to do with physiology and can only be useful in situations for which clinical outcome data have shown benefit of knowing the test result.

Prothrombin Time

Prothrombin time (PT) uses thromboplastin to activate the extrinsic clotting system at the time of recalcification and measures, in seconds, the time until fibrin clot formation. As with all clot-based assays, it does not measure cross-linking of fibrin, just fibrin formation, so it is impervious to the activity of factor XIII. The PT can be converted to a PT ratio by dividing the patient result by the laboratory mean PT value, in which case it is reported as a ratio (no units). Thromboplastins were originally extracted from animal brains but are now made mostly recombinantly. Each thromboplastin is assigned an international sensitivity index (ISI) based on a comparison with a WHO reference standard. The ISI will be different for each different analyzer on which the reagent may be used. The ISI also may vary from batch to batch and needs to be constantly reaffirmed. The INR is the PT ratio raised to the power of the ISI of the reagent being used. The INR was specifically developed

and is only validated for use in monitoring stable warfarin therapy, although pragmatically many laboratories use it interchangeably with the PT in many circumstances.

$$INR = (PT_{patient}/PT_{normal})^{ISI}$$

The PT is responsive to abnormalities in factor VII, the common pathway, and responsive to warfarin therapy, where the use of the INR obviates the interlaboratory variation and makes results across laboratories comparable. Because factor VII has a shorter half-life than the other vitamin K–dependent factors, the PT is often more sensitive in liver disease or vitamin K deficiency and will therefore prolong before the APTT. This is similar, but not as reliably, in disseminated intravascular coagulation (DIC).

Activated Partial Thromboplastin Time

The APTT uses a variety of activators to activate the clotting system via the contact factors of the intrinsic pathway in conjunction with phospholipid at the time of recalcification. The time to clot formation is measured in seconds. Unlike the PT, no correlation has ever been able to be formulated between the various APTT reagents (>300) available on the market, and direct comparisons between laboratories and reagents remain impossible. The APTT is responsive to factor deficiencies within the intrinsic pathway (factors XII, XI, IX, VIII) as well as the common pathway (factors X, V, II), as well as heparin therapy and lupus anticoagulants. Each reagent may have a different level of sensitivity to these three problems (factor deficiency, heparin, and lupus anticoagulant detection), and laboratories usually choose reagents that are most sensitive to the problems most relevant to the patient population. For example, maternity hospitals need good sensitivity to lupus anticoagulants, cardiac centers usually need good heparin sensitivity, and pediatric centers will demand sensitivity for congenital factor deficiencies. Today, there are many reagents available with good sensitivity across all three aspects. The APTT will usually be mildly prolonged with Von Willebrand disease (VWD) but not always, and if there is clinical suspicion, specific tests for VWD must be performed to exclude the diagnosis. Other coagulopathies to be considered in the setting of normal PT/APTT/platelet count include FXIII deficiency and platelet function defects. Factor XII deficiency will prolong APTT despite not being associated with a risk of bleeding.

If the APTT is prolonged, the next step is to determine whether it is due to factor deficiency or an inhibitor (heparin or lupus anticoagulant). The most common cause of an isolated prolonged APTT in the community is lupus anticoagulant, and the most common cause of an isolated prolonged APTT in hospitalized patients is heparin contamination. To determine the presence of an inhibitor or not, we use a mixing test, where the patient sample is mixed in a 1:1 ratio with normal plasma, and the APTT is repeated. The APTT now should be normal (full correction) if the problem is factor deficiency. This is because all APTT reagents are calibrated to not prolong until less than 50 percent of any given factor is present. Mixing 1:1 with normal plasma (by definition, each factor is 100 percent) means the resulting mixture must contain more than 50 percent activity of any given factor even if the patient's starting point was zero (e.g. severe hemophilia). Thus, anything less than full correction indicates an inhibitor, and then further tests can determine whether this is heparin related or a lupus anticoagulant.

Thrombin Time

The thrombin time uses bovine thrombin to convert fibrinogen to fibrin at the time of recalcification of the sample and records the time to clot formation in seconds. As such, it measures the integrity of fibrinogen and the presence of thrombin inhibitors such as heparin. In the setting of prolonged APTT and PT, this is very useful to identify where the problem is in the common pathway. Remember that the final common step of all clot-based tests is the conversion of fibrinogen to fibrin, so an acquired or congenital absence or dysfunction of fibrinogen will affect all tests.

Fibrinogen

Fibrinogen can be measured in many ways, and most coagulation analyzers provide a derived result calculated from the PT. The gold standard remains the Clauss technique, in which thrombin is used to activate fibrinogen, and the clotting time is compared to a calibration curve of a plasma with a known fibrinogen calibrated against an international reference standard. Fibrinogen is an important part of any coagulations screen in the bleeding patient because in terms of replacement therapy, a low fibrinogen usually indicates that cryoprecipiate is required compared to fresh-frozen plasma if there is coagulopathy but the fibrinogen is adequate.

Further Coagulation Assays

Most factor assays are based on the APTT or PT and involve the use of serial dilutions with factor-deficient plasmas in either one- or two-stage assays. They are complex and should be performed in experienced, specialized laboratories. Other tests involve activating the coagulation pathways at different points; for example, dilute Russell viper venom activates at factor X (dRVVT) and is particularly useful in determining presence of lupus anticoagulants. Specific chromogenic assays are useful in monitoring anticoagulants; for example, the anti-factor Xa assay is useful in monitoring heparin and low-molecular-weight heparin activity. It is important to remember that all these assays are subject to the sources of error discussed earlier and that preanalytical errors, as well as laboratory variation, are critical to consider in the interpretation of any results. While in acutely unwell patients clinical decisions must be made based on correlation of results and clinical details, in nonacute patients, much comfort is derived from seeing reproducible, consistent results, preferably with appropriate equally positive family testing over a prolonged time frame, before patients are labeled with any hemostatic abnormality.

Reference Ranges in Children

Key Messages

1. All laboratory parameters are only of value in distinguishing health from disease if the clinician knows what is normal for that particular patient and whether or not the parameter is affected by the disease in question.

2. Normal may vary with gender, ethnicity, comorbidities, and certainly age.

3. A reference range is usually the 95 percent confidence interval for the specific analyte in a specific population.

4. The reference-range determination requires some statistical assumptions about the distribution of normal values.

5. Normally distributed and skewed variables will require different methodologies in calculating accurate reference ranges.

6. By definition, 2.5 percent of subjects will be below a reference range and 2.5 percent will be above the reference range and yet be normal. These subjects may have results within the ranges that signify disease in other subjects.

7. Multiple methodologies are used in determining reference ranges, including testing relatively small numbers of healthy patients (presumed to be representative of a given population) versus determining means and standard deviations from very large numbers of clinically collected samples.

8. Most reference ranges will vary with the methodology (reagents and analyzer) used to determine the analyte, as well as the method used to collect the blood sample. The significance of this variation and the impact on clinical comparability of results vary according to the analyte in question, but reagent and analyte specificity is very pronounced for most coagulation assays.

9. Reference ranges are population measures, and as such, individuals may have significant disease and still be within the reference range for a relevant analyte. Knowledge of previous results and changes over time, even within the reference range, is often helpful.

10. Some analytes undergo minimal variation over time, and hence individuals are remarkably constant in their measured values when they are healthy, whereas other analytes have significant diurnal and even seasonal variations.

11. Some diseases are defined in relationship to the reference range of a single analyte (e.g. anemia by definition is a hemoglobin [Hb] concentration below the population-specific reference range), whereas other diseases are not.

12. In some cases, the trigger for clinical investigation or clinical intervention is far removed from the boundaries of the reference range.

13. Reference ranges are different from therapeutic ranges. Therapeutic ranges are target ranges for drug therapy that should correlate with clinical outcome data that support maximum efficacy for minimal side effects of the drug being monitored.

14. The failure to recognize the need for specific reference ranges for children of different ages has led many children to be misdiagnosed and poorly managed medically.

Introduction

The interpretation of any laboratory test depends on an understanding of what is normal for the parameter in question and what the significance of deviation from normal is in terms of disease processes. Gender differences for many parameters have long been understood, and increasingly, ethnic differences are being realized, especially in full blood examination (FBE) parameters such as Hb and platelet counts. Pregnancy, life at altitude, and extreme fitness are also well known to modify many hematologic parameters. However, age is arguably the most important modifying factor for hematologic measurements, and while the variation attributable to age continues throughout the entire life cycle, it is most marked and most clinically relevant during fetal, neonatal, and childhood. Of importance, many of these differences continue to evolve throughout adolescence so that it is true that even teenagers are not just little adults and should not be compared with adults when determining normality.

The age variations for hematologic parameters should be viewed as physiologic, and while the rationale for some of the physiologic changes (e.g. transition of postbirth Hb) are well understood, there are multiple other parameters, especially in the coagulation system, for which the physiologic significance of age-related change remains unknown. There are many parameters for which true age-related reference ranges spanning the entire pediatric age group, especially when one considers premature infants, are yet to be determined. Some of these parameters are very difficult to determine for a variety of reasons related to access to adequate blood volumes from healthy children (Are very premature infants ever actually healthy?). Another difficulty is that the natural transition of physiologic variables will vary from child to child (i.e. a value doesn't automatically flip to the next reference range on a child's birthday), so there will always be some blurred margins that will make clinical interpretation difficult because laboratories are bound to express variables with concrete boundaries. The appropriate interpretation of hematologic parameters in children often requires repeated tests over time to observe the pattern of change and whether it is consistent with the age-expected trend. Moreover, it often requires experience, an understanding of the underlying physiology and pathophysiology, and an ability to logically correlate clinical and laboratory data.

Clinical Significance of Reference Ranges in Children

The clinical significance of any parameter, whether within or outside the designated age-appropriate reference range, will depend on the parameter involved and the clinical situation. Take, for example, an APTT. In a critically ill child in pediatric intensive care, a result that is 1 or 2 seconds above the upper limit of the reference range is of no particular consequence. The rationale for doing a coagulation screen in the child was to determine the presence or absence of coagulopathy and the need for intervention, and in a nonbleeding child, a result that is slightly abnormal will not change the clinical decision process.

However, the implication of a result 1 to 2 seconds above the designated reference range has totally different consequences if the test was performed in an otherwise well child from the community in whom the question of a bleeding disorder has been raised. This could easily signify clinically significant Von Willebrand disease (VWD), and an accurate diagnosis is essential. Use of the wrong reference range could have adverse consequences for the child.

If we extend our example and say our community-based child is 4 years of age and our laboratory is using the PTT-A reagent (Diagnostica Stago, France) on an STA Compact Max analyzer (Diagnostica Stago), the 95 percent confidence interval for APTT results in this age group is 33 to 44 seconds (rounded to whole seconds). However, if the reagent being used for the APTT assay is CK-PREST (Diagnostica Stago), even using the same analyzer, the reference range encompassing 95 percent of the population is 30 to 35 seconds. Therefore, if one used the published reference range based on a CK-PREST analysis but the laboratory used the PTT-A reagent, then over 30 percent of children (assuming a normal distribution) in this age-group would be labeled as having a prolonged APTT when in fact they were perfectly healthy. Alternatively, if the laboratory used the adult reference range for an APTT (using the PTT-A reagent) and a STA Compact Max analyzer, which is 27 to 38 seconds (95 percent confidence interval rounded to whole seconds), once again, approximately 30 percent of children aged 1 to 5 years would be classified as abnormal if they were compared with this adult-specific reference range, even if their samples were analyzed using the same reagent and analyzer combination.

The true cost of this misclassification is startling. Children commonly have coagulation studies ordered because they are preoperative, and the surgeon is concerned about the past history ('My child bruises easily or has nose bleeds'), or because of a positive family history. Erroneous interpretation of an APTT as prolonged as a result of use of an inappropriate reference range leads to cancellation of surgery, multiple investigations, referral to specialist hematologists, and often overtreatment of the child – even blood product use to correct the 'prolonged APTT' – during the procedure. Similarly, children often have coagulation studies because of a positive family history of a bleeding disorder. Misclassification of the child due to nonspecific reference ranges can lead to a child being mislabeled as having a bleeding or thrombotic disorder when, in reality, he or she does not. This can have significant lifestyle and other implications for the child and family that can be problematic for many years to come. Reversing an already made 'diagnosis' is never easy. Finally, children thought to be at risk from physical or mental abuse will often have coagulation studies as part of their workup if they present with unusual bruising or injuries. Forensic medicine requires exact and explainable answers if justice is going to be achieved and 'atrisk' children protected.

Many clinical laboratories have not adequately determined age-related reference ranges specific to their analyzer–reagent combination, mostly because of cost and ethical difficulties, and this continues to support misdiagnoses and mistreatment of children.

However, interpretation of laboratory data in children is not as straightforward as just having determined age-appropriate reference ranges. There is often a second step in diagnosing disease. For example, if the lower limit of the reference range for factor VIII in a child is 59 percent based on a population study and a patient of appropriate age presents who, when using the same analyzer and reagent, has a factor VIII level of 50 percent, then it is unlikely that the patient has even mild hemophilia. This is so because, by definition, we define hemophilia by arbitrary plasma levels (<30 percent for mild hemophilia) or at least plasma levels that are thought to be associated with an increased risk of bleeding. In the absence of genetic studies, a definition of heterozygote states remains difficult. The dilemma is that for the laboratory tests to be clinically useful, we need to understand the level at which results define clinically relevant disease probably more so than the levels at which the results are outside the 95 percent confidence limits of the healthy population. The issue of results being outside the reference range versus being indicative of clinical disease is most problematic when considering the procoagulant proteins. One must always remember that a positive diagnosis of a hemostatic disorder should include the presence of a family history, a positive clinical phenotype, and reproducible abnormal laboratory results. The problem is that the clinical phenotype is much more difficult to define given the infrequency of thrombotic events, the family history is often equivocal in terms of the role of clinical precipitants of thrombosis, and yet the labeling of children as having a thrombophilic condition can have a significant impact.

For other parameters, optimal use of data can be even more confusing. Take, for example, mean corpuscular volume (MCV). Again, by convention, a MCV greater than the reference range may well signify significant disease (e.g. vitamin B_{12} or folate deficiency) or reflect an important change in the blood picture (e.g. reticulocytosis). However, age-related variation aside, our MCV is usually very constant for any given individual. So, if the appropriate reference range is 75 to 88 fl for a given analyzer and a patient who has previously had an MCV of 76 fl (tested on the same analyzer) now has an MCV of 86 fl, then this would signify a significant change for that person, even though both results are within the designated age-appropriate reference range. Early folate or B_{12} deficiency may well be present, and an appropriate clinical response would be to investigate further and manage appropriately. The response would be identical with movement of the MCV in the other direction, from 86 to 76 fl, which could signify developing iron deficiency. Alternatively, such a result might lead to the question of whether the two samples indeed came from the same individual or one was a case of 'wrong blood in the tube.' A high degree of suspicion is required to detect such errors.

In contrast, fluctuations of platelet counts within the spectrum of 150 to 400×10^9/liter are rarely of clinical significance, even if their magnitude represents an almost doubling (or halving) of the initial result. Strenuous exercise can cause a 30 to 40 percent fluctuation in platelet count, and it can vary by 20 percent across a normal menstrual cycle. The platelet count has diurnal variations of up to 5 percent, and there is considerable ethnic variation, with some recent studies suggesting a reference range of 100 to 400×10^9/liter being more appropriate for some racial groups.

The levels of some parameters in neonates are very low compared with adults, for example, protein C and antithrombin, and in fact, in premature infants, this may push heterozygote deficiencies below the detection limit for the assay (often 5 to 10 percent of adult values) such that even the distinction between heterozygote and homozygous deficiency is not possible on functional assays. Thus, there are a number of analytes for which, in the absence of immediate clinical drivers, one would recommend delaying testing until after the first year of life. Von Willebrand's factor is another of these determinants for the opposite reason – that infant levels are increased such that it is almost impossible to diagnose VWD prior to 1 year of age by standard assays. An appropriate question when faced with such difficulties is, 'Do I need to know now for this child, or can I delay testing to a time when the results are more readily interpretable?'

The challenge of when to accept that a result outside a reference range probably represents normal for that individual (as one of the 5 percent, by definition, who are outside the 95 percent confidence interval) and to reassure or simply observe versus when to be suspicious of disease and investigate further again depends on the parameter involved and the clinical status of the child. An isolated low Hb determination that is a few grams below the age-appropriate reference range in a thriving, healthy child is unlikely worthy of further investigation. However, an isolated MCV that is reduced may signify a thalassemic trait that will be of relevance for the child at some stage in his or her life. The timing of when is best to investigate is another question that will balance possible consequences versus pain and discomfort versus parental wishes versus opportunity. Clinical judgment supported by a knowledge of health and disease, as well as of normal growth and development, remains important.

Determining Reference Ranges

There have been few studies that have compared different methods of determining reference ranges. The question of determining the optimal numbers of patients required has been considered in a statistical sense and recommendations made, although whether these are correct across the range of parameters tested in hematology remains unknown. Determination of the age groups by which to bracket reference ranges is very difficult and involves statistical manipulation to try to identify the appropriate points of division. This is especially unwieldy in the first week of life. From a coagulation perspective, the results of assays change almost hourly, and there is huge variation based on samples obtained from cord blood versus peripheral venipuncture. Whether vitamin K prophylaxis should be a prerequisite for being 'normal' or not is also unknown, and the difference between breast-fed and formula-fed infants is also of unknown significance despite the differences in their vitamin K status. Thus, even with the best of intentions, many laboratories will have gaps in their knowledge as to what normal values are for some parameters.

Full Blood Examination

As discussed previously, specific numerical values of reference ranges will vary from analyzer to analyzer according to methodologic, sample, and patient population factors. Any numbers quoted subsequently are indicative only, and readers are referred to their own laboratories' data to verify the correct reference ranges for clinical use.

When considering the FBE, the greatest numerical difference between children and adults is seen in the WBC count and differential. The WBC count is significantly higher in children of all ages, until mid-adolescence, when it approximates adult counts. *Neutrophilia* is seen commonly, particularly in the neonatal age range, where the count may be up to 14×10^9/liter in a normal neonate.

A relative lymphocytosis is also common in normal children, where counts up to 11×10^9/liter are normal in children under 12 months of age, and elevated counts compared to adults also persist until mid-adolescence. Lymphocyte counts that may suggest lymphoproliferative disorders in adult patients are usually either normal or reflect common clinical and subclinical viral infections in children. Further and less commonly understood is the fact that morphologically normal lymphocytes in young infants often appear atypical or even 'blastlike.' Experience with pediatric blood films is required to avoid the unnecessary suggestion of leukemia in many children or the overcalling of specific viral infections associated with atypical lymphocytes.

RBC parameters also vary significantly between the various age ranges. Relative polycythemia is the norm in the early days of life in both the term and premature newborn. The normal hemoglobin concentration ranges from 135 to 220 g/liter in the first weeks of life. Hemoglobin concentration in normal infants then declines after birth to reach the physiologic nadir at approximately eight weeks of age (normal range 90 to 140 g/liter). Erythropoietin production is then reactivated, and the normal feedback mechanism that persists for the remainder of life is established. The impact of adverse neonatal events, prematurity, and hemolysis (due, for example, to maternal-fetal ABO incompatibility) may have a significant impact on the rate and extent of decline observed.

RBC size follows a similar pattern to the hemoglobin concentration. Fetal RBCs are macrocytic compared with adults, with the normal range of MCV typically reported at birth to be 100 to 120 fl, decreasing to 85 to 110 fl by one month and 70 to 90 fl by six months, before increasing again from early adolescence to reach normal adult values (80 to 97 fl) by late adolescence. As previously stated, exact reference ranges will vary according to analyzer and method of MCV determination.

Coagulation Assays

There are a multitude of studies reporting reference ranges for a variety of parameters related to coagulation testing in children. The studies are detailed in Table 4.1.

Some indicative results are shown in Tables 4.2 through 4.6. Clinicians should not carry these normal ranges with them in their heads but be aware that the results for any 'normal' neonate or child will be influenced by gestational age and postnatal age. Illness affects these data additionally. All results are analyzer and reagent specific.

Table 4.1 Studies reporting age-related differences in coagulation assays or proteins during childhood

Author	Year	Parameters reported	Age groups	N
Perlman	1975	PT, TT, APTT, fibrinogen, FDP, platelet count, hematocrit, FV, FVIII, plasminogen, hemoglobin	Healthy infants Small-for-dates infants Postmature infants	$N = 35$ $N = 26$ $N = 30$
Beverley et al.	1984	APTT, FII, FVII, FX, fibrinogen, α_2-antiplasmin, platelet count, MPV, megathrombocyte index, plasminogen	Cord blood Newborns (48 h)	$N = 80$
Andrew et al.	1987	PT, APTT, TCT, fibrinogen, FII, FV, FVII, FVIII, vWF, FIX, FX, FXI, FXII, PK, HMW-K, FXIIIa, FXIIIb, plasminogen, antithrombin, α_2-M, α_2-AP, C_1E-INH, α_1-AT, HCII, protein C, protein S	Day 1 newborn Day 5 newborn Day 30 newborn Day 90 newborn Day 180 newborn Adult	28 to 75 samples per age group
Andrew et al	1988	PT, APTT, TCT, fibrinogen, FII, FV, FVII, FVIII, vWF, FIX, FX, FXI, FXII, PK, HMW-K, FXIIIa, FXIIIb, plasminogen, antithrombin, α_2-M, α_2-AP, C_1E-INH, α_1-AT, HCII, protein C, protein S	Premature newborns (30 to 36 weeks' gestation) Day 1 Day 5 Day 30 Day 90 Day 180	23 to 67 samples per age group
Andrew et al.	1992	PT/INR, APTT, bleeding time, fibrinogen, FII, FV, FVII, FVIII, vWF, FIX, FX, FXI, FXII, PK, HMW-K, FXIIIa, FXIIIs, plasminogen, TPA, PAI, antithrombin, α_2-M, α_2-AP, C_1E-INH, α_1-AT, HCII, protein C, protein S (total and free)	1 to 5 years 6 to 10 years 11 to 16 years Adults	20 to 50 samples per age group
Reverdiau-Moalic et al.	1996	PT/INR, APTT TCT, FI, FII, FVII, FVII, FIX, FX, FV, FVIII, FXI, FXII, PK, HMWK, AT, HCII, TFPI, protein C (Ag, Act), protein S (free and total), C4b-BP	Fetuses 19 to 23 weeks' gestation 24 to 29 weeks' gestation 30 to 38 weeks' gestation Newborns (immediately after delivery) Adults	$N = 20$ $N = 22$ $N = 22$ $N = 60$ $N = 40$
Carcao et al.	1998	PFA100 Hb Platelet count	Neonates Children Adults	$N = 17$ $N = 57$ $N = 31$

Table 4.1 (*cont.*)

Author	Year	Parameters reported	Age groups	N
Salonvaara *et al.*	2003	FII, FV, FVII, FX, APTT, PT/INR, platelet count	Premature infants 24 to 27 weeks 28 to 30 weeks 31 to 33 weeks 34 to 36 weeks	$N = 21$ $N = 25$ $N = 34$ $N = 45$
Flanders *et al.*	2004	PT, APTT, FVIII, FIX, FXI, antithrombin, RCF, vWF, protein C, protein S	7 to 9 years 10 to 11 years 12 to 13 years 14 to 15 years 16 to 17 years Adults	124 per age group
Monagle *et al.*	2006	APTT (four reagents), PT/INR, fibrinogen, TCT, FII, FV, FVII, FVIII, FIX, FX, FXI, FXII, antithrombin, protein C, protein S, D-dimers, TFPI (free and total), endogenous thrombin potential	Day 1 Day 3 <1 year 1 to 5 years 6 to 10 years 11 to 16 years Adults	Minimum 20 samples per age group
Chan *et al.*	2007	Thromboelastography (TEG) (R. K. α, MA, LY30)	<1 year 1 to 5 years 6 to 10 years 11 to 16 years Adults	$N = 24$ $N = 24$ $N = 26$ $N = 26$ $N = 25$
Sosothikul *et al.*	2007	PT, APTT, fibrinogen, TAT, PC:Ac, TF, FVIIa, sTM, vWF (Ag and RCo), D-dimer, tPA, PAI-1, TAFI	1 to 5 years 6 to 10 years 11 to 18 years Adults	$N = 19$ $N = 26$ $N = 25$ $N = 26$
Mitsiakos *et al.*	2009	INR, PT, APTT, fibrinogen, FII, FV, FVII, FVIII, FIX, FX, FXI, FXII, antithrombin, protein C, protein S, APCr, tPA, PAI-1, vWF	Small-for-growth newborns Appropriate-for-growth newborns	$N = 90$ $N = 98$
Newall *et al.*	2008	PF4 and vitronectin	<1 year 1 to 5 years 6 to 10 years 11 to 16 years Adults	15 per age group
Ries *et al.*	1997	TAT, F1+2, PAP, D-dimer	1 to 6 years 7 to 12 years 13 to 18 years Adults	20 per age group
Boos *et al.*	1989	PIVKA II, FVII, FII, FII:Ag	Day 1, 2, and 3 neonates	$N = 57$ total
Attard *et al.*	2013	Immunological FII, FV, FVII, FVIII, FIX, FX, FXI, FXII, FXIII, plasminogen, protein C (total and free), protein S	Neonates (day 1 and day 3), 28 days to 1 year 1 to 5 years 6 to 10 years 11 to 16 years Adults	$N = 10$ (day 1) and $N = 10$ (day 3) $N = 20$ all other groups

Table 4.2 Age-Related APTT Reference Ranges Using a Variety of Commercial APTT Reagents on an STA Analyze

APTT result(s), commercial reagent	Age						
	Day 1	Day 3	1 Month–1 Year	1–5 Years	6–10 Years	11–16 Years	Adults
PTT-A	38.7 (29.8–54.5)	36.3 (28.4–69.1)	39.3 (35.1–46.3)	37.7 (33.6–43.8)	37.3 (31.8–43.7)	39.5 (33.9–46.1)	33.2 (28.6–38.2)
	N = 21 (10F/11M)	N = 25 (13F/12M)	N = 35 (3F/30M)	N = 56 (26F/30M)	N = 71 (27F/44M)	N = 54 (12F/42M)	N = 42
CK Prest	Not available	Not available	34.4 (31.1–36.6)	32.3 (29.8–35.0)	32.9 (30.8–34.8)	34.1 (29.4–40.4)	29.1 (25.7–31.5)
	–	–	N = 20 (3F/17M)	N = 22 (11F/11M)	N = 22 (12F/10M)	N = 39 (8F/31M)	N = 40
Actin FSL	Not available	Not available	37.4 (33.4–41.4)	36.7 (31.8–42.8)	35.4 (30.1–40.4)	38.1 (32.2–42.2)	30.8 (27.1–34.3)
	–	–	N = 20 (3F/17M)	N = 20 (10F/10M)	N = 21 (12F/9M)	N = 39 (9F/30M)	N = 40
Platelin L	Not available	Not available	36.5 (33.6–40.4)	37.3 (32.5–43.8)	35 (31.0–39.3)	39.4 (32.6–49.2)	31.3 (27.2–35.4)
	–	–	N = 20 (3F/17M)	N = 21 (11F/10M)	N = 22 (12F/10M)	N = 35 (7F/28M)	N = 38

M = males; F = females.

Table 4.3 Age-Related PT, INR, and Fibrinogen Reference Ranges Performed on an STA Analyzer

Coagulation tests	Age						
	Day 1	Day 3	1 Month–1 Year	1–5 Years	6–10 Years	11–16 Years	Adults
PT (s), neoplastine CI reagent	15.6 (15.2–16.0)	14.9 (13.2–17.4)	13.1 (11.5–15.3)	13.3 (12.1–14.5)	13.4 (11.7–15.1)	13.8 (12.7–16.1)	13.0 (11.5–14.5)
	N = 21 (10F/11M)	N = 25 (13F/12M)	N = 35 (8F/27M)	N = 43 (23F/20M)	N = 53 (22F/31M)	N = 23 (7F/16M)	N = 51
INR	1.26 (1.12–1.47)	1.20 (1.02–1.45)	1.00 (0.86–1.22)	1.03 (0.92–1.14)	1.04 (0.87–1.20)	1.08 (0.97–1.30)	1.00 (0.80–1.20)
	N = 21 (10F/11M)	N = 25 (13F/12M)	N = 35 (8F/27M)	N = 43 (23F/20M)	N = 53 (22F/31M)	N = 23 (7F/16M)	N = 51 (43F/8M)
Fibrinogen (g/liter)	2.80 (1.26–3.81)	3.30 (1.50–4.12)	2.42 (0.82!3.83)	2.82 (1.62–4.01)	3.04 (1.99–4.09)	3.15 (2.12–4.33)	3.1 (1.9–4.3)
	N = 22 (10F/12M)	N = 21 (10F/11M)	N = 34 (7F/27M)	N = 43 (23F/2OM)	N = 52 (22F/30M)	N = 21 (7F/14M)	N = 55 (47F/8M)

M = males; F = females.

Table 4.4 Age-Related Reference Ranges for Coagulation Factor Assays Performed on an STA Analyzer

Coagulation factors (%) (one-stage factor assays performed using STA-deficient plasma samples)	Age						
	Day 1	Day 3	1 Month–1 Year	1–5 Years	6–10 Years	11–16 Years	Adults
II	54 (38–73)	62 (47–74)	90 (62–103)	89 (70–109)	89 (67–110)	90 (61–107)	110 (78–138)
	N = 23 (13F/10M)	N = 22 (11F/11M)	N = 22 (7F/15M)	N = 67 (26F/41M)	N = 64 (23F/41M)	N = 23 (6F/17M)	N = 44
V	81 (39–120)	122 (86–169)	113 (94–141)	97 (67–127)	99 (56–141)	89 (67–141)	118 (78–152)
	N = 22 (13F/9M)	N = 22 (11F/11M)	N = 20 (6F/14M)	N = 75 (26F/41M)	N = 64 (23F/41M)	N = 20 (5F/15M)	N = 44
VII	70 (45–108)	86 (61–117)	128 (83–160)	111 (72–150)	113 (70–156)	118 (69–200)	129 (61–199)
	N = 22 (12F/10M)	N = 22 (11F/11M)	N = 20 (6F/14M)	N = 66 (25F/41M)	N = 64 (23F/41M)	N = 22 (6F/16M)	N = 44
VIII	182 (105–329)	159 (83–274)	94 (54–145)	110 (36–185)	117 (52–182)	120 (59–200)	160 (52–290)
	N = 20 (9F/11M)	N = 25 (12F/13M)	N = 21 (6F/15M)	N = 45 (26F/19M)	N = 52 (20F/32M)	N = 24 (6F/18M)	N = 44
IX	48 (23–76)	72 (40–125)	71 (43–121)	85 (44–127)	96 (48–145)	111 (64–216)	130 (59–254)
	N = 24 (11F/13M)	N = 23 (11F/12M)	N = 21 (5F/16M)	N = 44 (25F/19M)	N = 51 (19F/32M)	N = 25 (6F/19M)	N = 44
X	55 (39–78)	60 (43–83)	95 (77–122)	98 (72–125)	97 (68–125)	91 (53–122)	124 (96–171)
	N = 22 (12F/10M)	N = 22 (11F/11M)	N = 21 (6F/15M)	N = 66 (25F/41M)	N = 49 (20F/29M)	N = 24 (7F/17M)	N = 44
XI	30 (9–69)	57 (24–79)	89 (62–125)	113 (65–162)	113 (65–162)	111 (65–139)	112 (67–196)
	N = 20 (10F/10M)	N = 22 (11F/11M)	N = 22 (6F/16M)	N = 41 (24F/17M)	N = 50 (18F/32M)	N = 24 (5F/19M)	N = 44
XII	58 (29–85)	53 (13–97)	79 (20–135)	85 (36–135)	81 (26–137)	75 (14–117)	115 (35–207)
	N = 20 (9F/11M)	N = 21 (11F/10M)	N = 21 (7F/14M)	N = 39 (20F/19M)	N = 45 (17F/28M)	N = 22 (7F/15M)	N = 44

M = males; F = females.

Table 4.5 Age-Related Reference Ranges for Coagulation Inhibitors Performed on an STA Anlayzer

Coagulation inhibitors (%)		Day 1	Day 3	1 Month–1 Year	1–5 Years	6–10 Years	11–16 Years	Adults
				Age				
AT Stachrom ATIII		76 (54–99)	74 (34–108)	109 (72–134)	116 (101–131)	114 (95–134)	111 (96–126)	96 (66–124)
		N = 18 (9F/12M)	N = 22 (10F/12M)	N = 41 (8F/33M)	N = 49 (26F/23M)	N = 59 (25F/34M)	N = 26 (8F/18M)	N = 43
Protein C chromogenic Chromogenic–stachrom protein C		36 (20–48)	44 (19–72)	71 (31–112)	96 (65–127)	100 (71–129)	94 (66–118)	104 (74–164)
		N = 22 (9F/13M)	N = 21 (10F/11M)	N = 25 (5F/20M)	N = 42 (21F/21M)	N = 53 (21F/32M)	N = 25 (8F/17M)	N = 42
Protein C clotting Clotting–staclot protein C		32 (21–46)	33 (25–48)	77 (28–124)	94 (50–134)	94 (64–125)	88 (59–112)	103 (54–166)
		N = 20 (9F/11M)	N = 22 (11F/11M)	N = 24 (4F/20M)	N = 39 (16F/23M)	N = 50 (17F/33M)	N = 20 (6F/14M)	N = 44
Protein S clotting Clotting (functional)–staclot protein S		36 (17–50)	49 (32–70)	102 (29–162)	101 (67–136)	109 (64–154)	103 (65–140)	75 (54–103)
		N = 22 (13F/9M)	N = 24 (11F/13M)	N = 41 (8F/33M)	N = 49 (26F/23M)	N = 59 (25F/34M)	N = 27 (9F/18M)	N = 44

M = males; F = females.

Table 4.6 Age-related Reference Ranges for D-Dimers Using the Stago Liatest (Diagnostica Stago)

	Day 1	Day 3	1 Month–1 Year	1–5 Years	6–10 Years	11–16 Years	Adults
			Age				
D-dimers (µg/ml) Stago Liatest	1.47 (0.35–5.97)	1.34 (0.25–3.50)	0.22 (0.11–0.42)	0.25 (0.09–0.53)	0.26 (0.10–0.56)	0.27 (0.16–0.39)	0.18 (0.05–0.42)
	N = 20 (10F/10M)	N = 23 (12F/11M)	N = 20 (7F/13M)	N = 40 (19F/21M)	N = 39 (12F/27M)	N = 21 (6F/15M)	N = 32 (19F/13M)

M = males; F = females.

Neonatal Anemia

1. Clinicians must keep the normal ranges of red blood cell indices in mind before making the diagnosis of neonatal anemia.

2. Term or preterm infants with physiologic anemia of infancy do not require investigations or treatment.

3. Iron deficiency is not the cause of anemia in the first 6 months of life in healthy term infants.

4. Anemia of prematurity is frequently caused by iatrogenic blood sampling, and vigorous attempts should be made to limit laboratory draws in preterm infants.

5. While red blood cell transfusions are used primarily to treat anemia of prematurity, the role of recombinant erythropoietin in anemia of prematurity is not well established.

Introduction

Neonatal anemia is defined as hemoglobin/hematocrit concentration greater than 2 standard deviations below the mean for postnatal age. Fetal erythropoiesis starts in the yolk sac as early as 2 weeks of life, succeeded by the liver and, finally, in the third trimester, by the bone marrow, which remains the primary site of red blood cell production thereafter.

After birth, erythropoietin, produced by the kidneys, is an important regulator of erythropoiesis. Transition from fetal to newborn hemopoiesis exemplifies the many physiologic changes that need to take place for the fetus to successfully change from the relative hypoxic state *in utero* to an independent breathing unit. Hemoglobin, hematocrit, and red cell (RBC) count increase throughout fetal life. However, the size of the red cells (mean corpuscular volume [MCV]) decreases throughout gestation, while the mean corpuscular hemoglobin concentration (MCHC) does not change significantly. The preterm infant, however, begins with a lower baseline hemoglobin/hematocrit, and the discrepancy increases with decreasing gestational age at birth. It is important to keep the normal ranges of red cell indices with gestational age in mind before making the diagnosis of anemia in neonatal life.

Physiologic Anemia of Infancy in Term and Preterm Infants

After birth, there is an increase in oxygen available with increased oxygen-hemoglobin binding that results in a decrease in the hypoxic stimulus for erythropoiesis, and the hemoglobin/hematocrit consequently falls. In addition, the switch from fetal to adult hemoglobin further increases the oxygen delivery to the tissues with its reduced oxygen affinity, again downregulating erythropoietin and contributing to this decrease in hemoglobin. In healthy term infants, this 'physiologic' reduction in hemoglobin reaches a nadir at 8 to 12 weeks of life. Hemoglobin ranges between 90 and 110 g/liter and is termed *physiologic anemia of infancy* but it is not anemia in the strictest sense since this is normal. At this level of hemoglobin, erythropoietin production is stimulated, and erythropoiesis increases again. These healthy infants do not require investigation or treatment. The amount of iron is adequate for hemoglobin synthesis in the absence of dietary intake, and hence no additional iron supplementation is required.

In *anemia of prematurity*, preterm infants begin with lower baseline hemoglobin values, and this is more pronounced with decreasing gestational age at birth. Also, iron stores are transferred to the fetus during the late third trimester, and thus preterm infants are born with lower iron stores, predisposing them to iron deficiency. The physiologic nadir of hemoglobin occurs earlier and with a lower hemoglobin value than in term infants, at 3 to 8 weeks and 70 to 90 g/liter, respectively. Preterm infants are also at greater risk of developing pathologic anemia that may require intervention due to many factors including frequent iatrogenic blood sampling, decreased synthesis of erythropoietin in response to hypoxia, shortened RBC survival, and the rapid increase in RBC mass required to keep pace with rapid weight gain of such an infant.

Causes of Anemia in the Neonatal Period

Anemia can result from either decreased production of RBCs, increased destruction, or blood loss (Table 5.1).

Blood Loss

Blood loss anemia accounts for a small percentage of neonatal anemia. The most common causes include fetomaternal hemorrhage and iatrogenic losses secondary to blood sampling and birth trauma. Symptoms of anemia depend on the timing of the anemia, whether it is acute versus chronic, and the degree of volume depletion. Symptomatic infants may need RBC transfusion support, whereas asymptomatic infants respond to iron supplementation.

Decreased Production

This is an uncommon cause of anemia and usually associated with macrocytosis and dysmorphic features or skeletal defects. Diamond-Blackfan anemia is the only common cause and has specific diagnostic features and should be considered in the differential diagnosis in the appropriate clinical context. It is discussed further in Chapter 10. Viral and bacterial infections can cause bone marrow suppression and significant anemia. Parvovirus B19 infection, in particular, acquired transplacentally, can cause hydrops fetalis *in utero* or severe anemia (pure RBC aplasia) at birth. The parvovirus PCR will be positive in the neonate's blood and there will be serological evidence of recent infection in the mother, Nutrient deficiencies causing anemia in the neonatal period are rare.

Table 5.1 Causes of Anemia in Neonates Based on Pathophysiologic Mechanisms

Blood loss	Decreased production	Increased destruction

1. Fetal/*in utero*
   a. Fetomaternal
   b. Twin to twin
 2. During delivery
   a. Umbilical cord abnormalities such as vasa previa or velamentous insertion
   b. Placental abnormalities such as placenta previa or abruption
   c. Obstetric complications such as placental trauma, or umbilical cord rupture
 3. Birth trauma/ instrumentation Cephalhematoma, subdural, intraventricular, subgaleal
 4. Iatrogenic Frequent blood sampling
	1. Marrow failure Diamond-Blackfan anemia, congenital dyserythropoetic anemia or Sideroblastic anemia
	 2. Infections. Viruses/bacteria Parvovirus, CMV, HIV, syphilis, rubella, bacterial sepsis (*E. coli*), staph/strep
	 3. Nutritional/substrate deficiency Iron, folate, vitamin B_{12}
		1. Immune hemolytic anemia
		   a. RBC incompatibilities and alloantibody formation
		   b. Rh, ABO, minor blood group
		   c. Maternal autoimmune disorders
		   d. Medications, e.g penicillin, cephalosporin, valproate
		
		 2. RBC enzyme deficiency G6PD, pyruvate kinase
		 3. RBC membrane defects Spherocytosis, pyropoikilocytosis
		 4. Vitamin E deficiency
		 5. Infections, e.g. bacterial/viral infection might contribute to accelerated red cell destruction
		 6. Metabolic disorders, e.g. galactosemia
		 7. Hemoglobin disorders, e.g. alpha-thalassemia, unstable hemoglobinopathies (e.g. Heinz body hemolytic anemia)

Immune-Mediated RBC Destruction

The most common causes are Rhesus (Rh) and ABO blood type, although minor blood group mismatch also can occur. Immune-mediated destruction occurs because of antigen mismatch between maternal and fetal RBCs causing a humoral response and maternal transplacental passage of IgG antibodies causing RBC destruction. In Rh isoimmunization, sensitization occurs during a previous pregnancy with a Rh⁺ infant, fetomaternal hemorrhage, or procedures, with an increase in antibody production in subsequent pregnancies leading to significant anemia and hyperbilirubinemia. Because of the practice of administering anti-D antibody to Rh⁻ mothers to avoid sensitization, ABO incompatibility is now more common. It occurs in type A, B or AB infants born to mothers with type O blood type. The hemolysis seen with ABO incompatibility is less severe than that with Rh isoimmunization but can occur for a longer period and is not affected by birth order. Most infants do well with brief to no RBC transfusion support and have no long-term sequelae.

RBC Enzyme Deficiency

Glucose-6-phosphate dehydrogenase (G6PD) and pyruvate kinase deficiency can cause hemolysis in the neonate. Rare enzyme deficiencies are described but rarely seen. The hemolysis with G6PD deficiency is not usually severe but can be in the presence of oxidant stress such as that resulting from infection or medications. Testing for G6PD deficiency in the face of brisk reticulocytosis may give a falsely normal level.

RCB Membrane Defects

The range of cytoskeletal RBC membrane defects spans from hereditary spherocytosis (HS), hereditary elliptocytosis (HE), and hereditary pyropoikilocytosis (HPP) to Southeast Asian ovalocytosis (SEAO). Of these, HS is the most likely disorder to present in neonatal life with anemia and hyperbilirubinemia. A clinical diagnosis of HS can be made in infants with a family history of HS and the presence of spherocytes on blood smear, but definitive diagnosis is often deferred until later to avoid iatrogenic blood taking contributing to the neonatal anemia. Both HS and ABO incompatibility can have spherocytes on the blood smear, but in the latter, the Coombs test (direct antiglobulin test) is usually (although not always) positive.

Hemoglobin Disorders

These are rare causes of neonatal anemia and are the result of alpha or gamma defects leading to unstable hemoglobin and hemolysis. Deletion of three alpha genes causes hemoglobin H (Hb H) disease, whereas deletion of four genes leads to hydrops fetalis *in utero*. Most pregnant women who receive antenatal care in developed countries are screened for potential hemoglobinopathies in early pregnancy. The suggestion of thalassemia carrier status should lead to partner testing and, when appropriate, investigation of the fetus. Early detection of four-gene alpha-thalassemia (hydrops fetalis) is important because of the increased risk of maternal complications during pregnancy. Given the almost zero survival for affected infants, the diagnosis of hydrops fetalis *in utero* is usually considered a strong indication for termination of the pregnancy to reduce maternal risks.

Clinical Evaluation of Neonatal Anemia

Gestational age at birth, i.e. term or preterm, timing of anemia onset, and ethnicity should be taken into consideration to determine etiology and workup. The following points are important to note on history and physical examination:

- Family history of anemia, splenectomy/cholecystectomy, or recurrent RBC transfusions raises suspicion for RBC defects/hemoglobin disorders.
- Antenatal history of preexisting maternal hematologic conditions, medication use, or vaginal bleeding during pregnancy suggests these as the etiology of the anemia.
- On physical examination, evidence of tachycardia and an oxygen requirement may indicate a more acute anemia.

- The presence of exaggerated jaundice suggests hemolysis.
- Hepatosplenomegaly may indicate extramedullary hematopoiesis.
- Dysmorphic features/skeletal defects may indicate bone marrow failure or syndromic disorders associated with anemia.

Laboratory Evaluation in Neonatal Anemia

These tests should be carried out in a stepwise fashion to avoid unnecessary testing:

- Complete blood count, reticulocyte count, examination of the peripheral smear (including supravital staining for Heinz bodies). The blood film appearances and the presence or absence of increased reticulocytes are very important for determining whether the cause of the anemia is increased destruction (hemolysis) of blood cells, blood loss, or failure of production. This is critical for directing further investigations. Supravital staining will demonstrates Heinz bodies (denatured hemoglobin) suggesting alpha-thalassemias or oxidative hemolysis, as seen in G6PD.
- A simple test to detect fetomaternal hemorrhage is the Kleihaur-Betke test on the mother's blood sample to detect fetal cells. This should be done routinely on all infants with significant anemia because fetomaternal hemorrhage is often otherwise undetected, and the test is more accurate when performed immediately.
- If acute blood loss is suspected without any obvious source of bleeding, a cranial ultrasound should be done.
- Unconjugated hyperbilirubinemia in excess of age-related norms in addition to reticulocytosis makes a hemolytic process likely.
- The Coombs test (direct antiglobulin test) for immune-mediated RBC disorders is mandatory.
- Determination of evidence of parvovirus infection using maternal B19 serology and neonatal serology and PCR is needed in the presence of reticulocytopenia.

- Hemoglobin electrophoresis and subsequent DNA testing for alpha-thalassemia is necessary if Bart's hemoglobin is present (insoluble Hb with precipitates in RBCs and seen as 'golf ball cells' on supravital staining in three- or four-gene alpha-thalassemia deletions) or if the family history is suggestive.
- Bone marrow aspiration is appropriate if bone marrow failure is suspected.

Role of RBC Transfusions

RBC transfusions are given to maintain optimal tissue oxygen delivery and usually are prescribed for anemia of prematurity. Transfusion practices vary widely across institutions and countries and are based on expert opinion. While the optimal criteria for RBC transfusion remain unknown and require further investigations, most institutions have established guidelines that take into account

- Gestational age at birth
- Postnatal age of the infant
- Hematocrit
- Clinical condition and associated comorbidities such as cardiopulmonary disease
- Respiratory failure

Suggested guidelines for RBC transfusion based on hematocrit for anemia of prematurity are shown in Table 5.2.

There remain a number of controversies in transfusion practices in neonates. For example:

- *Restrictive versus liberal policy for transfusions.* Controversy still remains whether a restrictive policy should be used to minimize donor exposure. Few trials have tried to address the issue of whether preterm infants would be at risk of brain injury or neurologic damage if transfusion practices were restrictive in nature. Unfortunately, no definitive conclusions can be drawn, and currently, it is best to transfuse RBCs based on conventional policy.
- *Type of anticoagulant and preservative used to store RBCs.* Most transfusions are small in quantity and transfused over 3 to 4 hours and do not pose risks with regard to type of anticoagulant used and preservative solution in which the RBCs are suspended.

Table 5.2 Suggested RBC Guidelines for Transfusion for Neonatal Anemia

Hematocrit	Clinical situation
35% or less	Significant mechanical ventilation Severe cardiopulmonary disease
30% or less	Minimal mechanical ventilation Moderate cardiopulmonary disease
24% or less	Symptomatic anemia in the form of • Tachycardia • Tachypnea • Lack of weight gain despite adequate nutrition • Increase in episodes of apnea/bradycardia • Major surgery
21% or less	No symptoms

- *Duration of storage.* Previously, RBCs < 7 days of shelf life were advocated because of increased potassium, decreased in 2,3-diphosphoglycerate (2,3-DPG), and risks of additives in blood stored for longer periods of time. RBCs that have been stored for up to 42 days are now used to limit donor exposures in infants who require frequent transfusions. This is achieved by separating single adult donations into four Pedi Packs (smaller volume usually approximately 60 ml) so that the same donor can provide up to four transfusions to any individual infant over the course of 6 weeks.

- *Directed-donor donations. Directed donations* refer to the blood for transfusion coming from a relative of the infant (usually parent), who donates with a specific intended recipient. These have potential risks of alloimmunization and increased risk of transfusion-associated graft versus host disease. Gamma irradiation of all directed donations is essential. There are no data to suggest that directed donations improve safety or even reduce the risk of infectious complications of transfusion. In this context, many countries do not offer the service. A major concern is that parents who are not usual blood donors feel pressured into hiding their own potential risk exposures in order to be able donate to their child, and this makes the directed blood product actually less safe than random donor blood.

Recombinant Erythropoietin (r-HuEPO) in Anemia of Prematurity

The rationale for the use of r-HuEPO in preterm infants is that there is diminished synthesis of erythropoietin in response to hypoxia, although r-HuEPO causes an increase in reticulocyte, and RBC counts have conflicting results in studies aimed at demonstrating decreased RBC transfusion requirements. In addition to controversial data regarding its benefit in reducing frequency of transfusions, there have been concerns regarding risk of retinopathy of prematurity when preterm infants are exposed to EPO in the first week of life that are currently being investigated. There are additional concerns with respect to the risk of necrotizing enterocolitis (NEC). In conclusion, r-HuEPO may reduce the number of transfusions but does not completely eliminate them. Further work is required to clarify the safety profile of this therapy.

Supplemental Iron in Preterm Infants

Maternal stores of iron are transferred in the third trimester of pregnancy, and early preterm infants are thus born with low iron stores. Frequent blood sampling further compounds the issue. Between 25 and 85 percent of preterm infants develop evidence of iron deficiency during the first 6 months of postnatal life. Thus these infants benefit from supplemental iron. There is no clear understanding of the optimal time to begin this therapy, although times spanning from 2 to 10 weeks of postnatal age are often cited. Many nurseries commence iron therapy close to discharge. The optimal doses and duration of therapy are also unknown and may vary according to the gestational age, the use of iron-fortified formula, and the number of transfusions the infant received. However, total exogenous iron requirements of 2 to 4 mg/kg per day for 12 months is recommended.

Neonatal Abnormal Myelopoiesis and the Hematology of Down Syndrome

Key Messages

1. A unique transient leukemia is found in the neonatal period in infants with Down syndrome (DS), known as *transient abnormal myelopoiesis* (TAM). TAM is defined by mutation in the transcription factor *GATA1*. The incidence of this leukemia in infants with DS varies between studies – depending on the sensitivity of the *GATA1* assay – and may be clinically and hematologically 'silent.'

2. There may be clinical evidence of disseminated leukemia in TAM. Hematologic features include leukocytosis with blast cells, basophilia, myelocytes and neutrophils. Anemia is uncommon and the platelet count is not different from the platelet count of DS infants without TAM.

3. TAM usually resolves spontaneously within a few weeks.

4. The incidence of Acute Lymphoid Leukemia (ALL) and Acute Myeloid Leukemia (AML) are *both* markedly increased in DS. AML is a clonal evolution of TAM and the clone retains the *GATA1* mutation but the clone has additional molecular features. It is erythroblastic-megakaryoblastic lineage. The prognosis is good because it is sensitive to chemotherapy. The ALL of DS is almost exclusively of precursor B-cell lineage but the outcome is inferior to that for sporadic childhood ALL. In all children with DS, there is increased toxicity from applied treatment.

5. There are abnormalities of the blood counts of DS neonates and older children in the absence of these leukemias, including macrocytosis and lymphopenia.

Transient Abnormal Myelopoiesis (TAM)

Epidemiology and Diagnosis of TAM

TAM is a clonal, true but transient, leukemia of the neonatal period of DS that is always associated with *GATA1* mutations. Mutation is usually in exon 2 or 3 of the gene and causes transcription of a truncated protein that stimulates fetal DS megakaryocytic precursors. TAM requires the presence of *both* DS and *GATA1* mutations. It likely requires the specific features of the DS fetal liver hematopoietic microenvironment to exert its leukemogenic action because the *GATA1* mutation also does not cause leukemia in older children with DS. Note that TAM and AML can occur within the +21 cells of a patient with mosaic trisomy 21. In these children, the other features of DS may be clinically less apparent.

The incidence of TAM depends on how closely the clinician looks for it. Between 5 and 10 percent of DS neonates may have clinical or hematologic features, but with the use of next-generation sequencing to detect even tiny *GATA1*-mutated clones, this incidence may double as clinically silent TAM is detected. Some TAM is therefore clinically apparent (Table 6.1), some is apparent on routine blood testing (Table 6.1), and some is clinically silent and only apparent when a mutation in *GATA1* is specifically sought using molecular analysis. To reiterate, the diagnosis of TAM requires only the demonstration of a *GATA1* mutation in a neonate with DS. There need not be a clinical or hematologic abnormality.

Management of TAM

Most cases of TAM resolve spontaneously and no therapy is indicated. Usually the affected patient is followed in the hematology clinic every few months until the TAM is no longer apparent and the risk of subsequent AML has passed. Most features of TAM will have resolved within 6 months, but in some cases blast cells

Table 6.1 Clinical and Hematologic Features of TAM

Clinical features of TAM

Jaundice (common)

Hepatosplenomegaly (common)

Pleural and/or pericardial effusion (a relatively common finding in clinically apparent TAM)

Hepatic fibrosis (a classic but rare presentation of TAM)

Asymptomatic (hematologic features on blood testing or completely silent but *GATA1* mutation on screening)

Hematologic features of TAM

Leukocytosis: but note that some with TAM as defined by *GATA1* mutation will have a normal blood count, and leukocytosis is well recognized in DS neonates without TAM.

Blasts in blood: Note that blasts are present in most DS blood films, but the more present, the more likely it is that TAM is present (more than 20 percent always indicates TAM).

Blasts have megakaryoblast morphology (blebbed cytoplasm) and express myeloid and/or erythroid and/or megakaryoblast immunophenotype markers.

Neutrophilia: may also occur in DS without TAM.

Anemia: uncommon

Thrombocytopenia: common but not different from in DS without TAM

and hematologic abnormalities persist as an indolent myelodysplastic syndrome requiring appropriate treatment within the first year of life. Some TAM cases – perhaps 15 to 30 percent – have true AML within the first 5 years of life. The risk of leukemia is likely related to the size of the TAM clone. A higher risk of leukemia is reported in studies where TAM has been clinically diagnosed, and a lower risk is seen in the *GATA1*-mutation molecular studies. Where there is subsequent AML progression, then it retains the same *GATA1* mutation of the TAM clone, but there will also have been additional clonal evolution.

Some neonates with TAM require therapy and some patients will die. It should not be considered an entirely benign or incidental condition. The clinician must be aware, therefore, of the indications for treatment. There are recognized risk factors for death in neonates with TAM. Most infants with TAM-associated hepatic fibrosis will die. Other risk factors for an adverse outcome include hyperleukocytosis, massive and multiple effusions, cardiac failure not related to an independent structural abnormality, hepatic or renal dysfunction and significant organomegaly causing respiratory dysfunction. Many national collaborative groups have guidelines for treatment in TAM. When treatment is started, usually low-dose

cytarabine is given (POG9481 gave 10 mg/m^2 per dose or 1.2 to 1.5 mg/kg per dose twice a day for 7 days). The aim is to clear blasts and reduce the disease burden. The incidence of later AML may be reduced. The infants with liver fibrosis do not do well with therapy.

Acute Myeloid Leukemia of DS (ML-DS)

The risk of AML in DS is 150-fold increased in young children compared to age-matched non-DS children.. The AML of DS has its own World Health Organization (WHO) classification (ML-DS) because of its unique biology and presentation:

The leukemia:

- is always derived from cells responsible for TAM even if that TAM was clinically silent and not responsible for apparent clinical or hematological features;
- is erythroblastic/megakaryoblastic;
- always has the signature *GATA1* mutation of the TAM clone but this mutation alone is insufficient to cause ML-DS and additional events will have occurred and sometimes these events are those found in sporadic AML e.g. mutations in the RAS pathway or the TPO receptor or in the JAK-STAT signaling pathway;

Table 6.2 Hematologic Differences in the Newborn with DS in the Absence of TAM Compared to the Non-DS Neonate

Red blood cells
- Increased hemoglobin
- Increased mean corpuscular volume (MCV)
- Increased nucleated RBCs in the peripheral blood

White blood cells
- Leukocytosis
- Neutrophilia
- Increased basophils
- Increased peripheral blood blast cells
- Lymphopenia

Platelets
- Thrombocytopenia
- Giant platelets
- Circulating megakaryocytes

- presents clinically before the age of 5 years and there may be an indolent or myelodysplastic pre-phase that is otherwise uncommon in pediatric AML. The leukemia commonly presents as thrombocytopenia.

Treatment with conventional AML treatment has high remission rates and cure rates but is associated with high treatment-related toxicities, with death from such toxicity including infection exceeding that from disease. Therefore, reduced-intensity treatment regimens for ML-DS are adopted by many of the national leukemia collaborative treatment groups. These therapies are often based on cytosine because the clone is sensitive to this drug and it is relatively well tolerated.

Acute Lymphoid Leukemia of DS

ALL is also increased in incidence in children with DS but less so than AML. ALL in DS has particular biologic and clinical features, but in contrast to ML-DS, treatment failures occur both due to disease and to toxicity.

Biologically, DS-ALL is almost exclusively B-cell precursor in origin, and T-cell lineage disease is very rarely seen. The cytogenetic alterations rarely include those associated with good prognosis such as hyperdiploidy or t(12;21) and almost never those associated

with poor prognosis such as MLL gene rearrangement or the Philadelphia chromosome. The disease is biologically heterogeneous and does not have the characteristic molecular signature of AML in DS. There is a high proportion of 'normal cytogenetics' ALL. Recently, amplification of the cytokine receptor, CRLF2, has been identified in 60 percent of DS-ALL and is often associated with activating mutations within the CRLF2 itself or in its downstream signaling pathways including JAK2 and JAK1. This may have relevance for future treatment protocols of DS-ALL.

Clinically, ALL in DS does not occur in infancy. There is a high risk of disease relapse and there is significantly increased infection risk in children treated on standard treatment protocols. This infection risk occurs even in the lower-intensity phases of treatment, including maintenance therapy. These twin challenges of treatment failure and treatment toxicity must be recognized:

- Most national treatment groups recommend that children with DS are treated on national treatment protocols for all children with ALL and that the treatment of such children is minimal residual disease (MRD) based. Children with DS and 'risk-MRD' should receive intensified postinduction treatment as any other child with ALL.
- The increased risk of infection should be recognized in such children and reduced/managed by the use of antibiotic prophylaxis, the addition of prophylactic immunoglobulin where there is associated hypogammaglobulinemia and by more frequent medical review during treatment.

Hematologic Abnormalities That Are Not Associated with Leukemia in Children with DS

Recent studies have confirmed that the individual with DS may have specific hematologic abnormality compared to non-DS individuals of the same age. In the neonatal period, there may be abnormalities of RBC, WBCs, or platelets, and these are summarized in Table 6.2. In the older child, there is macrocytosis and reduction of T and B cells with lymphopenia. These findings suggest that the 'normal range' should be considered as different in children with DS.

Neonatal Thrombocytopenia

1. Thrombocytopenia is uncommon in term neonates but is a common hematologic problem in sick neonates in the neonatal intensive care unit.

2. Knowledge regarding congenital/inherited thrombocytopenia is expanding, and diagnosis is important for management and prognosis.

3. Timing of onset of thrombocytopenia and severity and presence of bleeding or thrombosis are useful guides in determining investigation and management.

4. Early-onset severe thrombocytopenia is secondary to fetal-maternal alloimmune thrombocyopenia (FMAIT/NAIT) unless proven otherwise.

5. Bleeding risk in neonates with thrombocytopenia are highest in the first week of life and in preterm infants, FMAIT/NAIT infants, and those with necrotizing enterocolitis (NEC) and sepsis.

6. Platelet transfusion practices vary between institutions and represent the most controversial area in neonatal transfusion medicine.

Introduction

Thrombocytopenia in neonates is defined as a platelet count of less than 150×10^9/liter and is present in 1 to 5 percent of all births. However one in four sick infants admitted to the neonatal intensive care unit will have platelet counts of less than 150×10^9/liter. Most of these neonates have mild to moderate thrombocytopenia, but up to 10 percent have counts of less than 50×10^9/liter and will require active investigation for etiology. Similar to the classification of neutropenia, thrombocytopenia is classified as mild, moderate, or severe. Although this classification is based on numerical counts, the platelet number does not always correlate with the severity of bleeding risk, which also depends on platelet function, ability of the bone marrow to produce new and more active platelets, and associated comorbid conditions.

Developmental Differences in Neonatal Megakaryopoiesis and Platelets

In fetal life, platelets first appear at 5 weeks of gestation and reach values of 150×10^9/liter by the first trimester. Thus, all newborns, regardless of their gestational age, have a platelet count that is similar to that of older children and adults. Megakaryopoiesis and platelet function in the newborn differ from adults in many respects. Compared with children and adults, newborns have higher thrombopoietin (Tpo) concentrations and increased sensitivity to low Tpo concentrations. The megakaryocyte progenitors have a rapid proliferative potential and undergo a full cytoplasmic maturation without polyploidization. However, in response to thrombocytopenia, the megakaryocytes increase in number but not size, and this is a developmental limitation to mount an appropriate response to thrombocytopenia.

Although platelets in healthy term infants are hyporeactive to platelet agonists, this is counterbalanced by higher hematocrits and mean corpuscular volume (MCV), increased platelet–vessel wall interaction, higher von Willebrand factor (vWF) concentrations, and predominance of longer vWF polymers such that there is a hemostatic balance. Presence of anemia, sepsis, maternal conditions such as diabetes and preeclampsia, and use of common medications in the neonatal intensive care unit (NICU) such as indomethacin and ampicillin may cause increased bleeding times, prolong closure times in platelet function screening assays such as the PFA100, and decrease platelet adhesion. The platelet hyporeactivity is greater in preterm infants than in term infants, and this is further pronounced by conditions and medications that are common in a preterm infant. Although preterm infants have adequate primary hemostasis, most physicians have lower thresholds for transfusion, especially in infants of less than 32 weeks' gestation in the first few weeks of life despite lack of bleeding symptoms.

Etiologies to Consider Based on Timing of Onset of Thrombocytopenia

The timing of onset of thrombocytopenia is an important consideration in diagnosis (Table 7.2).

Some causes may have antenatal onset. Early-onset thrombocytopenia (<72 h of birth) is predominantly due to antenatal and perinatal causes such as asphyxia and infections. In severe early-onset thrombocytopenia, FMAIT/NAIT is important to consider. In contrast, late-onset thrombocytopenia (>72 h of birth) is secondary to acquired causes such as infections or NEC.

Inherited Thrombocytopenia Presenting in the Neonatal Period

The platelet size, presence of skeletal defects, associated dysmorphology, and presence of other system involvement are helpful clues in the diagnosis of inherited/congenital thrombocytopenia presenting

Table 7.1 Classification of Congenital Platelet Disorders Based on Platelet Size

Disease	Platelet size	Inheritance	Gene	Features	Treatment/prognosis
Paris-Trousseau, Jacobsen	Large	AD	*FLI1* 11q23	Developmental delay, cardiac and facial defects, and predisposition to thrombosis	Supportive
GATA1-related disorders	Large	XL	*GATA1* Xp11	Hemolytic anemia ± globin-chain synthesis defect, erythropoetic porphyria	Supportive
Thrombocytopenia with absent radii	Normal	AR	*RMB8A* 1q21.1	Bilateral radial aplasia with presence of thumbs	Platelet transfusions Counts improve with age
Congenital amegakaryocytic thrombocytopenia	Normal	AR	*MPL* 1p34	Symptomatic with bleeding	High rates of major bleeding; usually requires bone marrow transplantation
Congenital thrombocytopenia with radioulnar synostosis (CTRUS)	Normal	AR	*HOXA11* 7p15-14	Radioulnar synostosis, sensorineural hearing loss	Possible evolution to aplasia
Familial platelet disorder and predisposition to AML	Normal	AD	*CBFA2* 21q22	Aspirin-like platelet defect, f/h/o AML/MDS	Leukemia/MDS in ~40 percent of patients
Wiskott-Aldrich	Small	XL	*WASP* Xp11	Severe immunodeficiency Eczema	High rates of major bleeding; usually requires bone marrow transplantation
X-linked thrombocytopenia	Small	XL	*WASP* Xp11	±Mild immunodeficiency	–

41

Table 7.2 Causes of Thrombocytopenia Based on Timing of Onset

Fetal	Early onset (<72 h of birth)	Late onset (>72 h of birth)
• Alloimmune • Congenital infections • Maternal autoimmune conditions, e.g. ITP, SLE • Aneuploidy • Severe hemolytic disease • Inherited thrombocytopenia	• Fetal hypoxia • Perinatal asphyxia • Perinatal infections • DIC • Alloimmune • Renal vein thrombosis • Inherited thrombocytopenia TAR/CAMT • Metabolic disorders, e.g. MMA • Autoimmune • Inherited thrombocytopenia	• NEC • Congenital infections • Maternal autoimmune • Metabolic • Inherited thrombocytopenia

in the newborn period. Table 7.1 lists congenital disorders based on platelet size and presence of other features.

Immune and Nonimmune Thrombocytopenia

Immune Thrombocytopenia

FMAIT/NAIT

The incidence is ~1:1000 live births and occurs because of antigen mismatch between parental human platelet antigens (HPAs). This results in maternal antibodies against a platelet-specific antigen present on fetal platelets that are inherited from the father. Allele frequency is specific for certain ethnic groups, with the most common mismatch occurring at the HPA-1a site in 75 percent of Caucasians. Less commonly HPA-5b and HPA-3b are implicated and result in a less severe phenotype. In Asians, HPA-4a is reported to be more common. HPAs are expressed on fetal platelets from the first trimester of pregnancy, and thrombocytopenia may occur before 20 weeks of gestation. Thrombocytopenia occurs in 50 percent of first pregnancies, with 10 to 20 percent of them complicated by intracranial hemorrhage (ICH). Seventy-five percent of ICH occurs before the birth of the infant. The hallmark of FMAIT/NAIT is severe early-onset thrombocytopenia with or without ICH. Platelet counts typically increase in the first week after birth, but occasionally thrombocytopenia persists for several weeks.

A head ultrasound is mandatory to rule out ICH in a severely thrombocytopenic infant with suspected FMAIT/NAIT. Because confirmation of diagnosis can take several days, therapy should be instituted based on clinical suspicion. There is no doubt that infants with suspected FMAIT/NAIT and low platelet counts should be treated even in the absence of clinical bleeding because of the high risk of ICH. However, there is lack of consensus as to the optimal first-line therapy. Much of the variation relates to pragmatic reasons and the availability of various platelet products in different countries/health services. The options for treatment include

- *Maternally derived platelet transfusions.* However, there are pragmatic and theoretical reasons against this approach. Maternal platelet collections are often difficult to organize in an immediate postpartum mother, especially if she has given birth away from a tertiary center, and take considerable time because the platelets harvested still need to undergo normal testing before being released for use. If using maternal platelets then they should be irradiated.

- More common practice is to use random donor platelets with intravenous immunoglobulin (IVIG) to maintain counts $>100 \times 10^9$/liter. If random donor platelets fail to achieve adequate increments (the increments might be poor, but they will at least deplete maternal antibody from the infant's circulation and usually prevent bleeding), then one can move to specific platelets negative for the antigens likely to be involved or based on the results of antigen testing in the parents.

- In some countries, the centralized blood banks hold as 'stock' the relevant antigen-negative platelets at the regional blood transfusion center. Thus, one can start rapidly with 15 ml/kg of HPA-1a,5b-negative platelets and measure the platelet increment. If the platelet count does not rise, then it is either not NAIT or the maternal antibody is directed at an antigen other than 1a or 5b. Random donor platelets might then be given with IVIG until testing is completed and specific antigen-negative platelets can be arranged.

There is no debate that subsequent pregnancies should be managed in a fetal medicine unit, and early booking is advised.

Diagnosis is established by detection of platelet-specific allo-antibodies in maternal serum and HPA genotyping detecting a mismatch in parental platelet antigens. Monoclonal antibody–specific immobilization of platelet antigen assay (MAIPA) is the gold standard for antibody identification. Polymerase chain reaction (PCR) with sequential primers is the method used for platelet antigen detection. These tests are particularly important to perform for counseling for future pregnancies. Recently, a risk-stratification approach has been applied in the management of pregnancies previously affected by FMAIT/NAIT to prevent the risk of ICH.

Autoimmune Thrombocytopenia

Performing a maternal platelet count is an important evaluation in early-onset thrombocytopenia in well infants. Thrombocytopenia is usually not severe, as seen in FMAIT/NAIT, and a maternal history of idiopathic thrombocytopenic purpura (ITP) or systemic lupus erythematosus (SLE) can be elucidated. Classically, in contrast to NAIT, the platelet count continues to fall after birth, reaching a nadir after several days. Predictors of severity of thrombocytopenia include severity of the underlying maternal illness, maternal platelet count during pregnancy(although the maternal platelet count at delivery is in no way predictive of the neonatal platelet count), and severity of the thrombocytopenia in an earlier affected infant. In severe cases, where treatment is required, the thrombocytopenia usually responds to IVIG.

Non-Immune-Mediated Thrombocytopenia

1. *Fetal hypoxia.* Thrombocytopenia is seen in infants with evidence of chronic fetal hypoxia such as intrauterine growth restriction (IUGR), maternal diabetes, and eclampsia secondary to suppression of megakaryopoiesis. This is rarely severe, and there is recovery of platelet count in a short period of time. Other abnormalities seen on blood counts concomitantly are polycythemia and neutropenia.

2. *Congenital infections.* Thrombocytopenia is seen in up to two-thirds of infants with cytomegalovirus (CMV) infections. Infants may have other sequelae of CMV, such as microcephaly, cataracts, hepatosplenomegaly, intracerebral calcifications, and chorioretinitis. Thrombocytopenia is rarely severe and does not cause bleeding symptoms. Thrombocytopenia also can be seen in other infections, such as rubella, herpes, enterovirus, and HIV.

3. *Neonatal infections.* Bacterial sepsis, particularly gram-negative septicemia, can cause platelet counts below 150×10^9/liter. Again, this is self-limiting and does not cause bleeding symptoms. Disseminated intravascular coagulation (DIC) leading to platelet consumption and NEC can result in severe thrombocytopenia and bleeding symptoms.

When Are Platelet Transfusions Indicated

There is no established cause and effect between platelet count and bleeding symptoms. Platelet transfusions are administered often to nonbleeding infants. There have been reports of adverse neonatal outcomes with platelet transfusions, although whether these outcomes are linked to the underlying cause of thrombocytopenia is not clear. Platelets are blood components most at risk of bacterial contamination because they are stored at room temperature. Another aspect to be considered with platelet transfusion is that transfusing adult platelets to neonates may disrupt the hemostatic balance and lead to a relative hypercoagulable state. When considering platelet transfusion, gestational age, postnatal age of the infant, perceived bleeding risk, and underlying etiology of thrombocytopenia should be factored into the decision-making process.

Role of Thrombopoietic Growth Factors in the Management of Neonatal Thrombocytopenia

Thrombopoetic agents have been approved by the Food and Drug Administration (FDA) for use in ITP in adults. Clinical trials for their use in children are ongoing. These agents have not been used in neonatal thrombocytopenia. Besides the cost, the limitation of their use in the setting of acute thrombocytopenia would be the latent period before increasing platelet counts.

Neonatal Bleeding Disorders

1. Healthy babies do not bleed or clot, and hence bleeding in a baby is always pathologic and requires investigation.

2. Distinguishing bleeding due to severe inherited bleeding disorders from that secondary to acquired bleeding disorders is important.

3. Management is specific and very different for the inherited severe bleeding disorders versus the acquired bleeding disorders, for example, cryoprecipitate for fibrinogen disorders and factor XIII concentrate for severe factor XIII deficiency.

4. A thorough family history is paramount because it will give helpful clues in identifying heritable bleeding disorders.

5. Interpreting coagulation profile/coagulation factor levels in a neonate can be problematic because levels may be physiologically low.

Developmental Hemostasis

Developmental hemostasis describes the physiologic changes in hemostasis taking place from the fetal to the adult period and is described in more detail in Chapter 2. The key concepts of developmental hemostasis must be considered before making a diagnosis of a bleeding disorder in the neonatal period. Hemostasis in the neonate is in balance such that healthy term babies do not bleed or clot. However, a number of inherited or acquired conditions can disrupt this balance, especially in sick babies, and lead to bleeding or thrombotic complications.

Bleeding in the Neonatal Period That Suggests a Bleeding Disorder

As mentioned earlier, healthy babies do not bleed or clot. Therefore, it is reasonable to consider a bleeding disorder workup in neonates in these clinical scenarios:

- Large cephalhematoma
- Oozing after venipuncture or heel sticks
- Oozing from the umbilical stump
- Prolonged bleeding following circumcision or other surgical procedures
- Intracranial bleeding

Inherited Bleeding Disorders Presenting in the Neonatal Period

Not all severe inherited bleeding disorders present in the neonatal period. Some may manifest in response to surgical/procedural challenges such as arterial/venipunctures or circumcision in neonatal males.

1. *Severe hemophilia (factor VIII or factor IX deficiency).* Bleeding manifestation in the neonatal period because of severe hemophilia is very distinct from the bleeding commonly seen in this condition in later infancy or childhood. Most babies with severe hemophilia present within 1 month of life. Bleeding from venepuctures/heelsticks or prolonged bleeding from circumcision is more common. Intracranial bleeding is usually subdural, intracerebral, or cerebellar. Hemarthrosis that is commonly seen in toddlers/children is rarely seen in the neonatal period.

2. *Rare factor deficiencies.* Severe coagulation factor deficiencies such as factors II, VII, X, and XI can present in the neonatal period but are rare.

3. *Fibrinogen and factor XIII deficiency*. These usually present with prolonged bleeding from the umbilical cord, and there is a risk of intracranial bleeding.

4. *Von Willebrand disease (vWD)*. Severe type 3 VWD is the only form of VWD that can be diagnosed in the neonatal period because von Willebrand factor (vWF) levels and high-molecular-weight multimers are increased in neonatal life, and bleeding does not occur with less severe types. The most common presentation is intracranial bleeding, and the mucous membrane bleeding typical of this condition in older children is rare.

Acquired Bleeding Disorders

The most common acquired bleeding disorders in clinical practice include vitamin K deficiency, liver disease/failure, and DIC. Table 8.1 highlights the differences and the laboratory tests that help to distinguish these disorders.

1. *Vitamin K deficiency*. Vitamin K is essential for synthesis of coagulation factors II, VII, IX, and X in the liver, which then become functionally active in coagulation. Babies are born with low vitamin K stores, and because of low quantities in breast milk, exclusively breast-fed babies are at risk of deficiency. Hence, all babies routinely receive vitamin K at birth. Bleeding secondary to vitamin K deficiency is usually because of nonadministration of vitamin K at birth either due to hospital system failure or parental refusal of the injection. Early vitamin K deficiency is related to maternal use of drugs that deplete vitamin K such as coumarins, anticonvulsants, or antituberculosis agents, and affected individuals present with ICH within 24 hours of life. Classical vitamin K deficiency bleeding occurs in the first week of life and presents as gastrointestinal or post circumcision bleeding or bleeding from venipuncture sites. Late vitamin K bleeding occurs between 3 weeks and 8 months of life and often progresses rapidly to ICH. Late vitamin K deficiency bleeding is almost totally excluded by parental vitamin K prophyalxis in the absence of severe liver disease. However, cases are reported when vitamin K supplementation is given orally, and this may relate to doses being missed.

2. *Liver disease*. Liver disease/failure causing coagulopathy and bleeding in a neonate is rare. The contributory causes include

   - Decreased synthesis of coagulation factors and impaired clearance of activated factors
   - Activation of coagulation and fibrinolytic pathways
   - Thrombocytopenia/platelet dysfunction

   Treatment is indicated only in the presence of bleeding and is aimed at correcting laboratory abnormalities.

3. *Disseminated intravascular coagulation (DIC)*. This is usually triggered in neonates by sepsis or asphyxia and causes activation of the coagulation system, leading to thrombin generation and widespread fibrin deposition and, ultimately, end-organ damage. The factors that tip the hemostatic balance toward bleeding complications versus thromboembolic complications are unclear, and it is common to have both manifestations in the same patient, with bleeding from invasive procedural sites and microvascular thrombosis causing organ failure. Treatment is largely directed toward correcting the inciting factor, supportive care, and correction of coagulation defects. In the absence of obvious triggers for DIC, the baby merits careful evaluation for hemangiomas (e.g. Kasabach-Merritt syndrome) or large arteriovenous malformations.

Points to Note in History Taking

Maternal History

- History of maternal bleeding disorders or trauma/surgically induced bleeding
- Use of any medications that could result in vitamin K deficiency
- Previous pregnancies and outcomes

Family History

- Ethnicity and consanguinity; e.g. factor XI deficiency is more common in the Ashkenazi Jewish population.
- Consanguinity for autosomal recessive bleeding disorders
- Determine whether there is a family history of bleeding disorders, especially hemophilia, before

Table 8.1 Key Differences That Help Distinguish Bleeding in Acquired Bleeding Disorders

	Vitamin K deficiency	Liver disease	DIC
Cause	Failure of vitamin K administration at birth	Viral infection, metabolic disorders	Sepsis, asphyxia, etc.
Type of bleeding	ICH, skin, or GI bleeding	±Bleeding, usually present with jaundice	Bleeding, if it occurs, is generalized or from procedural sites.
Factor VII	↓	↓	↓
Factor VIII	Normal	Normal or ↑	↓
Platelets	Normal	↓	↓
Treatment	Vitamin K injection, fresh frozen plasma (FFP)	Vitamin K, FFP, cryoprecipitate	Treat underlying cause; support with FFP, cryoprecipitate, platelets.

performing instrumental delivery, or post natal procedures such as circumcision.

Neonatal History

- History of birth trauma or instrumentation during delivery that could explain the bleeding
- Documentation of vitamin K administration at birth

Laboratory Investigations

It is reasonable to start with these investigations as baseline in a neonate suspected of having a bleeding disorder. Discuss with the hematology laboratory in advance of taking the blood.

- Complete blood count (thrombocytopenia)
- Prothrombin time/partial thromboplastin time. If prolonged, test for individual factor deficiencies based on prolongation of PT (FVII) or PTT (FVIII, FIX, FXI) or both (FV, FX, FII, fibrinogen). Failure to correct on mixing should raise the possibility of accidental unfractionated heparin overdose, which can be life-threatening in neonates (see Chapter 33). If the prolonged clotting tests fail to correct on mixing, heparin overdoses should be excluded before other coagulation inhibitors are considered.
- Von Willebrand testing (severe VWD) is only worthwhile in the setting of associated thrombocytopenia
- D-dimer, fibrinogen (DIC, hypofibrinogenemia)
- Thrombin time (hypo- and dysfibrinogenemia, heparin exposure)

- Clot solubility/factor XIII assay (factor XIII deficiency)

Pitfalls to Consider While Interpreting Laboratory Evaluations

Abnormal laboratory values should be confirmed, if possible, by repeat testing. Also, care needs to be exercised when interpreting factor levels after replacement with fresh frozen plasma (FFP)/cryoprecipitates or platelets because they may be falsely normal. Other things to consider:

1. *Blood sample collection.* Manual visualization of the blood smear to confirm thrombocytopenia because ethylenediaminetetraacetic acid (EDTA) can induce platelet clumping leading to pseudothrombocytopenia. Underfilling a sodium citrate tube can lead to falsely prolonged coagulation time.
2. Age-appropriate and analyzer/reagent-specific reference ranges in a laboratory should be established to interpret coagulation test results in a neonate.
3. It is difficult to evaluate for platelet function in neonates, and no uniform protocols exist. Testing should be avoided in the absence of known platelet function disorder or a family history.
4. Mild factor IX deficiency may be missed in the neonatal age range, and testing should be repeated when the baby is 6 to 12 months of age.

Therapeutic Options

1. *Fresh frozen plasma (FFP).* This should be considered in a bleeding neonate suspected of having a factor deficiency or with multiple factor deficiencies such as in DIC. It contains all factors, including labile factors V and VIII, but it is important to remember that it should not be used as a plasma expander in a bleeding neonate.

2. *Recombinant factor VIII/FIX concentrates*: If a diagnosis of severe hemophilia A (factor VII) or B (factor IX) is established, then infusion of specific factor concentrate will stop the bleeding fairly rapidly. Care should be taken to be judicious with factor replacement and to avoid any unnecessary or prolonged factor exposure because there is still a debate as to whether early exposure increases the risk of inhibitor development in severe factor VIII deficiency.

3. *Cryoprecipitate.* This is the product of choice for bleeding in a neonate suspected of having a fibrinogen disorder (afibrinogenemia or dysfibrinogenemia). It also contains factor VIII, vWF, and factor XIII but should be used only for bleeding suspected to be due to these deficiencies if disease-specific products are not available.

4. *Factor XIII concentrate.* Bleeding secondary to severe factor XIII deficiency is treated with a recombinant factor XIII product. Because it has a long half-life, only a single dose is sufficient to control bleeding. Monthly prophylaxis is usually adequate to prevent further bleeding secondary to severe factor XIII deficiency.

5. *Recombinant factor VIIa.* Clinicians sometimes use this off-label in a bleeding neonate when there has not been sufficient time to establish a definitive diagnosis and rapid control of bleeding is needed, e.g. severe ICH in an unstable baby. However, caution needs to be exercised because some babies may be in DIC with severe ICH and at risk of thrombotic complications if given a prothrombotic product.

Prenatal Diagnosis

This can be offered to families via chorionic villus sampling or amniocentesis with a known mutation for a severe bleeding disorder. Early diagnosis is useful because parents have the option to terminate the pregnancy or allow for early intervention. Advances in medicine also have made preimplantation diagnosis as well as embryonic biopsy to select an embryo unaffected by the mutation possible.

Neonatal Thrombotic Disorders

1. The neonatal period is the highest-risk period for venous and arterial thrombosis in childhood.

2. Central access devices are responsible for over 90 percent of neonatal thrombosis.

3. The most common spontaneous thrombosis in neonates is renal vein thrombosis.

4. The contribution of risk factors other than central access devices in neonatal thrombosis is unknown.

5. Thrombosis in the neonates can be associated with mortality and morbidity.

6. Thrombophilia testing in neonatal thrombosis should not be performed apart from specific circumstances, e.g. purpura fulminans.

7. Treatment of asymptomatic thrombi is controversial.

8. The extrapolation of anticoagulation principles from adults is least likely valid in the neonatal period.

9. Anticoagulation is particularly challenging in neonates for pragmatic reasons (i.e. vascular access, lack of subcutaneous tissue, variable vitamin K status).

10. Anticoagulation in neonates, especially small preterm infants, is particularly challenging because of risk of intracranial hemorrhage (ICH).

11. The long-term outcome of neonatal thrombosis is unknown.

Introduction

Thrombosis in neonates is very much a complication of tertiary care. Vascular access is responsible for almost all thromboses in neonates apart from spontaneous renal vein thrombosis. Presumably, many thromboses are asymptomatic, and their need for treatment remains very controversial.

The physiology of hemostasis is quite different in the neonate compared with adults and even older children. Coagulation proteins are independently synthesized in the fetus. Compared with adults, there are differences in the concentration of coagulation proteins, synthesis, and turnover in newborn babies. Moreover, there are also differences in the way the key hemostatic enzymes are regulated in the newborn.

Anticoagulation is difficult for multiple pragmatic reasons, whatever agent is used. Unfractionated heparin (UFH) is difficult to monitor because vascular access is usually very difficult to maintain, and the ability to run an UFH infusion without interruption is frequently limited. Low-molecular-weight heparin (LMWH) comes in pre-drawn-up syringes made for adult dosing, so accurately determining doses for infants weighing less than 2 kg can be very difficult. Further, LMWH may be problematic to administer in very premature infants with minimal subcutaneous tissue and may require significant dose reduction in the presence of renal disease. Monitoring tests are equally difficult to obtain. Vitamin K antagonists come in adult-sized tablets with no liquid preparation available. Reproducible dosing in this context is not easy because crushing tables and mixing into a fluid for feeding are required. Breast-fed infants have a relative vitamin K deficiency and tend to be exquisitely sensitive to warfarin. Formula-fed infants are resistant to warfarin given that all formulas are fortified with vitamin K. The optimal treatment strategies are not clear, and the long-term outcomes of thrombosis in neonates is also unclear, so treating neonatal thrombosis is unsatisfactory on many levels, and assessing the true risk-benefit ratio of treatment is not possible. This is an area of practice that needs considerable more research.

The most catastrophic thrombotic complication, purpura fulminans, which is due to homozygous protein C or S deficiency, usually presents in the newborn period.

Vascular-Access-Related Thrombosis

Central vascular access devices (CVADs) represent the most important risk factor in a majority of thrombotic events. Among CVADs, umbilical catheters and peripherally inserted central catheters (PICCs) are most frequently implicated. Thrombi associated with central venous lines are commonly located in the right heart, inferior vena cava (IVC), and hepatic veins. Other risk factors reported to be associated with thrombosis in the newborn include prematurity, intra-uterine growth restriction (IUGR), maternal diabetes, prolonged mechanical ventilation, hypoxic-ischemic encephalopathy (HIE), necrotizing enterocolitis (NEC), meconium aspiration syndrome (MAS), respiratory distress syndrome (RDS), prolonged hospital stay, sepsis, birth asphyxia, and congenital heart disorders. Whether these conditions simply represent the infants most likely to require medical intervention, particularly central vascular access, or whether these conditions somehow predispose to thrombosis in their own right is unknown.

Umbilical Artery Catheter (UAC)–Associated Thrombosis

The clinical presentation of UAC-associated thrombosis varies depending on the extent of the thrombosis and involvement of other arteries. Most such infants are clinically asymptomatic or have minor symptoms, whereas a smaller number have major symptoms. UAC-associated thrombosis may cause necrotizing enterocolitis secondary to mesenteric artery occlusion, embolic events to the lower limbs causing ischemia, or embolic events to the central nervous system (CNS) via a right-to-left shunt, such as patent foramen ovale. The incidence of major thrombosis-associated symptoms secondary to UACs is approximately 1 to 3 percent of infants. The gold standard test for the diagnoses of UAC-associated thrombosis is contrast angiography, but this is rarely feasible. There are many reports of UAC-associated thrombosis being first discovered at autopsy, suggesting that the diagnosis is frequently not made during life. Noninvasive imaging techniques such as Doppler ultrasound are most commonly used because of their ease of performance at the bedside. There are reports of failure of ultrasound to detect clinically relevant aortic thrombosis, but ultrasound techniques have improved dramatically over recent years, and there have been few recent studies.

Umbilical artery catheter tips are either positioned high (level of T5 to T10) or low (level of L3 to L5), and the position of umbilical artery catheters may affect the frequency of both thrombosis and intracerebral hemorrhage. While multiple studies have shown that low-dose UFH infusion prolongs patency of UACs, there are few data about the effectiveness of prophylaxis for major thrombosis or the risk of prophylaxis for intracerebral hemorrhage.

Umbilical Vein Catheter (UVC)–Associated Thrombosis

The frequency of asymptomatic UVC-associated thrombosis is almost 30 percent based on ultrasound, echocardiography (ECHO), or autopsy studies, but the symptomatic rates of thrombosis are only 1 to 3 percent. Once again, catheter placement technique is important is reducing the risk of thrombosis and the potential implications of thrombosis. UVCs should be placed beyond the ductus venosus. Portal vein thrombosis is the most common presenting thrombosis associated with UVCs, and while it may present acutely with abdominal distension and splenomegaly, it frequently presents as a late complication with evidence of portal hypertension including esophageal varices.

Central Venous Line–Associated Thrombosis

Symptomatic venous thrombotic events, almost always secondary to central venous access, can present with extremity swelling and/or thrombocytopenia. Vascular access dysfunction is another common presenting symptom. However, most often thrombi are detected during imaging for another indication. Diagnosis is established routinely by ultrasound or echocardiography.

Peripheral Artery Catheter–Associated Thrombosis

Peripheral artery catheter–associated thrombosis is not uncommon and usually presents with a cold and ischemic limb distal to the site of catheter insertion. Necrosis of the digit tips is frequent. Arterial puncture and catheter placement ideally should occur in arteries that are supported by dual supply, such as the radial/ulnar arteries and the dorsalis pedis/posterior tibial arteries. However, even when this is done, clinical ischemia can occur. Immediate removal of the catheter is always indicated to reduce the spasm component and to improve arterial flow. Further management of this entity is discussed in Chapter 31.

Treatment and Outcome of CVAD-Related Thrombosis

The optimal treatment or duration of treatment of thrombi is unknown. Most thromboses in newborns are treated with UFH or LMWH. Preterm infants require higher doses than term infants, and guidelines for doses and durations are available in literature based on case series, experience, and expert opinion. See Chapter 33 for more details. Supportive care and radiologic surveillance are preferred for the extreme preterm infants in whom risk of intraventricular hemorrhage (IVH) is high, especially in the first few weeks of life. Thrombolysis is reserved for life- or limb-threatening thromboses.

There are no prospective studies looking at short-term outcome based on treatment administered. Clinically, regardless of the treatment modality used, most neonatal thromboses get better symptomatically or resolve. A small percentage develop long-term sequelae of pulmonary hypertension or post thrombotic syndrome. Some infants die of the thrombosis, and at this stage, there are few data on which to predict the likely outcome for any individual child, other than the severity of the infant's overall health status and the degree of prematurity.

Renal Vein Thrombosis

Renal vein thrombosis (RVT) in neonates is the most common type of spontaneous venous thrombosis. The pathogenesis of this entity is not vascular access related, and studies indicate that the thrombotic process begins in the renal microvasculature and then extends out into the renal veins and potentially the IVC (in 50 to 60 percent of cases). This is important because it means that the kidney damage (which is usually the cause of acute death from renal failure or the cause of long-term consequences such as chronic renal failure [~3 percent] or hypertension [~20 percent]) is unlikely resolved by removal of the large vessel thrombosis within the IVC or renal veins, as would be achieved by thrombectomy. If treatment is required, then anticoagulation or possibly thrombolysis is more appropriate because these therapies can have an impact at the microvascular level. Approximately 25 percent of cases are bilateral, supporting the concept that this disease is related to something occurring within the renal parenchyma vasculature as distinct from large vessels.

The classic presentation of RVT in neonates is the triad of flank mass, hematuria, and thrombocytopenia. Further investigation usually reveals non function of the involved kidney, and the affected side usually evolves renal atrophy with hypertrophy of the non affected kidney as compensation. Obviously, bilateral disease more often progresses to renal failure.

Treatment is controversial because there are no data that conclusively show differences in the renal outcomes based on whether or not treatment is given. Recurrence rates are very low, and subsequent risk of other thromboses does not appear to be increased.

One approach to treatment is to treat unilateral RVT conservatively with observation and repeat imaging and support of renal function. Extension of the thrombus into the IVC may justify anticoagulation with UFH initially and LMWH subsequently (both therapies may need dose reduction based on renal function) for three months to reduce the risk of embolic phenomena. Bilateral RVT is usually treated more aggressively with anticoagulation owing to the risk of renal failure, and if renal function is deteriorating, then it may be an indication for urgent thrombolysis. The use of these agents is discussed in Chapter 33.

Neonatal Purpura Fulminans

Purpura fulminans is an acute, lethal syndrome of DIC characterized by rapidly progressive hemorrhagic necrosis of the skin due to dermal vascular thrombosis. Affected infants often look normal at birth and then over the subsequent 24 to 48 hours develop small ecchymotic areas that increase in a radial fashion, become purplish black with bullae, and then turn necrotic and gangrenous. The lesions occur mainly on the extremities but can occur on the buttocks, abdomen, scrotum, and scalp. The progression is often rapid and alarming. The syndrome is due to homozygous protein C (most commonly) or protein S deficiency or compound heterozygous states with undetectable plasma levels of the respective protein.

Despite the normal appearances at birth, up to 70 percent of affected infants will have cerebral or ophthalmic damage (or both) that occurred *in utero*. CNS imaging and formal ophthalmologic examination should be arranged as soon as possible. There may be a history of consanguinity, and interestingly, although both parents are usually heterozygotes for protein C or S deficiency, they almost never have a personal thrombotic history.

The diagnosis is based on the appropriate clinical picture, a very low or undetectable protein C/protein S level, heterozygous deficiency of the same protein in the parents, and ideally, identification of the molecular defect. The diagnosis can be more difficult with increasing prematurity because the normal levels of protein C and S can approach the lower detection limits of the assays, and in fact, heterozygotes may have undetectable levels in premature infants. However, the clinical picture is usually dramatic and unmistakable. Clinical differential diagnosis includes DIC from other causes, although rarely is the skin necrosis so florid and aggressive in a systemically well baby.

Initial therapy involves protein C replacement, and this can be achieved via 10 to 20 ml/kg of fresh frozen plasma (FFP) every 6 to 12 h, which is usually the form of therapy that is most readily available. Plasma levels of protein C achieved with these doses of FFP vary from 15 to 32 percent at 30 minutes after the infusion and from 4 to 10 percent at 12 h. Plasma levels of protein S (which is entirely bound to C4b) are 23 percent at 2 h and 14 percent at 24 h, with an approximate half-life of 36 h.

If the diagnosis is confirmed as protein C deficiency (much more common than protein S deficiency), then protein C concentrate can be used. Doses of protein C concentrate have ranged from 20 to 60 units/kg. Replacement therapy should be continued until all the clinical lesions resolve, which is usually at 6 to 8 weeks. In addition to the clinical course, plasma D-dimer concentrations may be useful for monitoring the effectiveness of protein C replacement.

The options for the long-term management of infants with homozygous protein C/protein S deficiency include long-term anticoagulation therapy, replacement therapy with either FFP or protein C concentrate, and liver transplantation. Protein C concentrate can be given subcutaneously. Central venous access should be avoided, if possible, due to the high incidence of aggressive large-vessel thrombosis. The natural history is of recurrent episodes of purpura fulminans and progressive damage of key organs unless optimal therapy can be maintained. Treatment is often not easy, and referral to a specialist center with experience is often required.

Acquired purpura fulminans is more common than congenital deficiencies in the neonatal period and is seen with infections, particularly group B streptococcal infections. Other acquired causes include DIC, warfarin therapy, severe liver dysfunction, and metabolic disorders, e.g. galactosemia.

Arterial Ischemic Stroke (AIS)/ Cerebrosinovenous Thrombosis (CSVT)

These entities are discussed in detail in Chapter 32.

Thrombophilia Testing in Newborns with Thrombosis

There are no data that really support changing the intensity or duration of treatment for vascular access–related thrombosis or RVT based on the presence or absence of thrombophilia testing. Further, the recurrence rates for thrombosis in neonates, in the absence of ongoing clinical factors, remain extremely small. Thrombophilia testing in the newborn is reserved for where homozygous deficiencies in protein S or C are suspected (i.e. neonatal purpura fulminans) or when large idiopathic thrombi occur. Even if testing is performed, it is important to remember the age-based differences in concentration of inhibitors of protein C or S and Antithrombin, and interpretation of results other than for exclusion of homozygous states is very difficult.

In situations where the neonate is asymptomatic but the parents have a known deficiency of one of these inhibitors and are requesting testing of their baby, deferral of testing until after 6 to 12 months of life is important because differentiation of normal from heterozygote deficiency is much easier at that time. Obviously, factor V Leiden and prothrombin gene mutation testing are genetic tests that are interpretable at any age, but there is rarely an indication for testing for these abnormalities in the newborn period.

10

Inherited Bone Marrow Failure Syndromes

Key Messages

1. For each inherited bone marrow failure (BMF) syndrome, there are clinical hematologic and nonhematologic features.

2. There have been enormous advances in our understanding of the molecular basis of these diseases in recent years. This pace of change is likely to continue and impacts on both the diagnosis and treatment of these disorders.

3. Acquired bone marrow failure (aplastic anemia) is distinguished from the inherited BMF syndromes by the absence of associated features and the absence of mutation in genes known to be responsible for heritable BMF. However, as the genetic basis of inherited BMT expands, some cases formerly considered to be acquired may be reclassified as genetic.

4. Treatment of these conditions is complex and requires specialist consideration.

5. Bone marrow transplantation has a role in the management of inherited BMF.

Introduction

This chapter introduces the bone marrow failure (BMF) syndromes, including Fanconi anemia (FA), Diamond-Blackfan anemia (DBA), dyskeratosis congenita (DKC), and Shwachman-Diamond syndrome (SDS). These are individually rare syndromes. Our understanding of the genetics and pathogenesis of these conditions has increased dramatically in recent years, and it is apparent that the individual syndromes are genetically as well as clinically diverse. Each syndrome will be considered under the headings of the hematologic manifestations, nonhematologic manifestations, diagnosis, biologic basis and treatment.

Fanconi Anemia

Fanconi anemia (FA) is a genetically and clinically heterogeneous disorder characterized by multiple physical congenital anomalies, hematologic abnormalities and a predisposition to hematologic and nonhematologic malignancy. The biologic foundation of the illness is mutation of one of the many genes that code for the proteins of the FA pathway, which is involved in DNA repair. The classic diagnostic test for FA is assessment of cellular hypersensitivity to DNA strand–strand cross-linking agents such as diepoxybutane (DEB) and mitomycin C (MMC).

The Hematologic Features of Fanconi Anemia

Hematologic manifestations represent the most prevalent pathologic manifestation of FA. The most obvious and predictable manifestation is bone marrow failure and hypoplastic/aplastic anemia. Most cases of FA have some degree of marrow failure by the age of 10 years and many patients will have aplastic anemia requiring transfusion support. In some, the onset of marrow failure may be in adulthood. The presence of FA as the underlying cause for a patient presenting with severe aplastic anemia (SAA) should be suspected where there is an associated physical abnormality, including short stature, and FA testing is mandatory for all patients presenting with aplastic anemia regardless of family history or associated features.

In addition to BMF, the presence of FA dramatically increases the risk of myelodysplasia (MDS) and acute myeloid leukemia (AML). The risk of AML is increased more than 500-fold in FA and the peak incidence is in the second decade of life. Although MDS or AML is usually preceded by a period of BMF, this is not always so. There are certain cytogenetic alterations that are typical in children with the MDS/

AML of FA, and they should be specifically looked for in children with known FA and should also alert the clinician to the likely underlying diagnosis of FA when found in a patient with apparently *de novo* AML. There are gains in 1q23-32 and 3q26. The latter might need to be looked for specifically using fluorescence in situ hybridization (FISH) techniques and is predictive of disease progression, usually appearing before monosomy 7 or deletion 7q, which are also commonly found in the MDS and AML of FA. The cytogenetic laboratory should be alerted when sampling the bone marrow of a suspected or known FA patient so that these cytogenetic changes can be specifically excluded.

The Nonhematologic Features of FA

Individuals with FA frequently have physical abnormalities that should be sought on examination of each new patient with aplastic anemia (AA) and that might alert the astute pediatrician to the presence of FA before BMF has developed. Not all FA patients have associated physical abnormalities, and laboratory testing for FA is therefore mandatory in all cases of AA.

The most common associated physical abnormalities are

- Short stature
- Associated skeletal abnormalities, frequently of the thumb and forearm. (The thumbs may be absent, smaller than normal, or duplicated. The radius may be absent or hypoplastic.)
- Skin pigmentation including café-au-lait patches
- Typical Fanconi dysmorphic facies, including microphthalmia
- Anomalies of the kidney (including single or horseshoe kidney), genitourinary tract, and heart

There is subfertility in individuals with FA. There might be increased osteoporosis.

The presence of FA increases the risk of solid tumors, including squamous cell cancers of the head and neck (especially the mouth) and cervical/gynecologic malignancies. The age at presentation of these cancers is later than the age at presentation of BMF and hematologic malignancy. In patients with known FA, these cancers should be specifically and regularly screened for so that intervention can be at an early stage of malignant change, be less damaging, and have a better chance of success.

Diagnosis of Fanconi Anemia

The diagnosis of FA should be specifically sought for

- In patients presenting with AA
- In patients with the characteristic physical anomalies, including short stature
- In patients with MDS or AML, especially with the characteristic chromosome changes of FA-associated hematologic malignancy, namely, 1q+ and 3q+

Diagnosis in the AA patient means that inappropriate immune-suppressant therapy is not employed in FA-associated AA, and the appropriate conditioning therapy for hematopoietic stem cell transplantation (HSCT) is given because intensive and standard conditioning regimens are likely to cause regimen-related toxicity that might be fatal. Diagnosed FA patients can be entered into a screening program for head and neck cancer and females for cervical and gynecologic cancers.

The classic diagnostic test for FA is based on the exquisite sensitivity of FA cells to DNA interstrand cross-linking agents such as DEB or MMC. These are the primary assays for FA.

- Occasional false-positive results might be obtained in other genetic disorders associated with DNA repair problems, including Nijmegen breakage syndrome.
- False-negative results might be obtained where there is somatic mosaicism. In somatic mosaicism, one FA-mutated allele in a single bone marrow stem cell becomes competent either through chance reversal of a point mutation or recombination between the two alleles carrying a heterozygous mutation so that one allele acquires both mutations and one loses the one that it did carry. The cell in the FA bone marrow that has acquired this normal allele will have an advantage over other FA cells in the bone marrow and will contribute more significantly to the peripheral blood cells, and those cells will not be sensitive to DEB or MMC because they bear a normal allele.

Where the clinical index of suspicion for FA is high and the DEB or MMC test is negative, then the test can be repeated on cultured fibroblasts because somatic mosaicism is not described in this tissue. There is no selective advantage to the FA fibroblast.

Reference laboratories will take the diagnosis of FA further. It is genetically heterogeneous with, to date, 15 different Fanconi genes. The exact elucidation of which is involved in a particular child can be achieved by

- Sequencing the genes individually in the order of the frequency in which they are found (*FANCA* most common; then *FANCG*, *FANCC*, and so on)
- Complementation analysis (A retrovirus is used to deliver *in vitro* a particular competent FA gene to the patient's cells. If the MMC sensitivity of the patient cells is corrected, then the retrovirus must have delivered the correct gene to that cell – e.g. a retrovirus bearing the correct *FANCA* gene will correct MMC sensitivity in a *FANCA* patient but not in a *FANCC* patient.)

The practicing pediatric hematologist usually will consult the family on two other issues. The family should be invited to register the case with the international FA registry and also to join the local (often national) patient support organization. This will support the family in coming to terms with a rare diagnosis and keep them (and the physician often!) abreast of updates in the biology and management of this condition.

Biologic Basis of Fanconi Anemia

Our understanding of the biology of FA has increased in recent years, and can be summarized as follows:

- To date, 15 FA genes have been identified: *FANCA*, *FANCB*, *FANCC*, and so on.
- That FA is so diverse was first identified by complementation analysis – fusing one FA patient's cells with another FA patient's cells sometimes corrected (complemented) the *in vitro* sensitivity to MMC or DEB. So fusing a *FANCA* cell with a *FANCB* cell will correct MMC sensitivity because it has nonmutated alleles of *FANCA* and *FANCB*, but fusing a *FANCA* cell with another *FANCA* cell will clearly not correct the MMC sensitivity.
- One of the FA genes, *FANCD1*, is the same as *BRCA2* gene, which is a recognized as a breast and ovarian cancer predisposing gene.
- These 15 genes encode for proteins that act together in complexes that constitute the FA/BRCA pathway that recognizes and repairs DNA interstrand cross-links, and this is illustrated in Figure 10.1.

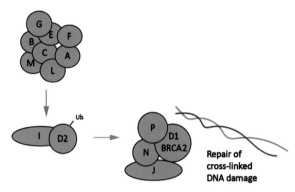

Figure 10.1 The FA complex and DNA repair.

- A key event is the mono-ubiquination of *FANCD2* and *FANCI* upon DNA damage.
- This mono-ubiquination is catalyzed by a group of 'upstream' FA proteins that include FANCA, -B, -C, -E, -F, -G, -L, and –M.
- The mono-ubiquinated FANCD2 and FANCI dimer then interacts with 'downstream' FA proteins that include FANCD1/BRCA2, FANCN, FANCJ, and FANCP.
- The whole complex ensures genome integrity.
- Cells that accumulate DNA damage will exit the cell cycle at the G_2M checkpoint, so using flow cytometry, increased cells are seen at this point in FA patients than in control individuals.
- Exit of cells from the cell cycle will lead to progressive BMF. Where there is a background of deficient hematopoiesis, then there is selective pressure on surviving stem cell for clonal escape. Such cells have additional mutations and will generate dysplastic and frankly malignant hematopoiesis.

Treatment of Fanconi Anemia

The principal treatment of the BMF of FA is allogeneic HSCT:

- Matched sibling donor HSCT is performed at diagnosis of BMF and with falling blood counts.
- Matched unrelated donor HSCT likely has higher toxicity and the procedure might be deferred a little – perhaps to transfusion dependence.
- HSCT results are better if performed earlier in the course of the disease rather than late in a heavily transfused, perhaps infected patient with accumulating comorbidities.

- The conditioning therapy is reduced compared to non-FA aplastic anemia. Fludarabine is used routinely as immune suppression and is well tolerated at full dose. Typically, cyclophosphamide is used with fludarabine, but the dose is usually much reduced compared to non-FA aplastic anemia (40 mg/kg total dose in HSCT for FA compared to 120 to 200 mg/kg in HSCT for idiopathic SAA). In some institutions, radiotherapy is still employed in the conditioning regimen when the donor is not a sibling.
- Usually, serotherapy is used as part of conditioning therapy even in sibling donor transplantation to reduce the risk of both rejection and graft-versus-host disease (GvHD). There is evidence that GvHD might increase the risk of head and neck cancers after transplantation.

After transplantation, there should be continued surveillance for head and neck cancer and, where relevant, for gynecologic cancer because successful HSCT does not reduce this risk and may even increase it, especially if there is chronic GvHD after transplantation or if radiotherapy has been used as part of the conditioning therapy for the transplant. Human papillomavirus (HPV) vaccination should be given to further reduce the risk of malignancy after HSCT.

Hematologic malignancy – MDS and AML – has a dismal prognosis where associated with FA. There is considerable toxicity with conventional treatments – AML treatments and HSCT – and there has been reported prolonged aplasia following chemotherapy treatment. There have been some reported cases of success using cytarabine-based AML treatments and reduced intensity HSCT performed during aplasia from chemotherapy. However, the optimal treatment of the AML and the optimal HSCT protocol remain to be defined and should be the subject of discussion between teams and with experts in the field for individual patients.

Other complications of FA should be managed in specialist multidisciplinary clinics. Orthopedic intervention might be needed. The use of growth hormone is controversial because it might accelerate malignant change. Androgens used even at low dose might help to sustain adequate blood counts. Transplantation from a matched donor is the first choice usually. Androgens – such as oxymethalone and danazol – are frequently virilizing. They might also increase the risk of liver tumors. Where no matched donor is available for a patient with FA and BMF, he or she might still be considered for alternate donor transplantation, such as haploidentical transplant.

Diamond-Blackfan Anemia

This is a clinically heterogeneous, usually autosomal dominant condition characterized hematologically by macrocytic, reticulocytopenic anemia that is usually evident from infancy. There is elevated red blood cell (RBC) adenosine deaminase (ADA), which is diagnostically helpful. There are often associated physical anomalies, including growth failure, and a number of affected individuals achieve transfusion independence with steroid therapy, whereas the remainder are managed with either RBC transfusion and iron chelation or HSCT. DBA is associated with malignant changes, including hematologic and solid tumors.

The biologic understanding of DBA has increased greatly in recent years. The genetic basis is due to mutations in genes that encode ribosomal proteins – the most common being *RPS19*. DBA is therefore a ribosomopathy, and the RBC precursor cell death (apoptosis) is mediated by p53 activation in the cell.

Hematologic Manifestations of Diamond-Blackfan Anemia

Most DBA cases present in infancy (but not at birth) with a reticulocytopenic, macrocytic anemia. The platelet count is variable but frequently elevated. On further investigation, there is elevated fetal hemoglobin, and a reference laboratory will identify that the RBC ADA concentration is elevated. The bone marrow is normocellular with a paucity of RBC precursors.

There is, however, an attenuated phenotype. The same genetic mutation may cause variable illness in different family members. Some might be phenotypically and hematologically completely normal, and some might have mild anemia only or macrocytosis of otherwise unexplained etiology. Pregnancy and puberty are particular times at which overt anemic DBA might be triggered. The distinction between affected and unaffected family members becomes particularly important in a family without a genetic marker in whom a sibling donor is being worked up. Transplantation of DBA donor marrow into a DBA recipient will not correct the hematologic abnormality of the patient.

In adults, the differential diagnosis of pure RBC aplasia might be considerable, but in children, the only common differential diagnosis is with transient erythroblastopenia of childhood (TEC). TEC usually occurs in older children (toddlers) and is transient. The anemia is normocytic (until the reticulocytosis that accompanies recovery), and the ADA is normal. Hemoglobin F (HbF) is similarly not raised until the stress erythropoiesis of recovery. The bone marrow is often sampled in early recovery phase, and there are sometimes plentiful RBC precursors present in the TEC marrow.

Hematologic malignancy is reported in DBA. There are cases of AML, ALL and MDS. The incidence is likely above the background population, but not increased to the same extent as such malignancy in FA.

Nonhematologic Manifestations of Diamond-Blackfan Anemia

It is common for there to be associated physical anomalies in DBA patients. The facial appearance – known as *Cathie facies* – is well recognized with widely spaced eyes and a snub nose. Abnormal thumbs are also classic, with the triphalangeal thumb being most common. These may be present in up to 50 percent of patients.

Growth failure is often present and may be contributed to by therapeutic steroids for the anemia. There may be other craniofacial anomalies, including cleft defects, and there may be other anomalies of the upper limbs.

For the newly diagnosed or suspected DBA patient, growth should be plotted on centile charts, the skeleton of the upper limb formally investigated, and cardiac and abdominal ultrasound performed to search for the sometimes associated cardiac and genitourinary abnormalities.

Non-hematologic malignancy is also reported in DBA and likely occurs above background incidence and earlier in life. However, such illness is not seen to the same extent as in FA.

Diagnosis of Diamond-Blackfan Anemia

The patient may present with the typical infantile macrocytic anemia. A marrow biopsy will reveal a paucity of RBC precursors, and the ADA concentration is raised. The HbF level is typically raised. A search for associated features should be formally undertaken.

Some cases will be diagnosed from those associated other features, and the presentation may be through the general pediatrician, neonatologist, or geneticist. Such a presentation may predate hematologic abnormalities or the hematologic changes may be subtle.

Finally, presentation may be within known kindred. The hematologic and non-hematologic manifestations of DBA within the same family and the same mutation are well recognized to be extremely variable. The ribosomal genes known to be associated with DBA should be screened in a reference laboratory.

The practicing pediatric hematologist will usually consult the family on two other issues, as for FA. The family should be invited to register the case with the international DBA registry and also join the local (often national) patient support organization. This will support the family in coming to terms with a rare diagnosis and keep them (and the physician often!) abreast of updates in the biology and management of this condition.

Biologic Basis of Diamond-Blackfan Anemia

This is a changing area of medicine. DBA is now known to be caused in many cases by mutation in one of the genes encoding for ribosomal proteins. The following points can be made:

- It is usually a mono-allelic mutation, which is consistent with the observed autosomal dominant inheritance pattern of DBA.
- Several different genes have been described to be mutated in different cases of DBA. It is genetically as well as clinically heterogeneous. The most common gene mutated is *RPS19*. Other ribosomal protein genes described to be affected are *L5*, *L11* and *S26*.
- A national reference DBA laboratory will screen known genes for mutation in a case of DBA. However, in about 50 percent of DBA cases, a mutation in one of the known genes cannot be identified, but this does not exclude the diagnosis of DBA.

DBA is therefore a ribosomopathy. Haplo-insufficiency of individual ribosomal proteins perturbs the precise stoichiometry of ribosomal biogenesis, and such an imbalance leads to the accumulation of p53, which has a central role in initiating apoptosis in the DBA erythroid precursor. The gene p53 acts as a cell-cycle checkpoint, and the *p53* gene is a known tumor suppressor gene, so loss of expression of *p53* is associated with constitutional cancer predisposition (the Li-Fraumeni syndrome).

Treatment of Diamond-Blackfan Anemia

There are three treatment strategies for the anemic patient with DBA:

- RBC transfusion with iron chelation
- Steroid therapy
- HSCT from an HLA-matched, unaffected donor

For the newly diagnosed infant, RBC transfusion support is usually indicated. Steroid therapy is often avoided in the first year of life so as not to impair growth when it might be expected to be at its maximal. For those failing steroid therapy, a regular transfusion program will remain the backbone of treatment. The components of such a program will be as for any such transfusion program: it should be regular. The median hemoglobin should be about 100 g/liter and the nadir about 80 g/liter. The blood selected might be phenotyped to reduce alloimmunization, and the annual use of RBCs be calculated. For those using excessive RBCs (>250 ml/kg per year), splenectomy may be considered. Iron chelation therapy will be required for children on such a regular transfusion program.

Steroids are effective in some cases of DBA. It remains unclear how they act. The following statements about steroids in DBA patients can be made:

- They have some effect in most but not all patients. About 20 percent of patients do not respond at all to steroids.
- In those who respond to steroids, the treating clinician will attempt to wean the steroid dose used to a minimum that maintains response but still retains the therapeutic benefit. Long-term steroid use is usually required and will have dose-dependent long-term side effects, including on growth, bone mineralization, and cataract formation.
- Prior to starting steroids, the clinician must be absolutely sure they are treating DBA and not TEC, and this requires either a clear abnormal ADA result or transfusion support for long enough to exclude TEC as a potential diagnosis.
- The maximal acceptable steroid dose is considered to be 0.5 mg/kg per day of prednisone, and this is often given on alternate days.

- About 35 percent of DBA patients on the international registry use steroids to maintain transfusion independence. The remainder either did not respond to steroids, the response was not maintained, or too high a maintenance dose was required to safely maintain the beneficial hematologic effect.

HSCT from an unaffected donor will correct the hematologic phenotype, including the risk of hematologic malignancy. HSCT will therefore obviate the need for transfusion support and iron chelation and will mean that long-term steroid therapy and its attendant toxicity are not necessary. The following points about HSCT in DBA must be noted:

- Care must be taken in selecting a family donor such that the donor does not have an attenuated, phenotypically milder DBA. This is easy, of course, where there is a genetic marker, but in the absence of such a mutation, the sibling should be carefully evaluated, including with a RBC ADA determination.
- HSCT carries short- and long-term toxicities. Many of the deaths reported to the DBA registries are associated with HSCT. Of course, DBA patients requiring HSCT are likely to be the more difficult cases. HSCT has generic risks of its own, and these should be carefully evaluated before accepting a DBA child for HSCT.
- The risks of HSCT are likely to be least in a child without comorbidity (e.g. iron overload) and with a well-matched donor. The best-matched donor will be an HLA-identical sibling. Few unrelated donor HSCT procedures have been done in DBA, but in general, the risks are much reduced than in the past, with better typing of donors and better matching of donors to recipients.
- The patient's condition should be optimized prior to HSCT. The iron overload in particular should be carefully evaluated and reduced with intensive chelation therapy.
- Transplantation will carry both short-term morbidity and mortality risk as well as long-term morbidity risk, including infertility.
- Different transplant programs will offer different preparative regimens. In general, the regimen should include serotherapy to reduce the risk of graft rejection and GvHD. Increasingly, reduced-intensity or reduced-toxicity regimens are employed in the transplantation of children with

DBA. There are some centers that will perform more DBA HSCT than others.

- Support for families undergoing HSCT will be available within the patient's support organization.

Dyskeratosis Congenita (DKC)

This is a clinically and genetically heterogeneous condition that is caused by mutation in the genes that encode for the proteins that maintain telomere length and integrity in hematopoietic stem cells. It is a rare condition, and no one hematologist will see many cases. The principal clinical manifestations are in the bone marrow, including aplastic anemia, and in the liver and the lung. These organs are affected to different extents, often even within the same kindred. The inheritance is variable. Both X-linked and autosomal recessive patterns have been described.

DKC and associated illnesses need to be diagnosed in central reference laboratories with experience in the illness, and the patients, too, should be seen in such centers. They also should be referred to national support organizations so that they can meet others affected by the same disease and learn about recent developments in this rapidly changing area of medicine.

Hematologic Manifestations of Dyskeratosis Congenita

The hematologic phenotype of DKC is variable:

- DKC may present as typical aplastic anemia with pancytopenia and a markedly hypocellular bone marrow trephine biopsy.
- A normal blood count with normal indices may be seen in an individual known to be genetically affected.
- Macrocytosis, a mild macrocytic anemia, or other cytopenias may be present. These may be progressive or relatively stable.

The diagnosis of DKC will follow from appropriate testing of the patient in whom clinical suspicion of the diagnosis was raised, usually from the presence of associated features or the family history. Children with DKC have a much increased risk – at least 100-fold – of AML compared to the background population. AML in these children will often have complex poor-risk cytogenetics including monosomy 7.

Nonhematologic Manifestations of Dyskeratosis Congenita

The diagnosis of DKC should be considered in newly diagnosed children with macrocytic anemia or aplastic anemia. Associated features should be looked for:

- The mucocutaneous triad:
  - Nail dyskeratosis and dystrophy with ridges
  - Leukoplakia of the mouth
  - Skin hypo- or hyperpigmentation with the characteristic 'plucked chicken' appearance
- There is also prominent involvement of the liver and lung:
  - There might be cirrhosis, portal hypertension, or steatosis. Abnormalities might be seen on imaging or biopsy and might have to be specifically elicited.
  - The classic lung pathology is idiopathic pulmonary fibrosis. There might be x-ray, computed tomographic (CT), or biopsy changes of such. The concurrence of such lung pathology and BMF is highly suggestive of DKC or a similar illness.
- There might be involvement of many other organ systems, including the gastrointestinal tract with diarrhea and bleeding.

There is a marked increased risk of oral cancer. A screening program should be implemented for this in known affected individuals so that it may be detected early and treatment might be expected to be more effective and less invasive.

Diagnosis of Dyskeratosis Congenita

This is a rare diagnosis. Diagnosis rests on three pillars:

- Clinical suspicion from associated nonhematologic features or from a family history
- The finding of shortened blood telomeres using flow-FISH technology in an experienced reference laboratory (The shorter the telomeres, the more likely is the diagnosis of DKC. Once the telomeres are less than the first percentile of the age-matched control population, then the diagnosis is likely.)
- The genes that are known to be mutated in DKC can be screened where the diagnosis is suspected. This also should be undertaken in a reference laboratory. Clinical findings should be correlated with genetic findings.

Biology of Dyskeratosis Congenita

DKC is a telomereopathy that arises from accelerated telomere loss from hematopoietic stem cells (HSCs). Understanding DKC is understanding telomere biology.

- Telomeres are long tracts of bland (not gene-encoding) DNA that cap eukaryotic chromosomes.
- When DNA is replicated by somatic cells, this telomere cap is shortened. The length of a telomere in any somatic tissue including blood is shorter in aged than in young individuals.
- When the telomere reaches a critical length, cell division will stop. This is known as the *mitotic clock*, and the limit to cell division that is related to critical telomere shortening is known as the *Hayflick limit*.
- Malignant cells have acquired various mechanisms to maintain telomeres with continuing replication, escaping the Hayflick limit.
- Some cells must preserve their telomeres during replication, and these cells include gonadal stem cells and tissue stem cells including HSCs. Maintenance of telomeres allows the extensive replicative potential of such cells, which allows them to provide a lifetime of blood cells to the organism.
- Telomeres are preserved by telomerase, which is a ribonucleoprotein enzyme complex that synthesizes telomeres. It has several components:
  - A reverse transcriptase
  - The telomerase enzyme that is encoded by the *TERT* gene
  - An RNA template that is encoded by *TERC*
  - A stablising protein, dyskerin, encoded by DKC1, found on the X-chromosome
- Many other proteins are involved in telomere stability, maintenance of integrity, and replication, and mutation of these genes will give rise to telomeropathies with some features shared with classical DKC.

Classic DKC arises from a mutation in DKC1, and is inherited in an X-linked recessive manner. There is loss of telomerase function. HSC telomeres shorten, and cells reach their replicative limit and exit the cell cycle, leading to HSC insufficiency and aplastic anemia. Clonal escape with alternative mechanisms of preserving telomeres is a step along the road to malignant hematologic disorders including AML.

TERC and *TERT* mutations cause disease that presents in both children and adults. Inheritance is autosomal dominant. Symptoms and signs and other organ involvement might be milder than in *DKC1* mutated disease. Mutations in many other genes have been described, and continue to be described, to cause disease, including in adult patients presenting with typical aplastic anemia. The genotype–phenotype relationship in telomereopathy requires much work for a clear interpretation of the significance of many mutations to an individual patient.

Treatment of Dyskeratosis Congenita

DKC is a variable disease, but is usually progressive. DKC is a multisystem disorder that requires multi-disciplinary management in a center with expertise in treating the condition. Aplastic anemia can be managed with BMT. The best HSCT results are with matched donors and with reduced-intensity conditioning in a patient without significant comorbidities. Successful HSCT will not correct the non-hematologic manifestations of the disease but will correct the predisposition to hematologic malignancy. Usually, serotherapy will be employed in the conditioning regimen to reduce the risks of graft rejection and GvHD.

The multidisciplinary team should include hepatologists and pulmonologists, who will systematically and regularly assess liver and lung function. A dental team also should be involved. There should be a screening program for mouth cancers.

Shwachman-Diamond Syndrome

Shwachman-Diamond syndrome (SDS) is a rare autosome recessively inherited multisystem disorder characterized by pancreatic exocrine failure, impaired hematopoiesis, and a predisposition to leukemia. SDS has recently been shown to be due to biallelic mutations in the Shwachman-Bodian-Diamond-syndrome (*SBDS*) gene. How this mutation mediates disease remains uncertain.

Hematologic Manifestations of Shwachman-Diamond Syndrome

The most consistent manifestation of SDS is neutropenia, which may be intermittent rather than constant. Other cytopenias are not uncommon and may be severe. Early onset of cytopenia is common. On testing, there may be RBC features of stress erythropoiesis, namely, elevated HbF and macrocytosis. Basophilic stippling may be prominent in the smear.

Marrow cellularity is not consistently hypocellular and may change. A good bone marrow biopsy core is required to accurately assess this.

The risk of AML is increased. Different subtypes are reported, but not M3. The risk is progressive and estimated by the chronic neutropenia registry to be 20 percent at 20 years and 40 percent at 40 years. The most common cytogenetic change will be that of monosomy 7 or 7q-. Isochrome 7q abnormalities have been described and have not been shown to be associated with progression to AML or MDS, unlike other abnormalities of chromosome 7.

Patients with SDS present with infection – usually bacterial or fungal – and pneumonia is common. Neutropenia will predispose, but there is evidence that SDS neutrophils are also dysfunctional. Abnormalities of T- and B-cell number and immunoglobulin levels are described and should be screened for in the SDS patient and will contribute to the increased infection risk.

Nonhematologic Manifestations of Shwachman-Diamond Syndrome

The hallmark of SDS is pancreatic exocrine failure:

- The pancreas is small and fatty on imaging.
- There is malabsorption of fat-soluble vitamins.
- Serum pancreatic trypsinogen is low, and stool elastase is low.

There may be hepatomegaly, and many patients will have elevated liver transaminases. Liver biopsy might demonstrate portal and periportal inflammatory cell infiltrates and some fibrosis or steatosis. Liver involvement is typically early in life and clears without sequalae. There may be hepatic complications of HSCT.

Skeletal dysplasia is seen in SDS related to abnormal development of the metaphyses. Metaphyseal dysostosis is present in many patients. Osteopenia is common.

Short stature is the norm. Cardiac abnormalities are also described. There may be cardiac decompensation during full-intensity conditioning for HSCT.

Diagnosis of Shwachman-Diamond Syndrome

The diagnosis rests on recognition of the clinical phenotype, multidisciplinary searching for associated features, and examination of the *SBDS* gene, which is known to be mutated in about 90 percent of cases. Patients should have the following tests:

- Complete blood count and film
- HbF determination
- Bone marrow aspirate, biopsy, and cytogenetics
- Imaging of the pancreas
- Stool elastase or serum trypsinogen determinations
- *SBDS* gene analysis

Diagnosed patients should be registered with family permission and should be referred to the relevant local or national support organization for children with this rare disease.

Biology of Shwachman-Diamond Syndrome

SBDS is a highly conserved gene in evolutionary terms. How mutations of *SBDS* mediate SDS is uncertain. The protein product of *SBDS* is present throughout the cell and thought to be involved in ribosome biosynthesis. *SBDS* also has been shown to function during mitosis to prevent genomic instability.

Management of Shwachman-Diamond Syndrome

Multidisciplinary management in a center with experience treating children with this rare disease is pivotal. HSCT from an unaffected HLA-matched donor will correct the hematologic and immunologic aspects of this disease. Experience is limited. Reduced-toxicity or reduced-intensity regimens are likely to have outcomes that are superior to full-intensity conditioning approaches. These children are brittle and likely more liable to experience drug-related toxicities. Serotherapy will reduce the risk of graft failure and GvHD after HSCT.

The rarity of the disease and the clinical heterogeneity mean that there is controversy about the exact role and optimal timing of HSCT. Delaying transplantation and allowing clonal hematologic illness will yield HSCT results inferior to those obtained in younger children without such comorbidities. HSCT is certainly indicated where cytopenia is interfering with quality of life or is risking life and where there is evidence of emerging clonal hematopoiesis.

Acquired Bone Marrow Failure Syndrome: Aplastic Anemia

Key Messages

1. Acquired bone marrow failure syndrome, or aplastic anemia (AA), is a rare and heterogeneous cause of pancytopenia in children.

2. The key clinical distinction is between inherited and noninherited disease. Bone marrow failure (BMF) may be the first evidence of an inherited syndrome, and Fanconi anemia is the most common disorder, and such a syndrome should be carefully excluded at presentation.

3. Most noninherited cases of AA are idiopathic and likely secondary to immune-mediated loss of hematopoietic stem cells.

4. Treatment of acquired AA is both supportive and specific. Specific management includes immunosuppressive therapy (IST) and allogeneic hematopoietic stem cell transplantation (HSCT), and treatment choices are based on the severity of the cytopenia and the availability of an HLA-identical donor.

Assessment of the Child with Aplastic Anemia

AA is peripheral blood pancytopenia (Hb < 100 g/liter, neutrophils < 1.5×10^9/liter, and platelets < 50×10^9/liter) that is caused by a hypocellular (empty) bone marrow that is neither infiltrated nor fibrotic. AA is rare (<5 cases per million per year) and is a far rarer cause of pancytopenia than hematologic malignancy.

Severity is assessed by both the peripheral blood count and the bone marrow trephine cellularity:

- Severe aplastic anemia (SAA) is defined as
  - Two of three of reticulocytes < 20×10^9/liter, platelets < 20×10^9/liter, and neutrophils < 0.5×10^9/liter
  - Less than 25 percent marrow cellularity
- Very severe aplastic anemia (VSAA) is defined as the same as SAA but the neutrophils are <0.2×10^9/liter.
- In non-severe AA, these criteria for SAA or VSAA are not reached.

Presentation of the Child with Aplastic Anemia

The clinical features of AA are those of pancytopenia, so lethargy, bruising/bleeding and fever are common. There is typically macrocytic anemia with reduced reticulocytes, and teardrop red blood cells (RBCs) may be prominent in the smear. There is a reduction in marrow cellularity with increased fat and there may be dyserythropoiesis. The marrow cellularity can be more accurately quantified on marrow trephine biopsy and the absence of infiltration and fibrosis should be confirmed in this biopsy. The bone marrow cytogenetics are usually normal in SAA, and the presence of clonal change such as monosomy 7 or 5q- should indicate the likelihood of a diagnosis of myelodysplasia (MDS) rather than aplasia.

Etiology of SAA: Excluding an Inherited BMF Syndrome

The key distinction for the clinician in the newly diagnosed child with SAA is between inherited and noninherited (acquired) causes. SAA can be the presenting manifestation of an inherited BMF syndrome. Alternatively SAA can evolve while children with an already diagnosed inherited BMF are being followed.

The most common of the inherited BMF syndromes is Fanconi anemia (FA), but SAA can be a feature of dyskeratosis congenita (DKC), Diamond-Blackfan anemia (DBA), Shwachman-Diamond syndrome (SDS), and congenital amegakaryocytic thrombocytopenia (CAMT). Pearson syndrome is a mitochondrial disorder that is associated with hypoplastic anemia, liver disease, and ringed sideroblasts. These disorders are dealt with more fully elsewhere in this book but the following might alert the clinician to the presence of one of these syndromes:

- The history might include a family history of AA or one of these syndromes and any genetic illness is more probable in a consanguineous family.
- The presence of other abnormalities on examination that are associated with these conditions. These might include the thumb abnormalities of FA, for example.
- The growth of all children presenting with SAA should be plotted because growth failure is commonly a feature of the inherited BMF syndromes.
- A diepoxybutane (DEB) or mitomycin C (MMC) test is mandatory in *all* newly diagnosed AA cases to exclude FA.
- The inherited BMF syndromes are genetically heterogeneous. Genetic (molecular) analysis of these genes is now possible and is considered in all presenting cases of AA. However, molecular analysis is often laborious and might be misleading. Taking time to carry out such an extensive analysis might delay appropriate therapy of acquired SAA and might be misleading because a correlation between molecular features and clinical features is not always possible.

Where there is a strong clinical suspicion of an inherited BMF syndrome, these further molecular and other diagnostic investigations should be undertaken but where there is no suggestion of such a diagnosis after careful history and examination and after a negative DEB or MMC test, then the child should be managed and investigated as having acquired AA.

Etiology of SAA: Investigation of Acquired Aplasia

In most cases of acquired AA, no cause is identified and the condition is labeled as *idiopathic*. Our understanding is that there is immune-mediated loss of hematopoietic stem cells (HSCs) leading to HSC insufficiency, hypoplasia, BMF, and pancytopenia. This underpins the immune-suppressant therapeutic approach. There is no diagnostic test for acquired SAA as such. There are several other recognized associations and causes of acquired SAA:

1. The diagnosis of acute lymphoid leukemia (ALL) might be preceded by hypoplastic or aplastic marrow change. Classically, the hypoplasia is accompanied by fever and, with resolution of fever, there is recovery of health and normal blood counts. Overt ALL is diagnosed several months later. There may be foci of ALL blast cells (TdT, CD19, CD10 positive) in the marrow aspirate and trephine biopsy.

2. Drugs may cause AA. Clearly, the most common cause in everyday practice is chemotherapy, where the effect is both dose related and expected. However, the effect may be idiosyncratic and the most well-known implicated drug is chloramphenicol.

3. AA is associated with liver disease. Autoimmune hepatitis is associated with SAA and may precede or follow the diagnosis. Similarly, SAA may follow liver transplantation. Viral hepatitis also may be associated with AA and screening for these viruses is part of the investigation of SAA, although the finding of liver disease or hepatitis virus does not alter management of the SAA.

4. The distinction between hypoplastic MDS and SAA is an important one because it influences management. This distinction depends on aspirate morphology and specific findings on the trephine biopsy and the cytogenetic analysis of the marrow aspirate:

    a. The presence of marked dysplasia beyond the erythroid lineage
    b. Fibrosis on the trephine biopsy
    c. The finding on the trephine biopsy of abnormally located immature precursor (ALIP) cells (Blasts are usually found adjacent to the bony trabeculae on the trephine and

ALIPs are found away from these marrow trabeculae.)

d. Cytogenetic alterations including monosomy 7 and 5q- (Other cytogenetic alterations may not so readily distinguish MDS from SAA because clonal hematopoiesis also may be a feature of SAA or become a feature of treated SAA.)

Supportive Care

The components of the supportive care of AA include transfusion support, antibiotic and antifungal prophylaxis, and hematologic growth factor treatment. In general, the following statements about transfusion support can be made:

- RBC transfusion should be given to keep the patient asymptomatic rather than to keep the hematocrit above an arbitrary level. Usually platelets are given to keep the patient above a certain threshold, which is often 10×10^9/liter unless there is fever or bleeding.

- All cellular blood products should be leukodepleted to reduce the risk of alloimmunization. In many countries, this is now routine practice.

- Where the patient is cytomegalovirus (CMV) negative or until the CMV serostatus of the patient is known, seronegative blood products should be given. It is not known whether CMV transmission is prevented by leukodepletion alone, but in some countries, including the United Kingdom, where leukodepletion is universally applied, selection of products for CMV-negative patients is no longer used. The reason for prevention of CMV transmission with blood products is that CMV status will adversely affect bone marrow transplantation outcomes.

- Irradiation of blood products is unnecessary in AA until immune-suppressant therapy or HSCT has been given as treatment.

- RBC transfusion will be associated with transfusion iron overload. If definitive therapy is associated with restoration of normal erythropoiesis, then this can be managed with subsequent venesection, but otherwise, pharmacologic iron-overload management will be needed. Deferiprone might be avoided because it is known to induce occasional idiosyncratic agranulocytosis.

All children with significant neutropenia ($<0.5 \times 10^9$/liter) usually will require antifungal prophylaxis and an azole is ordinarily chosen. Antibacterial prophylaxis is rarely helpful and likely will lead to resistance. There has been shown to be no role for routine growth factor in the management of idiopathic SAA.

Specific Therapies of Severe Aplastic Anemia

In general, both immunosuppressive therapy (IST) and hematopoietic stem cell transplantation (HSCT) have been applied in SAA and VSAA. Milder AA might be simply observed.

Both IST and HSCT are effective. They are each discussed in greater detail in the succeeding sections. They have advantages and disadvantages that are summarized in Table 11.1, and institutions and national groups should come to algorithms of SAA management such as that given in Figure 11.1, which is that for

Table 11.1 Advantages and Disadvantages of IST and HCT

Immunosuppressive therapy	Hematopoietic stem cell transplantation
Low treatment-related mortality	Higher treatment-related mortality • Increased by HLA mismatch • Increased by comorbidity
Slow restoration of blood counts	Rapid restoration of blood counts • Might favor in the presence of significant infection
Higher risk of treatment failure	Lower rate of treatment failure
Higher rates of later clonal hematologic illness (MDS, PNH)	Lower rates of later clonal hematologic illness Some HSCT-related late effects
HLA-matched donor not required	HLA-matched donor required; poorer rates using mismatched donors

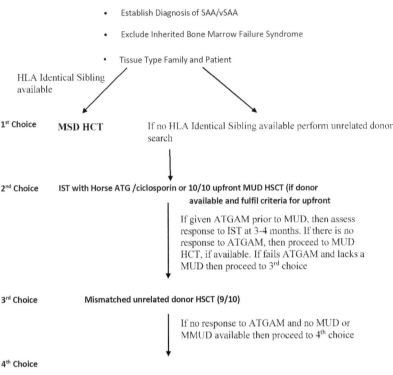

Figure 11.1. Algorithm for idiopathic pediatric SAA. This is the current UK algorithm for the management of SAA and details the different roles for MSD HSCT, MUD HSCT, IST with hATG and other agents.

- Establish Diagnosis of SAA/vSAA
- Exclude Inherited Bone Marrow Failure Syndrome
- Tissue Type Family and Patient

HLA Identical Sibling available

1st Choice **MSD HCT** If no HLA Identical Sibling available perform unrelated donor search

2nd Choice IST with Horse ATG /ciclosporin or 10/10 upfront MUD HSCT (if donor available and fulfil criteria for upfront

If given ATGAM prior to MUD, then assess response to IST at 3-4 months. If there is no response to ATGAM, then proceed to MUD HCT, if available. If fails ATGAM and lacks a MUD then proceed to 3rd choice

3rd Choice **Mismatched unrelated donor HSCT (9/10)**

If no response to ATGAM and no MUD or MMUD available then proceed to 4th choice

4th Choice

1. 2nd IST (Rabbit or Horse ATG)

2. Alemtuzumab (Investigational)

3. Eltrombopag (Investigational)

4. Haploidentical or Haploidentical ± unrelated donor umbilical HSCTs (Investigational)

(Investigational-recommended that this should be discussed at national MDT.)

the UK group. Individual patient decisions can be collectively discussed separately within these consensus guidelines by the group.

Immunosuppressive Therapy (IST)

The rationale for IST is that SAA is understood to arise following an immune-mediated depletion of hematopoietic stem cells (HSCs). IST will stop further HSCs depletion and allow repopulation of the bone marrow from the surviving, depleted HSC pool. Recovery from this pool imposes a replicative stress on those HSCs and their progeny, and there is an increased risk of clonal hematopoietic disorders, including MDS and paroxysmal nocturnal hemoglobinuria (PNH), following IST of SAA.

All studies in children have been performed using polyclonal horse-derived anti-T-cell immunoglobulin (hATG), and overall best response rates are about 60 to 70 percent. This product was marketed by

Genzyme as Lymphoglobulin. An alternative hATG is marketed by Pfizer as ATGAM, and a polyclonal rabbit-derived anti-T-cell product known as Thymoglobulin is marketed by Genzyme. These different ATG products are dosed differently and likely have different efficacy in SAA. ATG forms the backbone of IST in SAA, and the following statements can made:

- hATG is likely more effective than rabbit-derived ATG, and institutional practice should be to obtain and use such a product where possible for this indication.

- The response rates are improved by the addition of ciclosporin to the ATG, but the addition of other agents such as MMF, sirolimus, or granulocyte colony-stimulating factor (G-CSF) does not confer additional benefit. Ciclosporin is usually given for a year and then slowly tapered.

- The response rate can be slow and achieved over months rather than weeks. The response rate is

65

probably higher when treatment is applied sooner rather than later after diagnosis and to children with VSAA rather than AA.

- Some children do not respond to hATG. These children have a better outcome following unrelated donor HSCT than with a subsequent course of IST.
- There is a significant relapse rate (~20 percent following hATG) and a significant rate of later clonal hematopoietic disorders (which rises with time following therapy). Those who respond to hATG and subsequently relapse have a better chance of responding to a second course of hATG than those who failed hATG the first time, and usually the hATG product is changed for the second course, and the duration of ciclosporin therapy is lengthened.

Hematopoietic Stem Cell Transplantation (HSCT)

The rationale of HSCT in SAA is similar to that of IST in SAA. IST abrogates the immune-mediated depletion of HSCs. In HSCT, there is then donor HSC administration so that hematologic recovery proceeds from these infused, engrafting donor HSCs rather than from the depleted recipient HSC pool. There is therefore more rapid restoration of good blood counts following HSCT, and there is also a reduced incidence of later clonal hematologic disorders than following IST.

Matched sibling donor (MSD) HSCT has always been the treatment of choice for children with SAA or VSAA. Unrelated donor transplantation has traditionally been reserved for children who have either failed or relapsed following first-line treatment with IST. With better donor typing, unrelated donors are increasingly well matched to the recipient. The results of a well-matched unrelated donor HSCT in all indications are approaching MSD, and some institutions and national groups are using matched unrelated donor HSCT where there is a well-matched donor as the preferred initial therapy rather than IST.

The pre-transplant conditioning therapy comprises immunosuppressant drugs only. Usually these drugs will include cyclophosphamide, fludarabine, and T-cell-depleting serotherapy (such as ATG or alemtuzumab). The following points may be made:

- There are few late effects of HSCT because the conditioning therapy is light - growth is usually normal and fertility is preserved.
- The usual choice of donor HSCs is bone marrow because the risk of graft-versus-host disease (GvHD) is reduced with bone marrow as the donor source, and GvHD is of no benefit to the recipient in this disease. Results with cord blood in SAA have been poor historically.
- After HSCT, there is often mixed chimerism in the blood, so the recipient's surviving HSCs may make some contribution to hematopoiesis. This is usually of no consequence, and intervention is not indicated as long as bone marrow function is good, as assessed by transfusion need and peripheral blood counts.
- Usually the duration of ciclosporin therapy is longer than for transplants with other indications. This is to reduce the risk of later disease relapse from residual host (marrow-directed) immunity.
- The risk of HSCT is related to the closeness of the HLA match between the patient and the donor and the well-being of the patient. Matched sibling donor HSCT as soon as possible after diagnosis has always been the treatment of choice in SAA rather than IST because outcomes are good with well patients (not sensitized, not yet iron loaded, and usually without severe infections) with well-matched donors. Results from unrelated donors have improved as these transplants have proceeded earlier in the disease history and using better-matched, molecularly typed unrelated donors.
- Where there is a higher risk of graft rejection, such as for a mismatched donor or following a previous graft rejection, then the likelihood of donor cell engraftment might be increased by intensifying the immune suppression with the addition of total-body irradiation (often as a single low-dose fraction of 2 Gy) or total-nodal irradiation to the IST-based conditioning. The use of mobilized peripheral blood also will increase the likelihood of donor cell engraftment but will risk GvHD.

Sideroblastic Anemias

Key Messages

1. The sideroblastic anemias are a rare group of disorders in which ringed sideroblasts are present in the bone marrow smear. The ringed sideroblast is visible on iron (Perl's) staining of the erythroblast and represents pathologic iron accumulation in the red blood cell (RBC) mitochondria.

2. The childhood sideroblastic anemias (CSAs) arise from defective mitochondrial synthesis of heme or Fe/S clusters or from defective mitochondrial protein synthesis. There may be wider syndromic features, or the anemia may be the only manifestation. The severity of the anemia is also variable between different CSAs.

3. The sideroblastic anemias that the practicing clinician will encounter are X-linked sideroblastic anemia (XLSA), Pearson marrow-pancreas syndrome, and sideroblastic anemia with immunodeficiency, recurrent fever, and developmental delay (SIFD). Other CSAs are described but are often limited to small series or even single kindreds. The clinician will need expert assistance in unraveling these disorders.

4. ALAS2 catalyses the first step of heme biosynthesis, and mutation in the *ALAS2* gene gives rise to classic XLSA, where the anemia is mild and microcytic and the blood smear shows a dimorphic RBC population. There is iron loading prior to transfusion.

5. In Pearson marrow-pancreas syndrome, there is mitochondrial DNA deletion and defective mitchondrial protein synthesis. There are more general mitochondrial disease features and there is often pancytopenia, hypoplastic anemia, and sideroblastic anemia.

6. A recently described CSA, sideroblastic anemia with immunodeficiency (B-cell deficiency), recurrent fever, and developmental delay (SIFD) arises from a defect in the maturation of nuclear and mitochondrial transfer RNA.

Introduction

The sideroblastic anemias were named originally because of the appearance of ring sideroblasts within the erythroblast series on iron staining of bone marrow aspirates. They are a heterogeneous group of disorders that reflect mitochondrial dysfunction. Collectively, they remain very rare and the practicing pediatric hematologist may or may not see many such cases throughout his or her career. Hence, this chapter will focus only on the three major subtypes and remain relatively brief.

X-Linked Sideroblastic Anemia (XLSA)

This anemia arises from missense mutation in the first enzyme that catalyzes the first step in the synthesis of heme in the erythroblast mitochondrion:

- 5-Aminolevulinic acid (ALA) is formed by the condensation of glycine and succinyl-coenzyme A (CoA).
- 5-Aminolevulinic acid synthase (ALAS) is the enzyme. Its gene is carried on the X-chromosome, and the condition is X-linked.
- The anemia is microcytic and rarely severe enough to require transfusion. There is classically a dimorphic population of RBCs, and the RBC distribution width (RDW) on the full blood count (FBC) is greatly increased. It is responsive to pharmacologic doses of pyridoxine (vitamin B_6).
- Iron overload is significant in the absence of transfusion and might require management with

phlebotomy (if the anemia is mild) or pharmacologic therapy.

- XLSA is a rare illness. Patients should be seen in centers with expertise or cases should at least be discussed with such centers. Genetic analysis of the *ALAS* gene also should be carried out in reference laboratories and patients should be referred to national support organizations.

- There are other CSAs that arise from mutations affecting the catalytic functions of enzymes involved in Fe metabolism in the mitochondrion (heme biosynthesis and Fe/S biosynthesis). These anemias might be similar to XLSA but may not be sensitive to pyridoxine. There are small numbers of patients worldwide and reference laboratory expertise will be required for their elucidation.

Pearson's Marrow–Pancreas Syndrome

This is a mitochondrial illness caused by mitochondrial gene deletion – not always the same deletion – and many of the features are those of a mitochondrial illness. There is multisystem upset. There might be liver disease, myopathy and lactic acidosis. There is exocrine pancreatic failure.

In addition to the multisystem features of a mitochondrial disease, the following hematologic features should alert the clinician to Pearson's:

- The anemia is macrocytic and might be severe.
- The marrow is hypoplastic and pancytopenia may be present. There is an aplastic anemia.
- The erythroblasts show prominent toxic-type vacuolation.

Management is multidisciplinary and is not the sole realm of the hematologist. The aplasia has been found to be sufficiently disabling in a child, otherwise well enough from systemic features, for allogeneic hematopoietic stem cell transplantation (HSCT) to be offered , but this is not a common occurrence in Pearson's syndrome.

Sideroblastic Anemia with Immunodeficiency, Recurrent Fever, and Developmental Delay (SIFD)

This is a recently described condition with several kindreds across the world. It is also a multisystem disorder, and the mutation is in *TRNT1*, which encodes an enzyme responsible for adding the codon triple CCA to nuclear and mitochondrial transfer RNA (tRNA). This CCA binds the amino acid to the tRNA, which delivers it to the ribosome. The protein is highly conserved in evolution, indicating its importance. Mutations allow some protein action (they are missense or affecting splice sites, etc.), and gene knock-out animal models are lethal. The relationship between this observed mutation and the clinical phenotype is far from clear and will be the subject of further study. There is some heterogeneity in clinical presentation, but in general, this is a severe disease. Most children with SIFD in the original series have died of the disease.

- There is multisystem disease, as might be expected with a mitochondrial illness.

- There is prominent developmental delay, retinopathy, and cardiac involvement but the kindreds variably exhibit different manifestations.

- There is a B-cell maturation arrest and panhypogammaglobulinemia, but this is not responsible for the recurrent fever syndrome and it persists even if immunoglobulin replacement therapy is given.

- The sideroblastic anemia is iron loading like the CSA of XLAS.

Intriguingly, several children with SIFD have been given allogeneic HSCT, and this completely corrects hematologic, immunologic and fever manifestations of the disorder and appears to prevent early death. Early reports suggest that HSCT also might ameliorate other aspects of the disorder, although more HSCT experience in the disorder is required before more exact conclusions can be drawn.

13

Iron Deficiency

Key Messages

1. Iron deficiency is common in infants from 6 months to 2 years of age and is usually associated with insufficient dietary intake of iron. Early introduction of cow's milk and failure to transition to solid foods at an appropriate age are the most likely causes.

2. Iron deficiency is also common in menstruating teenage girls.

3. If iron deficiency is diagnosed during infancy or in menstruating teenagers and the history is typical, then therapy can begin without further investigation.

4. Serum ferritin is the most useful blood test for iron deficiency, not withstanding being an acute-phase reactant. A serum iron determination is unhelpful in making the diagnosis of iron deficiency.

5. In Western society, where helminth infestations are rare, other than infants and menstruating teenagers, iron deficiency is not usually seen in children, and further investigation for a source of blood loss is always appropriate.

6. The anemia of iron deficiency is often very well tolerated, and children may be clinically asymptomatic despite severe anemia.

7. For any child with iron deficiency, even if not anemic, three months of iron therapy is always required to adequately replace iron stores.

8. In infants, considerable effort is required to support the parents to correct the diet, and this is critical if permanent cure is to be achieved.

9. In infants, iron deficiency has the potential to cause long-term neurocognitive impairment and so should be treated aggressively.

10. Most children will respond adequately to oral iron, and it should be first-line therapy in all children unless there is a contraindication such as the presence of inflammatory bowel disease. Intramuscular iron administration is painful and stains the skin, and is rarely, if ever, indicated. Intravenous iron administration is useful, and careful choice of iron preparation and rate of infusion can reduce the risk of anaphylaxis.

Regulation of Iron

Our understanding of the physiology of iron metabolism has increased in recent years. Some of this is relevant to clinical pediatric hematologists. The salient points are as follows:

- The regulation of iron intake into the body is at the level of absorption. Iron is absorbed in a *controlled* way by enterocytes. This iron replaces that lost from the body in an *uncontrolled* way, such as in bleeding or in sloughing of the gut epithelium. There is no mechanism for controlled loss of iron from the body. There is therefore no mechanism for the body to lose iron when it is administered parenterally, such as the iron within a RBC transfusion.

- The amount absorbed is relatively low compared with the dietary intake. Iron leaves the enterocyte and enters the circulation via ferroportin, the only known cellular iron exporter in vertebrates. This protein is also expressed in other iron-handling cells such as the macrophages of the reticuloendothelial system, where old RBCs are destroyed and their iron recycled.

- Ferroportin is also the receptor for hepcidin, which negatively regulates its production. Hepcidin is produced in the hepatocytes of the liver and acts to control iron metabolism in a negative manner, reducing the export of iron from the gut (reducing absorption) and release from the reticuloendothelial macrophage. Hepcidin downregulates ferroportin, which exports iron from these iron-handling cells.
- Hepcidin is decreased in iron deficiency anemia, hemolytic anemia, and anemias with ineffective erythropoiesis (e.g. thalassemia and congenital dyserythropoietic anemia) and is maintained when iron is replete.
- Inappropriate hepcidin contributes to several diseases:
  - Hepcidin excess contributes to the anemias of inflammation and chronic kidney diseases and can also cause a rare iron-refractory iron deficiency anemia.
  - Hepcidin deficiency or inaction contributes to hereditary hemochromatosis, the iron-loading anemias, and the hepatic iron overload with hepatitis C infection.

Normal Iron Requirements and Iron Metabolism in Children

Iron is crucial for the formation of hemoglobin, so it is particularly relevant for RBC production. Approximately 65 percent of total-body iron is in hemoglobin, and 15 to 30 percent is stored in the form of ferritin. Iron stores are transferred from mother to fetus predominantly in the third trimester, so premature infants will readily become iron deficient if not supplemented appropriately. Iron supplementation should begin in infants born prior to 33 weeks' gestation by 4 weeks of chronological age once enteral feeds have been established. Preterm infants have a daily requirement of 2 to 3 mg/kg per day of elemental iron, which can be met by supplementing feeds until there is adequate dietary iron intake, usually between 6 and 12 months of corrected age. Regardless of gestational age, low-birth-weight infants, in particular, those weighing less than 1800 g, have inadequate iron stores at birth and should receive similar iron supplementation until 6 months of age.

Table 13.1 Age-Related Daily Iron Requirements

Age	Iron requirement
Preterm, low birth weight (LBW), 1 to 12 months	2–4 mg/day
Term, 0 to 6 months	0.2 mg/day
Term, 6 to 12 months	11 mg/day
1 to 3 years	9 mg/day
4 to 9 years	10 mg/day
9 to 13 years	8 mg/day
14 to 18 years	Boys: 11 mg/day Girls: 15 mg/day

In contrast, term infants are almost never iron deficient during the first 6 months in the absence of blood loss (iatrogenic or pathologic). Most infant formulas are iron fortified, so they contain similar amounts of available iron as breast milk. Thus, either breast milk or formula is suitable for infants in terms of iron needs. Standard cow's milk, goat's milk, and soy milk have low iron content and should not be offered to infants younger than 12 months of age. Cow's milk often also induces an enteropathy, which will increase iron loss as well. By 6 months, infants should be weaned onto iron-rich solids. Most early infant foods such as cereals are iron fortified. The age-related daily iron requirements are summarized in Table 13.1.

Epidemiology of Iron Deficiency in Children

Iron deficiency is the most common nutritional deficiency in the world, and the World Health Organization (WHO) estimates that iron deficiency anemia (IDA) affects one-quarter of the world's population, predominantly infants and women. Anemia due to iron deficiency is one of the 10 most important factors contributing to the global burden of disease. More individuals worldwide have IDA than any other condition.

In the United States, approximately 10 percent of toddlers have iron deficiency, and 2 to 3 percent have IDA. Up to 16 percent of teenage girls have iron deficiency, and 3 percent have IDA. Socioeconomic status has a strong inverse correlation with the frequency of iron deficiency and IDA.

Children with iron deficiency are at risk of detrimental long-term neurologic, developmental, and behavioral effects. Iron deficiency has been linked to poorer cognitive and motor function, including lower development assessment scores as well as socioemotional behavior difficulties. A meta-analysis of 17 randomized, controlled trails in children showed that iron supplementation had a modest effect on improving mental development indices; this effect was most noticeable in those who had IDA.

Thus, early identification and aggressive treatment of iron deficiency are important to maximize the child's long-term potential. A high index of suspicion should be maintained for iron deficiency, and opportunistic dietary history screening should be performed on all children presenting for medical intervention. The classic history of failure to transition to solids after 6 months and ongoing high breast milk or formula intake should arouse suspicion and appropriate analysis of full blood count and serum ferritin. Persistence of milk or formula intake greater than 600 ml/day after 12 months of age is often associated with iron deficiency. Similarly, any child who has started cow's milk prior to 12 months of age should be screened.

Menstrual histories in teenage girls are notoriously difficult in terms of accurately assessing blood loss, and given the additive impact of reduced meat intake in this population, one could argue for opportunistically screening any menstruating teenage girl who presents for medical review for iron deficiency with full blood count and serum ferritin.

Other children at high risk for iron deficiency who deserve investigation include those with celiac disease, inflammatory bowel disease, known bleeding disorders, those having major surgery associated with blood loss, or those with any chronic disease with reduced dietary intake and chronic iatrogenic blood sampling.

Premature and low-birth-weight infants are at particular risk of iron deficiency and, as described earlier, should be routinely supplemented. Minimization of iatragenic blood loss is important in the management of all small children. Based on the local epidemiology, some countries advocate for routine screening for iron deficiency. For example, the American Academy of Pediatrics recommends universal laboratory screening for iron deficiency at approximately 1 year of age.

Clinical Presentations of Iron Deficiency

The classic clinical presentations of iron deficiency in children include

1. Incidental presentation in a child presenting for unrelated medical issues

2. Symptomatic IDA
3. Behavioral abnormalities such as pica

Incidental Presentation

Many children have full blood examinations performed when presenting for unrelated medical issues, such as trauma or fever. Even in the absence of such routine investigations, unexplained pallor or tachycardia noted on routine examination should always raise the suspicion of underlying IDA. If a full blood count is performed, the finding of a hypochromic microcytic picture, with or without anemia, raises the possibility of iron deficiency. The major differential diagnosis is thalassemia minor, and the RBC count (often elevated in thalassemia minor and reduced in iron deficiency) may provide a clue. In the setting of acute fever, serum ferritin may be falsely normal due to the acute-phase response, but if the dietary history is suggestive of iron deficiency, then it is reasonable to make a presumptive diagnosis and begin therapy. If the diet is appropriate or unclear, then follow-up with a serum ferritin determination when the child is clinically well can be used to confirm the diagnosis. Alternatively, confirmation of a thalassemia minor state can be done with appropriate testing for beta- and alpha-thalassemia, respectively.

Symptomatic IDA

The presenting symptoms of IDA include pallor, tiredness, and lethargy, the manifestations of which will vary with age. In infants and toddlers, poor feeding, breathlessness, and edema (i.e. cardiac failure) may be signs of more severe anemia. In older children, exercise intolerance, sleepiness, or just poor concentration may be the presenting clinical symptoms. Exertion associated palpitations may be noted, almost always in the setting of baseline tachycardia. Regional ischemic symptoms are rare in children.

IDA usually develops slowly over a prolonged period of time and thus is often very well tolerated by children, especially infants. Incidental presentations of children with hemoglobin levels as low as 10 g/liter are well described. Many children with hemoglobin levels of 40 to 50 g/liter will be described by parents as normally active. Often it is an acute intercurrent viral infection that precipitates the clinical presentation as the metabolic demands of fever and infection alike push the cardiac compensation toward failure. While some studies have reported associations between iron deficiency and febrile seizures, breath-holding spells, and even cerebral sinovenous thrombosis, more studies are required to prove a causal relationship.

Behavioral Abnormalities

Pica refers to a desire to eat non-food-related substances such as paper, dirt, Velcro, and ice. Preference for ice is specifically referred to as *pagophagia*. Pica is a relatively common presenting feature of iron deficiency in childhood, and questions to this effect should be part of all screening dietary histories. Often such children present to allied health practitioners and child psychologists because the parents are concerned about the behaviors, and the biologic basis of the behavior is not appreciated. These behaviors are highly associated with iron deficiency and often resolve within days of starting iron supplementation, well prior to resolution of hematologic abnormalities. Nonspecific irritability, sleep disturbance, and concentration or learning issues are also often described by parents of children with iron deficiency, and such disorders often resolve with the introduction of adequate iron replacement prior to resolution of hematological abnormalities.

Diagnosis of Iron Deficiency

The investigations required for the diagnosis of iron deficiency depend on the age and clinical circumstances of the child. Such investigations vary from no blood tests at all to complex diagnostic algorithms. As described previously, in the appropriate age group, and if the dietary history is suggestive, it may be reasonable to do no laboratory investigations whatsoever to make a presumptive diagnosis of iron deficiency and start therapy accordingly.

Similarly, in children in whom incidental abnormalities are found on full blood examination, if the history then supports a dietary deficiency or association with menstrual bleeding, no further investigations are required, and therapy can be started. For community-based children without major underlying disease, a serum ferritin determination is the only required confirmatory test. As noted earlier, serum ferritin is an acute-phase reactant, and if it is normal despite a suggestive clinical situation, repeating the serum ferritin determination when the child is well is reasonable.

Full iron studies, including serum iron, transferrin saturation, and total iron-binding capacity, rarely add to the diagnostic decision making in otherwise well children and are unnecessary investigations for most children. In particular, the serum iron level has tremendous diurnal fluctuation and should never be used in considering the diagnosis of iron deficiency. The only time serum iron is helpful is to monitor compliance with iron therapy or when concerned about potential iron overdose. Many children are falsely labeled as iron deficient based on low serum iron measurements, and the measurement often causes confusion and unnecessary alarm for parents.

In children with major underlying diseases and persistent inflammatory markers, the ferritin level can be unreliable, and in these children, consideration of full iron studies with perhaps the addition of soluble transferrin receptor measurement can be helpful. Serum transferrin receptor concentration increases with increased severity of iron deficiency. However, normative data for these parameters, especially in younger age groups, are lacking. Serum transferrin receptor concentration results differ based on the assay system, and the results of different assays cannot reliably be compared.

Another relatively new test for iron deficiency is zinc protoporphyrin measurement because zinc protoporphyrin also increases in iron deficiency. The assay involves direct measurement of the fluorescence of zinc protoporphyrin in a hematofluorometer. The simple test requires a small sample size and has the advantage that it can reliably detect iron deficiency even after treatment has been started because it takes a number of weeks for the iron-deficient RBCs to be replaced with new iron-replete RBCs. However, just as for transferrin receptor measurements, the zinc protoporphyrin level increases in the anemia of chronic disease as well as in iron deficiency.

Bone marrow iron stains are said to be the gold standard measurement for determining the adequacy of iron stores, but they are rarely, if ever, used in children unless there are coincidental indications for bone marrow examination. Age-related normative data are also lacking, and appropriate positive controls for the iron stains are important to include in this testing.

For children in whom the cause of iron deficiency cannot be determined by dietary or menstrual history alone (most commonly children outside the usual demographics for iron deficiency in children), then investigation of the gastrointestinal tract is usually most helpful. Fecal occult blood sampling needs to be done on multiple occasions over a period of time. Investigation of causes of iron malabsorption (especially diseases of the duodenum and proximal small intestine) often requires upper gastrointestinal tract endoscopy, as well as serology for celiac disease. Investigation of causes of blood loss, including cow's milk enteropathy, other enteropathies, and inflammatory bowel disease, may require lower gastrointestinal endoscopy. Rarer causes including Meckel's diverticulum may require nuclear medicine scans. Hereditary hemorrhagic telangiectasia may be very difficult to diagnose, and genetic testing is now often most helpful.

Treatment of Iron Deficiency

There are three major principles of therapy for iron deficiency in children:

1. Blood transfusion is rarely necessary and should be given only when there is an urgent need to replace oxygen-carrying capacity in severe decompensated anemia.
2. Full replacement of iron stores with pharmacologic iron therapy for an adequate duration is essential. This can usually be achieved with oral iron therapy.
3. Treatment of the underlying cause (i.e. dietary, menstrual loss, or other) is required to prevent relapse.

Blood transfusion is rarely required. The only indications for blood transfusion in children with iron deficiency are cardiac decompensation such that urgent restoration of oxygen-carrying capacity is required or the presence of a comorbidity that makes cardiac decompensation likely such that there is insufficient time for iron-replacement therapy to work (e.g. if imminent surgery is required or a child develops an intercurrent illness that will likely precipitate cardiac decompensation in the presence of significant anemia). The indications for transfusion in all children are discussed in Chapter 34.

Furthermore, because iron deficiency anemia is slowly developing and compensatory mechanisms include maintenance of intravascular volume, the risk of fluid overload when transfusing children with iron deficiency is real. If children do require transfusion, then aiming for a moderate increase in hemoglobin level, purely to enable cardiac stability, rather than full correction to normal hemoglobin and slow transfusion with careful monitoring of fluid and respiratory status is recommended.

Once a child is iron deficient, it is unlikely that he or she will be able to replenish his or her iron stores without pharmacologic iron therapy. Over-the-counter multivitamins do not have sufficient iron content for the treatment of iron deficiency anemia. Different iron preparations will have different elemental iron concentrations, and doses should take into account the degree of anemia and weight of the child. The recommended dosing (in terms of elemental iron) is 3 to 6 mg/kg per day in two to three divided doses. Oral iron is best administered on an empty stomach, with absorption enhanced by taking with fruit juice that is high in vitamin C. Absorption is inhibited by tannins (tea) and calcium (milk), so oral iron therapy should not be taken with either of these drinks.

Most countries have oral liquid iron preparations available that usually contain 6 mg of elemental iron per milliliter. Thus, 1 ml/kg would be the maximum daily dose. Capsules that contain Spansul preparations may be sprinkled onto foods, and these commonly contain 270 mg of ferrous sulfate, or approximately 90 mg of elemental iron. Thus, one capsule is the maximum daily dose for a 15-kg child. Smaller children would require the use of fractions of capsules for each daily dose, and this is often fraught with difficulties. Most iron tablets contain 325 mg of ferrous sulfate, or approximately 105 mg of elemental iron and so are suitable for older children. Teenagers may require up to two to three tablets per day.

Poor compliance of iron supplementation is common, and considerable effort should be expended to maximize compliance. Gastrointestinal disturbance as a side effect of oral iron is frequently discussed, although the evidence supporting it from randomized trials is not strong. In general, ongoing encouragement, starting at low doses and increasing weekly, or dividing the total daily dose into two or three doses is usually effective.

Irrespective of the presence of IDA, once iron deficiency is present, at least 3 months of iron-replacement therapy is required. Shorter durations of therapy are associated with higher relapse rates and inadequate resolution.

Most children can be adequately treated with oral iron preparation. Parenteral iron therapy should be considered in children with persistent iron deficiency despite oral therapy. Indications for intravenous iron administration include contraindications to oral iron such as inflammatory bowel disease, poor compliance or tolerability of oral iron preparations, malabsorption, chronic renal disease requiring erythropoiesis-stimulating agents, and ongoing iron losses that exceed iron absorption, such as gastrointestinal bleeding or menorrhagia. Intravenous iron administration should be considered in patients requiring rapid iron repletion (e.g. in those undergoing nondeferrable surgery within 2 months). Intramuscular iron administration is never indicated in children. The injections are painful and can lead to permanent skin staining. There would appear to be no advantages over the use of intravenous iron unless the healthcare setting does not support safe intravenous access.

Intravenous iron is available as iron polymaltose, iron sucrose and ferric carboxymaltose. There is very limited experience with ferric carboxymaltose in younger children. These iron formulations have different iron concentrations, maximum doses, dilutions, and rates of administration. They are not interchangeable with regard to any of these parameters, and it is important to refer to the specific product information.

To calculate the required total dose of intravenous iron, one must calculate the patient's total-body iron deficit. Multiple infusions may be required because each iron formulation has a maximal iron dose per infusion. Iron polymaltose is the only iron formulation in which it is possible to correct the total-body iron deficit in one infusion.

The appropriate iron dose may be calculated by the Ganzoni formula:

$$\text{Iron dose (mg)} = \text{body weight (kg)} \times [\text{target}$$
$$\text{Hb} - \text{actual Hb (g/liter)}] \times 0.24 + \text{iron depot}$$

where iron depot is 15 mg/kg for those weighing less than 35 kg and 500 mg for those weighing 35 kg and above.

Allergic and anaphylactic reactions to intravenous iron (especially iron polymaltose) are well reported; therefore, it should only be given in facilities that are able to adequately manage anaphylaxis. Premedication with steroids and antihistamine may be considered. Drug extravasation can cause irreversible skin staining.

In one sense, management of iron deficiency in children is easy because oral iron therapy represents a simple therapy. However, the underlying cause must be managed, or relapse is certain. In infants with dietary insufficiency, support of the parents to adequately correct the diet is essential. This is often very difficult. Limiting daily milk intake, introducing appropriate solids, and managing resulting toddler behavioral responses often require real commitment by parents and all involved in feeding the child. Dietary correction needs to be attained within the 3-month treatment period if the child is to become independent of oral iron supplements. This may be particularly difficult in children with developmental mental health problems such as autism. Failure to substantively change the diet will inevitably lead to relapse, and given the cumulative effect on neurocognitive development, this is less than ideal.

In menstruating teenagers, management of the underlying menorrhagia, combined often with improved dietary intake of iron, is also essential. Ongoing, uncontrolled blood loss will see any iron replacement therapy inadequate. Gynecologic consultation to investigate and manage menorrhagia is almost always required in girls in whom menorrhagia has led to iron deficiency. Management of local uterine issues, hormonal manipulation, or management of bleeding disorders may be required. Transexamic acid is often effective when taken during the first five days of each menstrual period irrespective of the initial cause of the menorrhagia. Ongoing monitoring of the effectiveness of these measures is also critical to ensure that iron deficiency does not relapse following adequate iron replacement.

Finally, in children with underlying gastrointestinal causes of iron deficiency (e.g. celiac disease or inflammatory bowel disease), successful therapy of the primary disorder is important to prevent relapse of iron deficiency.

Follow-Up of Iron Deficiency

After commencement of oral iron therapy, there is usually an immediate improvement in any behavioral components, even prior to hematologic recovery. In children with significant anemia, a reticulocytosis is often seen in 3 to 5 days and is useful for ensuring normal absorption of iron and compliance with therapy. Failure to respond to adequate iron with a reticulocytosis response may indicate the need for immediate investigation for malabsorption syndromes. Documentation of initial adequate response, especially in children with severe anemia who are being managed as outpatients, is important. Once compliance and response are confirmed, further monitoring should be minimized. The hemoglobin is usually two-thirds back to normal after about 3 weeks of therapy and fully normalizes within 2 months. Thus, for children with anemia, another FBE at 4 to 6 weeks of therapy is reasonable. The mean corpuscular volume (MCV) will usually normalize within 3 months, and failure to do so might indicate a coexisting thalassemia minor. The ferritin level should be normal by the end of 3 months of therapy. In children with no anemia, there is no need for further testing until the end of the treatment period.

However, following completion of 3 months of oral iron therapy, documentation of full resolution of iron deficiency is important. Testing includes repeat FBE to demonstrate normalization of hemoglobin and MCV, as well as repeat serum ferritin determination to demonstrate normalization of iron stores. Failure of normalization usually is secondary to poor compliance or the presence of an unrecognized cause of iron malabsorption or loss. Thus, in children in whom the initial assessment was that the iron deficiency was likely due to poor diet, there may now be an indication to further investigate the gastrointestinal tract.

Once iron therapy has ceased, ongoing monitoring of FBE and ferritin levels at 3- to 6-month intervals for at least 12 months is required. Relapse of iron deficiency in children who have presumed to be iron deficient due to diet alone should trigger reconsideration of the need to comprehensively investigate causes. This presumes that the dietary deficiency was corrected successfully.

After intravenous iron replacement, 3 months should be given for full correction of the FBE parameters. Measuring the ferritin level much before that time is likely unhelpful due to the initial high peak attained. Ongoing monitoring to ensure that underlying causes are now controlled, or in cases where ongoing iron loss cannot be controlled, to determine the optimal timing of future intravenous iron replacement therapy is also recommended.

Iron Toxicity in Children

Whenever oral iron therapy is prescribed for children, parents must be made aware of the dangers of iron overdose. Iron should be stored safely and out of reach of children. Once iron therapy is no longer required, any remaining supplies should be discarded appropriately.

The severity of iron toxicity depends on the amount of elemental iron ingested; doses of 40 mg/kg of elemental iron or higher are typically associated with serious toxicity. Symptoms of iron poisoning typically occur within 20 minutes of ingestion. Initial symptoms within the first 6 hours following iron ingestion include nausea, vomiting, diarrhea, and abdominal pain. Absence of symptoms within 6 hours implies that toxicity is unlikely. There is often a quiescent period between 12 and 24 hours when symptoms transiently resolve before overt toxicity becomes apparent. Subsequently, there is evidence of systemic toxicity, including tachycardia, hypotension, hypovolemic shock, and metabolic acidosis. Hepatotoxicity may be seen and typically occurs within 48 hours. Early recognition of iron overdose and aggressive management can be lifesaving.

Disorders of Vitamin B₁₂ and Folate

1. Vitamin B_{12} and folate are essential hematinics but are also essential vitamins for most tissues.

2. Most presentations of vitamin B_{12} and folate deficiency in children are secondary to dietary insufficiency and in breast-fed infants due to maternal vitamin B_{12} deficiency

3. Inborn errors of metabolism are less common but important causes of clinical deficiency. Transcobalamin II deficiency, which is autosomal recessive, can present in an identical fashion to deficiency secondary to maternal vitamin B_{12} deficiency.

4. Vitamin B_{12} deficiency in infancy is uncommon but important because it is one of the few reversible causes of failure to thrive (FTT) and developmental regression.

5. Any child who presents between 6 months and 3 years of age with FTT, developmental regression, and any hematologic abnormality should have vitamin B_{12} and folate deficiency excluded as a matter of urgency.

6. A blood film with any degree of cytopenia, macrocytosis, hypersegmented neutrophils, or a combination of these abnormalities should raise the prospect of vitamin B_{12} or folate deficiency and lead to immediate follow-up with the clinical team.

7. Children with vitamin B_{12} or folate deficiency in the 6-month to 3-year age group often present nonspecifically, and by the time the diagnosis is made, rapid deterioration can ensue. Urgent intervention can make a significant difference in the long-term neurologic outcome.

8. Laboratory investigation can be confusing, and clinicians should be aware of the difference between serum vitamin B_{12} and active vitamin B_{12} laboratory measurements.

9. Determinations of serum homocysteine and urinary methylmalonic acid are critical investigations to demonstrate the presence of intracellular vitamin B_{12} or folate deficiency and in cases of inborn errors of metabolism are useful in differentiating the potential mechanism.

10. Folate deficiency is very rare in childhood but is seen commonly in infants fed goat's milk, which is deficient in folate.

Introduction

Megaloblastic anemia in childhood is a rare but important condition. The importance stems from the fact that in the young infant age group, marked neurologic impairment is common, and delays in diagnosis can significantly worsen the long-term neurodevelopmental outcome. Thus, urgent recognition and intervention are required. This demands a high degree of clinical suspicion and a high degree of proactive intervention from the hematologist because an abnormal blood film in this age group may be the first clue to the potential diagnosis.

The physiology of vitamin B_{12} and folate metabolism is well known but remains a mystery to most clinicians who have done their best to forget the complex metabolic pathways that seemed so important in medical school. However, even if the complex intracellular pathways cannot be visualized, a basic understanding of the absorption and delivery pathways of these two important nutrients is required to anticipate the patients who are likely to suffer from malabsorption or dietary deficiencies.

The laboratory testing for vitamin B12 deficiency in particular is often confusing, and there remain some questions about the interpretation of active vitamin B$_{12}$ assays in neonates. The introduction of organic acid screening into newborn screening protocols in some countries now means that many infants are having elevated methylmalonic acid detected early in life while asymptomatic. These advances in laboratory methodology are changing the way vitamin B$_{12}$ and folate problems are detected in childhood.

Physiology of Vitamin B$_{12}$ and Folate

Vitamin B$_{12}$ is not found in plants, so dietary sources include meat, fish, dairy products, and eggs. As such, strict vegans readily become deficient in vitamin B$_{12}$ unless they take specific steps to supplement their diet. The recommended daily dietary intake is 2 µg for adults, with increased requirements during pregnancy and lactation. Infant requirements are 0.1 µg/day. The average body stores are 2 to 5 mg for adults, with over 50 percent located in the liver, so deficiency tends to develop very slowly. Many infants with deficiency do not present until the second 6 months of life.

Once vitamin B$_{12}$ (bound to animal protein) is ingested, it is cleaved off in the stomach and proximal small intestine, where it then is bound to intrinsic factor. The intrinsic factor–vitamin B$_{12}$ complex travels to the distal ileum, where it binds to specific receptors leading to vitamin B$_{12}$ absorption into the bloodstream. In plasma, the bulk of vitamin B$_{12}$ is bound to haptocorrin, which is a carrier protein only. A small proportion binds to transcobalamin II, which facilitates receptor-mediated uptake into the cells as required. Hence, children with transcobalamin II deficiency will have normal serum vitamin B$_{12}$ measurements, which reflect the haptocorrin binding, despite their severe intracellular deficiency.

Once inside the cells, vitamin B$_{12}$ is a coenzyme in two important cellular reactions:

- In the methionine synthesis pathway within the cytoplasm, vitamin B$_{12}$ is a coenzyme for methionine synthase, and failure of this pathway leads to increased homocysteine, which can be measured in the plasma.
- Within the mitochondria, vitamin B$_{12}$ is a coenzyme for methylmalonic acid mutase, which leads to the production of succinyl CoA. The failure of this pathway leads to accumulation of methylmalonic acid, which can be measured as part of a urinary organic acid screen.

Thus, elevated serum homocysteine and urinary methylmalonic acid levels are evidence of cellular vitamin B$_{12}$ deficiency irrespective of the serum vitamin B$_{12}$ levels. Specific metabolic defects in the vitamin B$_{12}$ metabolism pathway may favor elevation of one or the other metabolite preferentially. Deficiency of vitamin B$_{12}$, whether dietary deficiency, absorption or transport failure, or metabolic abnormality, affects metabolically active tissues, and hence, symptoms are often reflected in the gut mucosa, bone marrow, and the brain, although eventually almost every organ will become dysfunctional.

Folate is present in many foods of both plant and animal origin, but substantial losses can occur during cooking and storage. However, dietary deficiency in children is very rare unless they are fed goat's milk alone, which is deficient in folate. Goat's milk–based formulas are supplemented with folate and therefore not a problem. Other than that, children are usually significantly malnourished in general before they suffer from folate deficiency. The average daily requirement for folate is approximately 3 µg/kg, with children having slightly higher requirements than adults. Because folate deficiency in mothers was associated with neural tube defects in the past, many pregnant women take folate supplements throughout pregnancy. Some countries also now have folate-fortified staple foods such as bread to reduce the risk of folate deficiency in the community. Children with chronic hemolysis of any etiology may have higher folate requirements and are generally deserving of additional supplementation (0.5 to 5 mg weekly is usually sufficient). The absorption of folate is less well understood than that of vitamin B$_{12}$ but appears to occur in the proximal small bowel by both a specific receptor and nonspecific pathways. Within the plasma, folate circulates mostly unbound, although albumin may bind some folate. Folate is used in a number of cellular reactions, and deficiency can lead to an excess of methionine and homocysteine.

Hematologic and Clinical Manifestations of Vitamin B$_{12}$ and Folate Deficiency

The classic hematologic changes in peripheral blood films are macrocytosis, hypersegmented neutrophils, and varying degrees of cytopenia. Any cell line may be more or less affected, and while pancytopenia is common, a high index of suspicion should be had for any abnormality on the blood film if the clinical picture is suggestive. Alternatively, a left shift with increased numbers of neutrophil precursors with abnormal morphology can be seen. While macrocytosis is typical, clinicians should remember that most individuals have a relatively stable mean corpuscular volume (MCV), so changes in MCV (that are not age related) flag a problem, even if the actual MCV is still within the 'normal' range. The true diagnosis of megaloblastosis is a bone marrow diagnosis, in which dyshemopoiesis is obvious in all cell lines, with giant forms, disordered nuclear appearances, and classic nuclear cytoplasmic asynchrony. The bone marrow may appear proliferative, and this has been mistaken for myeloid malignancy. Thus, the clinical presentation of the hematologic manifestations may include the presentation of anemia, thrombocytopenia, and neutropenia/neutrophil dysfunction as isolated abnormalities or in combination. Often the blood picture is identified incidentally during a full blood examination (FBE) performed for intercurrent viral infection or nonspecific reasons.

In addition to the hematologic abnormalities – and of more concern – is the neurologic deterioration associated with megaloblastic anemias of childhood. Especially in young children, there is often neurodevelopmental regression, with loss of developmental milestones such as smiling, vocalization, head control, and purposeful movements. There may be reduced tone (although tone may be increased), seizures, and abnormal movements that may range from jitteriness to true choreoathetoid movements. This picture is often associated with failure to thrive or weight loss, and there may be a multitude of other symptoms, including signs of gastrointestinal dysfunction and skin rashes. Glossitis or mouth ulceration is common. The development of these symptoms is often slowly progressive over months, and it is not uncommon for children to have presented on multiple occasions for medical assessment – with mothers stating that something is wrong with their baby and they just cannot put their finger on it – before the diagnosis is eventually made. Megaloblastosis is one of the few reversible causes of neurologic regression in infancy and hence the need for a high index of suspicion. The long-term outcome appears to be related to the depth of deterioration reached, so early diagnosis and treatment offer a far better prognosis.

In older children, the clinical presentation can be variable, and the neurologic manifestations can vary from seizures, to poor school performance, to specific neuropathies, and even to psychiatric-type presentations. Again, a high index of suspicion is required for any child with suggestive hematologic features in the presence of any neurologic or nonspecific clinical features.

Etiology of Megaloblastosis in Childhood

Megaloblastosis has different etiologies depending on the age of the presenting child. Folate deficiency is extremely rare, and most clinical presentations are due to vitamin B$_{12}$ deficiency unless infants are fed on pure goat's milk, which is severely deficient in folate (goat's milk–based formulas are supplemented with folate and therefore not a problem). The ages at which the different causes of vitamin B$_{12}$ and folate deficiency usually present clinically are shown in Table 14.1.

Cobalamin metabolic defects are rare and are labeled cobalamin A through G according to the exact enzyme deficiency in the pathway. Diagnosis may be suspected by earlier presentation or positive family history in previous children. The exact diagnosis

Table 14.1 Causes of Vitamin B$_{12}$ and Folate Deficiencies and Age at Usual Clinical Presentation

Age at presentation	Effects
Vitamin B$_{12}$ deficiency	
<6 months age	Cobalamin metabolic defects
6 months to 3 years	Maternal vitamin B$_{12}$ deficiency in breast-fed infants Transcobalamin II deficiency Malabsorption syndromes Cobalamin metabolic defects
5 to 10 years	Immerslund-Grasbeck syndrome Juvenile pernicious anemia
10 to 18 years	Juvenile pernicious anemia Early-onset adult-type pernicous anemia Strict veganism
Folate deficiency	
1 to 36 months	Dietary deficiency (goat's milk)
>3 years	Dietary deficiency

requires metabolic analysis, usually of skin fibroblast culture, and is only performed reliably by a small number of laboratories around the world.

Transcobalamin II deficiency is autosomal recessive and often presents with neurologic regression, failure to thrive, and hematologic abnormalities in the second 6 months of life, that is, in an identical fashion to children with dietary deficiency due to maternal vitamin B$_{12}$ deficiency. Thus, formula-fed infants with the relevant clinical presentation are likely transcobalamin II deficient because all infant formulas are supplemented with vitamin B$_{12}$, so dietary deficiency in these infants is rare.

Dietary deficiency due to maternal deficiency of vitamin B$_{12}$ is common in infants whose mothers who are strict vegans, whose mothers have undiagnosed pernicious anemia, or whose mothers have a malabsorption syndrome. Often the mother has had a number of children in close succession, breast feeding in between, and has simply run out of vitamin B$_{12}$ for the presenting child. While, classically, pernicious anemia has been said to be associated with infertility in affected women, this is clearly not the case, and many of the mothers are asymptomatic.

Malabsorption syndromes in children that are associated with vitamin B$_{12}$ or folate deficiency include celiac disease, cystic fibrosis, and various causes of short gut syndrome. The presentations of these diseases are usually quite different, but there are reports of megaloblastic features being the initial presenting symptom.

Immerslund-Grasbeck syndrome is a rare condition in which selective vitamin B$_{12}$ malabsorption from the gut is associated with proteinuria. While familial in nature, it does not usually present until later in childhood.

Juvenile pernicious anemia is the absence of intrinsic factor and is not common. Adult-type pernicious anemia, or auto immune antibodies against intrinsic factor and gastric parietal cells, is also not common but is reported in teenagers.

Diagnosis of Vitamin B$_{12}$ and Folate Deficiency in Childhood

There are two major aspects to the diagnosis. First is the need to confirm vitamin B$_{12}$ or folate deficiency, and second is identification of the cause. The FBE

and, in particular, the blood film are very helpful in raising suspicion of the condition but in themselves are not necessarily diagnostic. The bone marrow appearance is more specific, but there is rarely an indication for doing a bone marrow aspirate these days because the following assays and tests usually can be done quickly in most laboratories to assist in the diagnosis.

In terms of vitamin B$_{12}$, traditional testing has included a serum vitamin B$_{12}$ determination. Over the years, there have been numerous problems with these assays technically and in terms of interpreting the results, with large variations in normal results and often an indeterminate range that could be associated with physiologic variation or pathologic deficiency. In recent times, the development of holotranscobalamin (holoTC) measurements or 'active' vitamin B$_{12}$ assays has improved the diagnostic sensitivity. These assays measure the component of plasma vitamin B$_{12}$ that is bound to transcobalamin II and therefore available for active transport into cells. The method is probably more robust and less variable than traditional serum vitamin B$_{12}$ measurements, although reference ranges for all ages of children are not yet established, and there remains some doubt about the clinical significance of values in the low-normal range. Children with vitamin B$_{12}$ deficiency from maternal vitamin B$_{12}$ deficiency or malabsorption (including Immerslund-Grasbeck syndrome or any form of pernicious anemia) will have low serum vitamin B$_{12}$ measurements and low HoloTC measurements. However, children with transcobalamin II deficiency will have normal serum vitamin B$_{12}$ measurements but low holoTC measurements. Children with metabolic defects of intracellular vitamin B$_{12}$ metabolism will have normal serum vitamin B$_{12}$ measurements and normal holoTC measurements.

An important adjunct to the diagnosis of vitamin B$_{12}$ deficiency is therefore the demonstration of intracellular deficiency of vitamin B$_{12}$, which is achieved by demonstrating elevated serum homocysteine levels and/or elevated urinary methylmalonic acid (MMA). Taking samples for these measurements prior to replacing vitamin B$_{12}$ can be very useful in confirming the diagnosis. For all dietary, absorption, and transport pathologies of vitamin B$_{12}$, both parameters will be elevated. For cobalamin defects, the increase in homocysteine or MMA depends on the exact defect.

With respect to identification of the cause, the clinical situation and age of the patient will determine the relevant investigations. In infants, measurement of maternal vitamin B$_{12}$ level and subsequent investigation of a cause for any maternal deficiency (e.g. dietary history, autoantibodies to exclude pernicious anemia, investigation for potential malabsorption syndromes) is usually required. Transcobalamin II deficiency can be confirmed by measuring transcobalamin II levels or by genetic testing for the relevant known mutations. Malabsorption syndromes in infants should be identifiable by other clinical features, but appropriate investigations such as endoscopy and biopsy, celiac serology, or sweat tests may be required. Cobalamin metabolic defects require specialist investigation.

In older children, a search for proteinuria or appropriate testing to exclude autoantibodies should be conducted. The presence of antibodies to gastric parietal cells and intrinsic factor is common in adult-type pernicious anemia. Parietal cell antibodies are found in other autoimmune disorders and also in up to 10 percent of healthy individuals, making the test nonspecific. However, around 85 percent of patients with pernicious anemia have parietal cell antibodies, which means that they are a sensitive marker for the disease. Intrinsic factor antibodies are much less sensitive than parietal cell antibodies, but they are much more specific. They are found in about 50 percent of patients with adult-type pernicious anemia and are very rarely found in other disorders. Elevated serum gastrin is found in approximately 90 percent of patients with pernicious anemia, but it also may be found in other forms of gastritis, and often endoscopy is required to differentiate causes of gastritis. In teenagers with adult-type pernicious anemia, appropriate investigation for other autoimmune disease is probably worthwhile. Juvenile pernicious anemia will be negative for all the autoantibody assays.

Folate deficiency should be suggested by the dietary history. Measurement of RBC folate is the preferred diagnostic assay because plasma folate tests merely reflect recent ingestion. Homocysteine is elevated in folate deficiency, whereas MMA remains normal.

Treatment of Vitamin B$_{12}$ or Folate Deficiency

Especially in infancy, treatment of vitamin B$_{12}$ or folate deficiency should be regarded as a medical emergency, and replacement therapy should be initiated as soon as possible. Delays of hours can potentially make a difference in the long-term neurologic outcome.

While the optimal dose and duration of initial replacement therapy are unknown, there seems to be little adverse effect from giving an excess of the missing nutrient. For vitamin B$_{12}$, 1000 µg given intramuscularly (IM) daily for the first week, until the cause of the vitamin B$_{12}$ deficiency is known, seems reasonable. Hydroxycobalamin should be used rather than cyanocobalamin because if the child turns out to have a cobalamin metabolic defect, some will not respond to cyanocobalamin. In cases of maternal deficiency, once the mother has been treated adequately, the child can continue to breast feed and, after initial replacement therapy, should need no further specific treatment. If the infant has a malabsorption syndrome, specific treatment is required, but ongoing supplementation also may be required. In children with transcobalamin II deficiency, ongoing twice to three times weekly IM injections may be required because the principle of treatment is to drive plasma levels so high that adequate vitamin B$_{12}$ simply diffuses into cells. While correction of the hematologic abnormalities seems relatively easy to achieve, the exact amount of vitamin B$_{12}$ required to normalize brain development is unknown. These children may require high-dose vitamin B$_{12}$ for life, and adequate doses cannot be achieved through oral vitamin B$_{12}$ supplements alone.

The vitamin B$_{12}$ deficiency that presents later in life usually requires lower maintenance vitamin B$_{12}$ doses, although high-dose daily treatment in the initial phase of treatment is not unreasonable. The various types of pernicious anemias probably only require monthly or even 3-monthly 1000-µg injections in the longer term. As with all conditions, homocysteine and MMA may be useful monitoring assays.

Adequate folate supplementation can be achieved with 5 mg orally daily until sufficient modification to the dietary intake has been made to guarantee ongoing sufficient intake. Many clinicians give vitamin B$_{12}$ (single IM injection of 1000 µg) at the start of folate replacement therapy as well, just in case there is combined deficiency and to avoid the potential for worsening symptoms of subacute combined degeneration of the cord. Likewise, many clinicians add oral folate therapy when treating vitamin B$_{12}$ deficiency on the basis that it will do no harm and may be of benefit.

Outcome of Vitamin B$_{12}$ or Folate Deficiency

The hematologic abnormalities associated with vitamin B$_{12}$ or folate deficiency correct rapidly and easily with replacement therapy. The more important outcome relates to the degree of neurologic recovery. This seems to relate to the degree and duration of impairment in the first place. Even for dietary deficiencies in which there is no ongoing biochemical pathology, reported outcomes vary from severe deficits (unable to perform activities of daily living, constant seizures), to specific learning deficits, to no apparent abnormalities. All children diagnosed with vitamin B$_{12}$ or folate deficiency require ongoing developmental follow-up and probably neuropsychological assessment at key points during their schooling progression.

Hemolytic Anemia

1. Hemolytic anemia in children is usually acute and potentially life threatening, so it should always be regarded as a medical emergency.

2. In general, any child presenting with hemolysis should be admitted to the hospital and monitored closely until the tempo of the hemolysis is understood, irrespective of the initial hemoglobin measurement.

3. Transfusion support is the mainstay of treatment for acute hemolysis, and early transfusion is usually recommended.

4. Transfusion should never be delayed because of diagnostic uncertainty. It is always better to have a living child in whom the diagnosis is uncertain than a dead child who has had a full diagnostic workup.

5. The blood film is a critical part of the workup of any hemolytic episode.

6. Haptoglobin and lactate dehydrogenase (LDH) determinations are usually unnecessary in children with hemolysis and do not add to patient management.

7. For inherited hemolytic syndromes, which often recur intermittently, parental and patient education is vital.

8. Parvovirus is a potential cause of transient aplasia in children with underlying hemolytic anemia.

9. Folate supplementation is recommended for all children with hemolytic anemia.

10. Gallstones in children should always raise the possibility of an underlying hemolytic disease.

Introduction

Hemolysis refers to the increased breakdown of red blood cells (RBCs) or shortening of RBC survival from the usual 120 days. The destruction of the RBCs leads to increased production of unconjugated bilirubin, which leads to clinical jaundice when the bilirubin concentration rises to greater than 60 to 70 µmol/liter. As the RBC survival decreases, the bone marrow responds by increasing RBC production, so there is increased reticulocytosis and, in more severe cases, the presence of nucleated RBCs in the peripheral blood (with or without a nonspecific left shift). The bone marrow can usually increase RBC production six- to eightfold to keep pace with cell breakdown, thus giving a compensated hemolytic anemia. It is only when RBC survival is less than approximately 20 days that the marrow can no longer meet demands, and an uncompensated hemolysis develops leading to anemia. Any coexisting hematinic deficiency leads to failure of compensation more readily. If the RBC breakdown occurs intravascularly, then hemoglobin may be excreted in the urine (hemoglobinuria), leading to dark urine.

Hemolysis in children can develop exceeding rapidly, with hemoglobin dropping from normal values to life-threatening anemia within hours. Thus, in any child presenting with anemia, the first requirement is to confirm or exclude hemolysis so as to determine the likely urgency of ongoing management. In broad terms, this is referred to as distinguishing *aregenerative (slowly developing) anemias* from *regenerative anemias* (hemolysis and blood loss) that have the potential to deteriorate rapidly. The presence of anemia, reticulocytosis, and elevated serum bilirubin levels is usually sufficient to confirm hemolysis. Reduced haptoglobins and elevated LDH are less reliable measures in children and rarely add to the diagnostic process, so they are usually not worth ordering. The blood film may show polychromasia and is most helpful in guiding further investigations, which should be aimed at determining the cause of the haemolysis. Neonatal RBC alloimmunization and post-transfusion-related hemolysis are discussed in Chapters 5 and 35 respectively.

Diagnosis of Hemolysis

Having confirmed a hemolytic process (i.e. anemia with increased reticulocytosis and serum bilirubin), the next step is to consider the underlying cause. In simple terms, hemolysis can be considered as either intrinsic or extrinsic to the RBCs. RBCs have no nucleus, and hence, intrinsic causes must be due to membrane, hemoglobin, or enzyme abnormalities (Table 15.1). Extrinsic causes can be considered immune or nonimmune (Table 15.2). Of the nonimmune causes, separation into microangiopathic causes of hemolysis versus other causes is also helpful. Thus, the classification of acute anemias in childhood is simple with relatively few decision points. While there remain some rare causes of hemolysis, this simple classification will deal with almost all causes encountered clinically.

Thus, the blood film is useful in guiding subsequent investigations. If hereditary spherocytosis is suspected, the traditional osmotic fragility testing is now mostly replaced by the eosin-5-maleimide binding test (E5M or EMA), a relatively specific flow cytometric test (approximate sensitivity 90 percent and specificity 95 percent) that can be done on less than 0.5 ml of blood, including capillary samples, within hours. If hemoglobin problems are suspected, then rapid sickle preparations or hemoglobin electrophoresis is usually diagnostic. If unstable hemoglobins are suspected, either heat instability or isopropanol testing is required. If glucose-6-phosphate dehydrogenase (G6PD) deficiency is suspected, then G6PD assay is the most useful test. It may be falsely normal during acute hemolysis because reticulocytes have higher levels of G6PD even in deficient patients. Investigation for less common and rare causes is usually fruitless in the acute setting, and such disorders can be diagnosed in the fullness of time.

Once again, the blood film is useful in guiding subsequent investigations. A direct antiglobulin test (DAT) or Coombs test is warranted in almost all first presentations of hemolysis to exclude immune causes. Remember that some drugs may causes immune hemolysis (as well as precipitate G6PD), so

drug history is important in all children with hemolysis. Microangiopathic causes need only be investigated in the presence of RBC fragmentation on the blood film. Thrombotic thrombocytopenic purpura (TTP) and hemolytic-uremic syndrome (HUS) usually are found in association with other clinical features, including renal or neurologic symptoms. Disseminated intravascular coagulation (DIC) is usually seen in very sick children, most commonly precipitated by sepsis. Wilson disease rarely presents as primary hemolysis, and preexisting liver disease is more common. Malaria should be preceded by history of travel to an affected area.

Initial Assessment of the Child with Suspected Hemolysis

There are three major principles to the initial assessment of a child with suspected hemolysis:

1. Confirm hemolysis.
2. Assess severity of anemia.
3. Determine underlying cause of hemolysis.

As described earlier, the most useful investigations to confirm hemolysis are the full blood examination, serum bilirubin determination, reticulocyte count, and blood film. Occasionally, autoimunne hemolytic anemia (AIHA) has a low reticulocyte count because the antibody destroys reticulocytes as well. Determining the presence of hemoglobinuria associated with intravascular hemolysis is important both for confirming hemolysis and also assessing severity. Subsequent investigations relate to determining the cause of the hemolysis.

Hemoglobin is required for oxygen delivery, and thus, assessing the oxygen delivery capacity is critical in the assessment of any child with anemia. As described in Chapter 1, tissue oxygen delivery (ml/min) = cardiac output (liters/min) × Hb (g/liter) × oxygen saturation (%) × 1.34 ml/g (constant: amount of oxygen per gram of normal Hb), where cardiac output is the product of heart rate and stroke volume. The clinical implications of this equation are also described in Chapter 1. However, the heart rate is arguably the most critical component of the assessment of a child with acute hemolysis because it is a guide to cardiac compensation. The hemoglobin directly provides a measure of anemia. Be aware that in patients with intravascular hemolysis, the measured hemoglobin may be falsely elevated if there is

Table 15.1 Description of Intrinsic RBC Causes of Hemolysis

Site of intrinsic problem	Most common	Less common	Really rare	Causes jaundice at birth	Causes intermittent hemolysis during childhood	Blood film features of common abnormality during acute hemolysis	Intravascular hemolysis
Membrane	Hereditary spherocytosis	Hereditary pyropoikilocytosis	–	Common	Common	Spherocytes	No
Hemoglobin (Hb)	Sickle cell disease (SCD) or thalassemia	Unstable Hb	Methemoglobin	Rare	Common	Sickle cells (SCD), target cells, Hypochromic microcytosis (thalassemia)	Yes
Enzyme	G6PD deficiency	Pyruvate kinase	Other enzymes	Common	Common	Blister and bite cells	Yes

Table 15.2 Extrinsic Causes of Hemolysis

Extrinsic cause	Pathophysiology	Blood film features in acute hemolysis	Diagnostic tests	Intravascular hemolysis
Immune	Warm (IgG) Cold (IgM) PCH	Spherocytes (IgG) Agglutination (IgM) Specific PCH features	Direct antiglobulin test (DAT)	IgM and PCH only
Microangiopathic	Mechanical intravascular hardware hemangioma DIC TTP/HUS	RBC fragmentation Thrombocytopenia (DIC, TTP/HUS)	–	Yes
Infective	Malaria	Parasitemia	Thick and thin films Rapid diagnostic tests (antigen tests)	Yes
Metabolic	Wilson disease	Acanthocytes	Serum ceruloplasmin	Yes

substantial free plasma hemoglobin. Clues to this include examining the blood sample for plasma color and the finding of a patient who seems more tachycardic and hypoxic than expected for a given hemoglobin level. Also, the RBC count is reduced out of proportion to the reported hemoglobin level. Similarly, acute intravascular hemolysis, especially due to G6PD, can be associated with methemoglobin formation, which has reduced oxygen affinity (hence changing the constant in the tissue oxygen equation). This would also indicate severe hemolysis that would benefit from early aggressive transfusion therapy.

In summary, the useful investigations in the acute setting should be guided by the appearance of the blood film, but a DAT is always required. Immune-mediated hemolysis often can be particularly aggressive, and immunoglobulin G (IgG)–mediated hemolysis will benefit from steroid therapy. Therefore, this should never be missed. E5M and G6PD determinations and hemoglobin electrophoresis (HbEP) are also reasonable front-line investigations. Relevant investigations for the remaining extrinsic causes should be guided by appropriate details from the history and examination. Further investigations for rarer causes generally should be left for a later date because waiting for initial investigation results to be negative before embarking on more comprehensive investigation delays transfusion, and all-inclusive investigation at initial presentation prior to transfusion wastes time and resources because the most common causes are covered by the simple investigations just detailed.

Initial Management of the Child with Hemolysis

All children presenting with an acute hemolytic episode should be admitted to the hospital until the tempo and severity of the hemolysis are understood. This is irrespective of whether the patient has had previous episodes and whether those were severe or mild. Initial hemoglobin level and matching heart rate should be noted, and transfusion should be given as clinically required. Given the potential for the hemoglobin level to deteriorate rapidly, one would not usually allow the child to become unwell in any way. Aggressive transfusion to stabilize the hemoglobin level is usually warranted. Occasionally, multiple transfusions over a number of days are required, and close and repeated monitoring of such patients is critical. In such cases, post-transfusion hemoglobin measurements as well as regular timed measurements are often required to assist in determining optimal volumes for each transfusion. Oxygen therapy is of no value because the RBCs remaining in circulation are fully oxygenated unless there is methemoglobin. If the DAT is positive for IgG, then steroid therapy should be started, usually at a dose of 1 mg/kg oral prednisolone. In cases of autoimmune hemolysis, it is often necessary to give least-incompatible units of blood

85

because the antibodies cross-react with all donors. Delays in transfusion to search for perfectly compatible blood should be avoided unless the child has been previously multiply transfused and is known to have alloantigens. If the child is initially stable, then monitor for increases in heart rate. (It is suggested that the physician write specific instructions to nursing staff that an increase in heart rate of 20 to 25 percent should trigger a medical review of the patient based on an assessment that whatever the current state is, a 20 to 25 percent deterioration would trigger considering transfusion). Remember that in the absence of fever, increases in heart rate will occur in inverse linear relationship with decreases in hemoglobin level and hence can be used to detect clinically relevant deterioration even before repeat blood tests are performed. Regular (6-hourly) hemoglobin checks will also assist in determining the tempo and usually, after the first 24 hours, the behavior of the hemolysis remain relatively consistent. If over 24 hours the child has remained stable without requiring transfusion, then depending on geography, social situation, and parental understanding, the child often can be supported as an outpatient with daily review. However, if there is any doubt about clinical course or ability to return to the hospital quickly, ongoing hospitalization is required until the child is stabilized.

Specific Causes of Hemolysis and Their Acute and Chronic Management

Hereditary spherocytosis has an incidence of approximately 1 in 2000 people. Seventy percent are autosomal dominant, usually with a parent known to be affected; thirty percent are autosomal recessive. Neonatal jaundice is very common and must be differentiated from ABO blood group incompatibility, which also causes spherocytes on neonatal blood films in otherwise well babies. Patients usually have chronic compensated hemolysis with acute exacerbations related to viral illness. Parvovirus can induce aplastic crisis, in which anemia is of slower onset and without increased hyperbilirubinemia and reticulcytosis, although the latter is noted in the recovery phase. Early cholelithiasis is common. Splenomegaly is usually clinically detectable after 12 months of age, and the spleen can get quite large. Definitive treatment is splenectomy. Indications for splenectomy include frequent transfusion requirements over a number of years, multiple life-threatening hemolytic episodes,

perceived risk of splenic trauma related to lifestyle (contact sports), and cholelithiasis requiring cholecystectomy. Splenectomy is delayed until after 5 years of age if at all possible, and partial splenectomy may be effective. Appropriate presplenectomy vaccinations and postsplenectomy antibiotic prophylaxis are recommended. Most children, however, do not require splenectomy and only intermittent transfusion support. Weekly folate supplementation of 0.5 mg (<1 year of age) or 5 mg (older children) is routine.

Hereditary pyropoikilocytosis is a rare disorder that is considered a homozygous form of autosomal recessive hereditary elliptocytosis. It usually presents in neonatal life with jaundice and anemia and a characteristic blood film with marked poikilocytosis. Transfusion support is often required. It usually becomes less severe with age, and older children become asymptomatic. Parental blood films might be abnormal.

Unstable hemoglobins are rare causes of hemolysis. The blood film findings are often nonspecific, although Heinz bodies are often obvious on supravital staining. HbEP is often normal, and unstable hemoglobin is only detected on specific heat instability or isopropanol testing. Of the 146 described unstable hemoglobin variants, Hb Koln is the most common, and is a beta-chain abnormality, thus usually does not present until after 6 months of life. Patients usually have a chronic compensated hemolysis with acute exacerbations. Regular folate supplementation is worthwhile. Transfusion support is necessary as indicated clinically. Splenectomy is sometimes required as definitive treatment. Hb Poole is an unstable fetal hemoglobin that may cause hemolysis in the newborn period. Diagnosis is difficult because both heat stability and isopropanol testing use fetal hemoglobin as their positive control given that fetal hemoglobin is more unstable than adult hemoglobin normally. The condition is usually self-limiting, so extensive diagnostic efforts are usually not justified.

G6PD deficiency is one of the most common single-gene mutations that cause disease in humans. While it is X-linked, girls commonly present with clinically significant hemolysis as well, so gender should not dissuade the diagnosis. Neonatal jaundice is very common. Occasionally, neonates with jaundice have initial blood films consistent with oxidative hemolysis but turn out not to be G6PD deficient, and the cause of this is unclear. Most children with G6PD deficiency present with classic favism, that is, hemolysis on exposure to fava or broad beans. Fresh beans in springtime are more potent, and it is not uncommon to see a cluster of hemolytic patients at this time of year. While many children have severe hemolysis on first and all exposures to fava beans, some appear very random in their response to exposure. Whatever the situation, once diagnosed, the family should be counseled to avoid exposure ever again. Families should be reassured that all other beans and vegetables are safe and that unjustified dietary exclusions should be avoided. Some children also have acute hemolysis with viral infections as their most frequent presenting problem. While there is a known list of drugs that can precipitate hemolysis in G6PD-deficient patients, including sulfur drugs and some antimalarials, in pediatric practice, these are infrequent problems. Routine neonatal vitamin K is safe and should be given as per usual. Napthalene (moth balls) is a known precipitant, and baby clothes previously stored with naphthalene should be avoided. Often blood tests when the child is well reveal no abnormality, although some patients do have evidence of chronic, compensated hemolysis in between acute episodes. Parental education about an appropriate response to acute pallor, jaundice, or lethargy is critical, as is true in all hemolytic anemias, and this should be a major aim of follow-up after any acute episode. There seems little value in routine annual blood tests in well children, and one could argue about the value of routine clinical review once the parents are well educated, except in those in whom there is evidence of chronic compensated hemolysis. Acute episodes can be severe, and the proportion of blister or bite cells on blood film does not predict severity. Marked hemoglobinuria with or without methemoglobin formation is a hallmark of severe episodes. Aggressive transfusion support may be required, but the crises are usually short-lived. Folate supplementation at least transiently around acute episodes seems logical. G6PD assay is diagnostic but may be normal in the setting of acute reticulocytosis. Repeat assays when the hemolysis has settled, but at least 3 months post-transfusion, will clarify the diagnosis. Splenomegaly is not a feature, and these children should be reassured and encouraged to live normal lives but with the relevant diet and drug restrictions.

Pyruvate kinase deficiency is an uncommon autosomal recessive cause of hemolysis. Although there is racial variance in the incidence, in a mixed Western society, the prevalence is rare. Neonatal jaundice is common, and a chronic hemolysis, either compensated or, occasionally, transfusion dependent, usually ensues. Acute exacerbations with illness do occur. Folate supplementation is appropriate. Transfusion support as indicated clinically, either acutely or to support growth and development if chronic anemia exists, is recommended. Side effects of chronic hemolysis, such as large splenomegaly and cholelithiasis, are possible. Splenectomy is not curative, but it usually greatly reduces the severity of the anemia.

Autoimmune hemolytic anemia (AIHA) is common in children, but unlike in adults, it is most often an isolated phenomenon and not related to other autoimmune, malignant, or inflammatory conditions or drugs, although all of these are possible.

Warm AIHA (IgG) is most often precipitated by nonspecific viral infection. Hemolysis is often severe and can be prolonged. Warm AIHA is steroid responsive, so oral prednisolone 1 mg/kg should be commenced immediately, as well as initial transfusion support. Usually all cross-matches will be incompatible due to the strong autoantibody, but transfusion should proceed regardless, unless preexisting alloantibodies are also demonstrated. Once the hemolysis has settled, prednisolone can be weaned slowly. Failure to settle with prednisolone or inability to wean prednisolone can occur, and in such patients, steroid-sparing alternative therapies must be considered. Azothiaprine, mycophenolate mofetil (MMF), and rituximab have been used. Splenectomy is often recommended in chronic AIHA. Children presenting with AIHA from IgG antibodies appropriately invoke high anxiety from experienced pediatric hematologists and should be managed with a great deal of caution.

Cold AIHA (IgM) is most commonly associated with *Mycoplasma pneumoniae* infection. DAT is positive for complement only. The hemolysis can be severe but usually settles relatively quickly. The hemolysis is intravascular, so hemoglobinuria is common. Steroid therapy is of no value, so the treatment of choice is transfusion support. There is commonly agglutination on the blood smear, and such agglutinates might occur in the absence of clinical hemolysis. The blood may need to be warmed prior to its automated analysis so that the agglutinates disaggregate.

Paroxysmal cold hemoglobinuria (PCH) is a specific type of AIHA in which the IgG antibody fixes complement and causes intravascular lysis (the family describe black – coke-coloured – urine). The antibody, known as the *Donath Landsteiner antibody*, characteristically binds in the cold peripheral circulation but lyses in the warm central circulation. It is much more commonly seen in the winter and in colder countries. There may be a relative reticulocytopenia, and there is typically erythrophagocytosis by neutrophils in the blood smear as well as red cell agglutination. The DAT is positive for complement. It may follow Epstein-Barr virus (EBV) infection, although a number of viral infections are associated with it. The hemolysis can be mild or severe, and transfusion support and keeping warm is the mainstay of treatment of this self-limiting illness.

Chapter 16

Infections in Hematology Patients and the Hematologic Features of Infectious Disease

Key Messages

1. Infection and hematology go together.
2. Looking after patients with primary hematologic illness involves commonly preventing and treating infectious disease in those individuals. The cells of the blood form a vital part of the defense of the organism against infection, so abnormalities of the blood will often mean that this defense is weaker
3. In the presence of infection, the appearance of the blood might be different and might be used to specifically contribute to the diagnosis of a specific infection.

Infection in Children with Hematologic Illnesses

Children with hematologic illnesses get infections. Their immunity to infection is reduced by both the disease itself and the treatment of the disease. Such infections are responsible for much of the morbidity associated with hematologic illness and are also responsible for significant mortality. Infection may be with opportunistic organisms and may be bacterial, fungal, viral or another opportunist in origin. The types of infections and the specific organisms are influenced by the hematologic disease itself and the type and intensity of treatment given.

Infection is intimately linked with hematology. A well-functioning clinical hematology unit will have infection management at its heart. Protocols will vary between institutions, and various guidelines and reviews are published. However, in each center, the protocols must exist for the following (governance will require that staff know and follow such protocols and that such adherence is audited regularly):

- Prophylaxis and therapy of bacterial infection
- Prophylaxis, diagnosis and therapy of fungal disease (preemptive or empirical therapy as well as therapy of documented infection)
- Prevention, prophylaxis, diagnosis, and treatment of viral infection especially during hematopoietic stem cell transplant (HSCT)
- Prophylaxis and therapy of *Pneumocystis jiroveci* infection
- Strategies for the management of varicella-zoster virus (VZV), including postexposure prophylaxis, herpes simple virus (HSV) and measles infection
- Strategies for vaccination in children receiving cancer chemotherapy and for those who have undergone HSCT

Prophylaxis and Therapy of Bacterial Infection

- Most studies support the use of prophylactic oral antibiotics in children who have severe and prolonged neutropenia to reduce the incidence of bacteremia. Drugs used include ciprofloxacin, other quinolones, and trimethoprim-sulfamethoxazole.
- Prompt treatment with appropriate parenteral antibiotics saves lives in neutropenic children with fever. The antibiotics chosen should be institutional and given empirically to the neutropenic child presenting with fever. Examples include monotherapy with piperacillin-tazobactam or meropenem or either of these two drugs combined with an aminoglycoside. The center must audit both the antibiotic sensitivity of the bacteremic isolates from its neutropenic children and the interval between presentation with fever and subsequent administration of the antibiotic.
- The empirical antibiotic therapy can be adjusted once the specific sensitivity of a blood culture isolate is known.

- Antibiotics should be continued until the fever is resolved and for a defined period (7 to 14 days) in those with positive blood cultures.
- In certain circumstances, consideration might be given to removal of the Hickman line. A persistently positive line-drawn blood culture despite antibiotic therapy or infection with a particular organism such as *Klebsiella*, *Pseudomonas* or *Staphylococcus aureus* might prompt such consideration.
- Hospitalization and prompt initiation of empirical broad-spectrum intravenous antibiotic therapy have dramatically reduced infection-related morbidity and mortality. The intensity of this approach, however, is not without undesirable sequelae. Prolonged antibiotic exposure and hospitalization are potent risk factors for the emergence of resistant microorganisms and secondary infection. Inpatient therapy is also associated with inferior health-related quality of life for children with cancer, and hospitalization is significantly more expensive. It may be possible to step down to outpatient parenteral or oral antibiotics or even give oral antibiotics only in certain circumstances ('low-risk' febrile neutropenia). This is an evolving field and practice is changing in this direction.

Prophylaxis, Diagnosis, and Therapy of Fungal Infection

- The risk factors for invasive fungal infection (IFI) are duration and depth of neutropenia, mucosal tissue damage induced by chemotherapy, use of steroids (>0.3 mg/kg per day prednisolone or equivalent) and – for *Candida* infection – the presence of a Hickman line (see Table 16.1).
- IFI is seen most commonly in acute myeloid leukemia (AML), in relapsed acute leukemia, and following allogeneic transplantation. The most common organisms are *Candida* and *Aspergillus*. The former is usually line associated and the latter is usually pulmonary in origin, although dissemination to other sites is seen in about a third of cases. *Mucor* is a mold that is relatively resistant to drug treatment.
- A prompt diagnosis of IFI will make treatment more effective. Strategies will include either or both of (1) screening high-risk patients with twice-

weekly serum galactomannan determinations (this is a cell wall component of *Aspergillus* and can be detected using a sensitive assay) and (2) imaging using computed tomography (CT) of the chest in high-risk patients with prolonged febrile neutropenia. Even non-typical infiltrates might be indicative of IFI. An abnormal CT scan might be followed by bronchial lavage of the area to try to identify the specific pathogen.
- Antifungal prophylaxis should be given to high-risk patients. Drugs used include the azoles – itraconazole, posiconazole and voriconazole (preferably with monitoring of drug levels with these agents) – liposomal amphotericin, and an echinocandin such as caspofungin or micafungin.
- *Empirical* antifungal therapy has been a common practice in neutropenic children with persistent fever despite appropriate empirical antibacterial therapy. In adult oncology practice and increasingly in children, empirical therapy is being replaced by *preemptive* (diagnosis-driven) therapy of early-diagnosed fungal infections using galactomannan and CT imaging. This restricts the use of antifungal drugs.
- *Candida* infection is usually treated with liposomal amphotericin or fluconazole. Hickman lines should be removed. *Aspergillus* is treated with voriconazole or liposomal amphotericin. Additional disseminated sites of infection should be looked for with CT scanning. *Mucor* treatment requires a combination of surgery and higher-dose liposomal amphotericin.

Virus Infection during Allogeneic Stem Cell Transplantation

Virus infection is common in allogenic transplantation because of the removal of recipient T-cell immunity during the conditioning therapy (to reduce the risk of allograft rejection). The infection risk persists until the recipient immune system has generated an equivalent T-cell repertoire and this will be longer where T-cell-depleting serotherapy has been included in the conditioning or where there is significant graft-versus-host disease (GvHD).

Management of such virus infection is crucial to the outcome of the transplant because virus infection may be responsible for significant morbidity and mortality. Exposure to new virus is reduced by the relative

Table 16.1 Key Questions for the Clinician Concerning Invasive Fungal Infection (IFI)

What are the risk factors for fungal illness?

What fungal organisms are commonly seen?

Who is at greatest risk and should receive prophylaxis? And with what drugs?

How is IFI diagnosed? And how can it be diagnosed earlier?

What is empirical and preemptive therapy?

What drugs are used in therapy of IFI? What is the role of surgery and line removal?

isolation of children in the early post-transplant period. Most institutions keep children away from school at this time. Early diagnosis of infection with polymerase chain reaction (PCR)–based assay of respiratory secretions in symptomatic children will allow early diagnosis and therapy of influenza or respiratory syncytial virus (RSV) infection.

HSV prophylaxis is routine in the transplant patient. This will also serve as VZV reactivation prophylaxis. Immunoglobulin replacement is often used and might reduce the risk of virus infection.

Children who have been exposed to cytomegalovirus (CMV), adenovirus, Epstein-Barr virus (EBV), and human herpesvirus 6 (HHV6) prior to transplantation are at risk of reactivation of these viruses after transplant. This is so because the memory T-cell repertoire that controls these viruses from reactivating in all of us has been removed. Screening the blood for these viruses will detect them during an asymptomatic phase prior to clinical illness. Where children have been exposed to CMV prior to transplantation and are seropositive, using a seropositive donor might reduce the risk of post-transplant CMV reactivation and illness because some immunity to the virus is transferred with the transplant as donor immunity becomes established in the recipient.

The strategies for reducing viral infection after transplantation are summarized in Table 16.2.

Pneumacystis jiroveci Infection

Pneumocystis pneumonia (PCP) is a life-threatening infection in immunocompromised children with quantitative and qualitative defects in T-lymphocytes. At risk are children with lymphoid malignancies, HIV infection, corticosteroid therapy, transplantation and primary immunodeficiency states. It is a fungal infection but was formerly thought to be protozoan.

Infection is diagnosed in a suspected case by PCP PCR of respiratory secretions. The clinical presentation is fever, cough, breathlessness and hypoxia. There is an interstitial infiltrate on chest x-ray and this is predominantly perihilar. Various drugs are used in prophylaxis and treatment of PCP (Table 16.3). In severe PCP, therapy may be associated with a decline in clinical condition and an added steroid is an important therapeutic adjunct in this situation.

Management of Varicella-Zoster and Measles Exposure in Susceptible Children

Chickenpox caused by VZV can produce a severe illness in children who are immune suppressed because of treatment for a malignancy. It is routine practice to screen such children at diagnosis using serology for evidence of previous exposure. Those who were previous exposed need no post-exposure prophylaxis (PEP). Those who are seronegative and significantly exposed (they must themselves be in direct contact with the case of VZV) receive PEP either with varicella-zoster immunoglobulin (VZIG) or a course of aciclovir. There is no randomized trial evidence that demonstrates superiority of one approach over the other. It is similarly routine practice to offer measles immunoglobulin to exposed seronegative oncology children.

Vaccination after Chemotherapy or HSCT

Children who have completed cancer chemotherapy or have undergone HSCT and now have discontinued immune suppression are candidates for revaccination. There may be a consensus national practice. In general,

Table 16.2 Strategies to Reduce Viral Infection in the Post-Transplant Recipient

Primary antiviral prophylaxis with aciclovir for HSV/VZV and with regular immunoglobulin infusion

Isolation of children from non-family members while immune suppressed after transplantation

Screening of respiratory secretions in symptomatic children for viruses for which therapy exists, including influenza and RSV

Regular screening of the blood for the 'reactivation' viruses – CMV, EBV, adenovirus, and HHV6 – and institution of drug therapy when these viruses are found – ganciclovir/foscarnet/cidofovir for CMV and HHV6, rituximab for EBV, and cidofovir/ribavirin for adenovirus

Reduction of immune suppression in the presence of significant virus infection; In certain circumstance, virus-specific and donor-derived cytotoxic T cells can be derived and used to rapidly reconstitute virus-specific immunity in the infected post-transplant patient.

Use of a CMV-seropositive donor for a CMV-seropositive recipient so that engrafted immune donor cells have retained CMV 'memory' for reactivated CMV; Use of a CMV-seronegative donor for a seronegative recipient will reduce risk of CMV transfer with donor cells in transplantation to a CMV-naive recipient.

Table 16.3 Drugs Used in the Treatment and Prophylaxis of PCP

Treatment of PCP	Prophylaxis of PCP
TMP-SMX: TMP: 15–20 mg/kg per day + SMX: 75–100 mg/kg per day – preferred therapy; use alternatives where toxicity is seen (e.g. rash)	$150/750$ mg/m^2 per day: • Three times weekly in two divided doses on consecutive days or single dose three times a week on consecutive days • Two divided doses daily • Two divided doses three times a week on alternate days • For adolescents/adults: one double-dose tablet orally daily or three times weekly
Pentamidine: 4 mg/kg per day	300 mg nebulized 3-weekly in older children
Atovaquone Clindamycin-primaquine Dapsone-trimethoprim Limited pediatric data and used only in milder infections	–

- All children who are immune suppressed because of active chemotherapy or recently completed chemotherapy should receive the influenza vaccination each winter.
- Children who have undergone HSCT should undergo a complete revaccination program beginning 12 to 18 months after transplantation. They should have normal T- and B-cell numbers and be off immune suppression and without active GvHD. Live vaccination should not be given until 24 months after the transplant.
- Children who have received leukemia therapy should have a single booster set of immunizations to those they had received pretreatment at about 6 months after completion of treatment.

Infections That Affect the Blood

Many infections affect the blood. Hematology is part of the routine investigation of all sick children. However, this section reviews four infections in which hematologic changes are particularly prominent and where the clinical hematologist might be consulted. The hematology of HIV infection is reviewed in Chapter 23.

Table 16.4 Possible Therapeutic Interventions in Post-Transplant Lymphoproliferative Disease (PTLD)

Administration of the monoclonal antibody directed at B cells (rituximab) to reduce B-cell proliferation

Reduction of the dose of calcineurin inhibitor (ciclosporin or tacrolimus) in solid-organ transplantation-associated PTLD to encourage EBV-directed T-cell tumor surveillance

Congenital immune deficiency and EBV PTLD will require HSCT for restoration via transplant of a competent immune system. The PTLD might not need to be fully in remission prior to such an approach, and reduced-intensity conditioning (RIC) transplantation might be appropriate.

Screening of HSCT recipients for the asymptomatic EBV viremia that will precede PTLD. Those with a rising level or a level above a certain threshold will receive rituximab.

Ex vivo expanded EBV-specific partially HLA-matched T cells derived from a third party can be administered to a patient without T-cell function (after HSCT or a patient with a congenital immune deficiency) to restore EBV-directed surveillance of EBV-associated B-cell proliferation

Chemotherapy of the B-cell tumor

Hematology of Pertussis Infection

Leukocytosis and lymphocytosis are features of this bacterial infection. There is an association between outcome and degree of leukocytosis. Predominantly, the leukocytes are mature lymphocytes. Many physicians will advocate hydration where there is leukocytosis and exchange transfusion where the white blood cell (WBC) count is greater than $100 \times 10^9/$ liter.

Hematology of EBV Infection

EBV is discussed further

- As a reactivation virus during HSCT in Chapter 39 and
- As a cause of hemophagocytic lymphohistiocytosis (HLH), even in the absence of genetic mutation driving the HLH episode, in Chapter 23.

EBV immortalizes B cells and is a cause of B-cell tumors in immune-compromised patients, in whom T-cell surveillance of such EBV-related B-cell proliferation is impaired. The resulting lymphomas may be part of congenital T-cell immune deficiency or part of T-cell lymphocytopenia after HSCT, or part of T-cell immune suppression after solid-organ transplantation and use of calcineurin inhibitors. The tumor is known as *post-transplant lymphoproliferative disease* (PTLD). There may be accompanying or preceding EBV viremia. A reflection on the etiology of PTLD leads to an understanding of the possible therapeutic interventions in this illness (Table 16.4).

Acute EBV infection with seroconversion is one of the causes of infectious mononucleosis. There may be numerous atypical lymphocytes and leukocytosis. There may be associated hemolytic anemia. The monospot test might aid rapid diagnosis and detects the heterophile antibodies directed at other mammalian RBCs during acute EBV infection. Specific EBV serology including the IgM antibody will lead to a more exact diagnosis.

Hematology of Malaria

Malaria is a truly devastating disease and more common than most of the conditions dealt with in such detail in this book. The parasite spends much of its life in the RBC, and it is not therefore surprising that there are effects on RBCs, WBCs, platelets, and the coagulation system. These effects are most pronounced in *Plasmodium falciparum* infection because it parasitizes all RBCs while *P. malaria* infects only old RBCs and *P. vivax* and *P. ovale* infect only reticulocytes.

Its hematologic features are complex but might be summarized as follows:

- *Anemia*. This can be severe, particularly in children and pregnant women and is a significant cause of mortality. Its severity indicates that it is due not simply to hemolysis of infected RBCs but of non-infected RBCs too. There also may be some suppression of hematopoiesis. It is managed by RBC transfusion and occasionally by exchange transfusion where there is severe parasitemia.
- *Thrombocytopenia*. This is a persistent feature of severe malaria. It is likely a consequence of

93

endothelial damage and platelet sequestration and consumption. The mean platelet volume is raised and there are increased reticulated platelets.

- WBC cell counts are typically low or normal in malaria. Leukocytosis is rare and may represent concurrent or associated infection rather than malaria itself.
- Splenomegaly is frequent in malaria and may be huge.

Hematology of Parvovirus Infection

Parvovirus is cytopathic to RBC precursors. The marrow at the time of infection shows giant and vacuolated early pronormoblasts. In acute infection, there is an associated reticulocytopenia of 7 to 10 days' duration. In those with shortened RBC survival – chronic, inherited hemolytic anemia – this reticulocytopenic period is accompanied by symptomatic anemia, whereas in those with normal RBC survival it will go clinically unnoticed.

Parvovirus infection may be chronic in the immune-compromised host, post-HSCT, HIV infection, or the acute lymphoid leukemia (ALL) maintenance therapy patient, and there may be continuing reticulcytopenic anemia. It may be a cause of severe fetal anemia and hydrops in vertically acquired infection by the fetus during pregnancy. It should be distinguished from Diamond-Blackman anemia. It has been described to be a triggering infection for HLH. It also has been described as associated with the presentation of ALL in children.

Sickle Cell Disease

Key Messages

1. Sickle cell syndrome is a heterogeneous group of disorders with variable phenotypic severity.

2. Early detection of sickle cell anemia and initiation of penicillin prophylaxis and immunization against encapsulated bacteria decrease mortality and morbidity.

3. Recurrent vaso-occlusive crises (VOCs) are the most frequent acute sickle cell complication.

4. Hydroxycarbamide ameliorates severe frequent episodes of VOC and acute chest syndrome (ACS).

5. Transcranial Doppler (TCD) screening starting at an early age detects those with high risk for acute stroke and those who may benefit from regular blood transfusions.

6. Education and regular comprehensive care have increased survival in sickle cell anemia.

Embryonic, Fetal, and Adult Hemoglobin

The four embryonic hemoglobins synthesized in the yolk sac–derived primitive erythroid cells are hemoglobin Gower-1 and -2 and hemoglobin Portland-1 and -2 (Table 17.1). After the first 10 to 12 weeks of development, the fetus's primary form of hemoglobin switches from embryonic hemoglobin to fetal hemoglobin. At birth, fetal hemoglobin comprises 50 to 95 percent of the infant's hemoglobin. By 6 months, the switch from fetal hemoglobin to adult hemoglobin is complete, and quantitative hemoglobin disorders such as beta-thalassemia major are clinically manifest (see Figure 1.3). Certain genetic abnormalities can cause the switch to adult hemoglobin synthesis to fail, resulting in a condition known as *hereditary persistence of fetal hemoglobin* (HPFH).

Hemoglobin Disorders

Mutations in genes for any of the hemoglobin subunits alpha and beta can cause decreased production of globin chains (quantitative disorders, e.g. thalassemia) or production of abnormal globin chains with altered function (qualitative disorders, e.g. sickle cell syndrome). The latter will be discussed in this chapter, and the following list touches on some of the hemoglobin variants of which hemoglobin S (HbS), hemoglobin C (HbC), and hemoglobin E (HbE) are the most prevalent. HbE disease will be discussed with Thalassemia in Chapter 21.

- *Hemoglobin S.* Sickle cell mutation results from the substitution of glutamic acid to valine at the sixth position of the beta-globin chain causing formation of sickle hemoglobin. This is the predominant hemoglobin (>50 percent) in the different genotypes collectively referred to as *sickle cell disease* (which are described later). The alpha chain is normal, whereas both the beta chains are abnormal. Those who have one sickle mutant beta gene and one normal beta gene have *sickle cell trait*, which is clinically benign. There are four African haplotypes and one Arab–Asian haplotype, and these relate to the historical spread of the underlying genetic mutations. Different haplotypes may be associated with different severity/phenotype of disease, and in Africa, most patients with sickle cell disease in specific regions are homozygotes for the local haplotype, although in Western countries patients are often compound heterozygotes. Sickle cell mutation confers resistance to *Plasmodium falciparum* malaria.
- *Hemoglobin C.* The hemoglobin C mutation in the beta-globin gene results in substitution of glutamic acid to lysine at the sixth position. In the homozygous and heterozygous states, hemoglobin C also confers protection against *P. falciparum* malaria. Hemoglobin C disease causes a microcytic

Table 17.1 Human Hemoglobins

Embryonic hemoglobins	Fetal hemoglobins	Adult hemoglobins
Gower-1 ($\zeta_2\epsilon_2$)	Hemoglobin F ($\alpha_2\Upsilon_2$)	Hemoglobin A ($\alpha_2\beta_2$)
Gower-2 ($\alpha_2\epsilon_2$)		Hemoglobin A2 ($\alpha_2\delta_2$)
Portland-1 ($\zeta_2\Upsilon_2$)		
Portland-2 ($\zeta_2\beta_2$)		

Table 17.2 Sickle Cell Syndromes with Genotypes, Frequency, and Severity

Genotypes	Frequency	Clinical severity
HbSS	60–65%	HbSS > HbSβ0 > HbSC > Hb S+ > Hb S other
HbSC	25–30%	
HbS β0^a/HbSβ^{+a}	5–10%	
HbS O Arab/hemoglobin D	<5%	

^{a} β0 and β+ indicate no production of beta-globin and decreased beta-globin production, respectively.

hemolytic anemia and splenomegaly, and target cells are a diagnostic feature on the peripheral smear. Hemoglobin C trait is a benign condition.

- *Hemoglobin E.* Mutation in the beta-globin chain resulting in substitution of glutamine to lysine at the twenty-sixth position causes hemoglobin E disease. This is a mild hemolytic anemia with splenomegaly. Hemoglobin E trait is benign. Hemoglobin E is extremely common in Southeast Asia and in some areas equals hemoglobin A in frequency.

- *Hemoglobin D.* Hemoglobin D mutation results in substitution of glutamine to glycine at position 121. Homozygous hemoglobin D causes mild hemolytic anemia. This variant is found in Los Angeles (United States) and Punjab (India).

- *Hemoglobin O.* Hemoglobin 0 mutation results in substitution of glutamine to glycine at position 121. In the homozygous state, hemoglobin O is asymptomatic, whereas the compound heterozygous state (hemoglobin O Arab/beta-thalassemia) causes a moderate microcytic anemia with splenomegaly.

Sickle Cell Syndromes

Sickle cell syndromes are the different genotypes where one of the beta-globin gene mutation is a sickle cell mutation and comprises of HbSS, HbSβ0, HbSC, and HbSβ+. HbSS and HbSβ0 are clinically more severe than HbSC and HbSβ+. Hb S other (i.e. Hb S with hemoglobin O or hemoglobin D and Hb S hereditary persistence of fetal hemoglobin [HPFH]) are less common forms of sickle cell syndrome. Sickle cell anemia represents homozygous sickle mutation HbSS and HbSβ0 and accounts for most of the sickle cell syndromes (Table 17.2).

For the remainder of this chapter, the pathophysiology, clinical features, and management apply to the genotypes HbSS and HbSβ0 (i.e. sickle cell anemia).

Pathophysiology

Substitution of glutamine for hydrophobic valine causes polymerization of hemoglobin when deoxygenated under hypoxic conditions and the deformation of RBCs to sickle cells (Figure 17.1). The rate and extent of Hb S polymerization determine disease severity. These rigid sickle cells have a shortened lifespan and lack flexibility to cross microcapillaries, causing both extravascular and intravascular hemolysis, vaso-occlusion, and abnormal erythrocyte–endothelial cell interactions. Hypoxia-induced sickling and hemolysis increase cell-free hemoglobin in the circulation, which depletes nitric oxide (NO) and in recent years has been thought to contribute to pulmonary hypertension. Thus, vaso-occlusion with ischemia and hemolytic anemia are the two mechanisms that are central to the pathophysiologic process in sickle cell anemia.

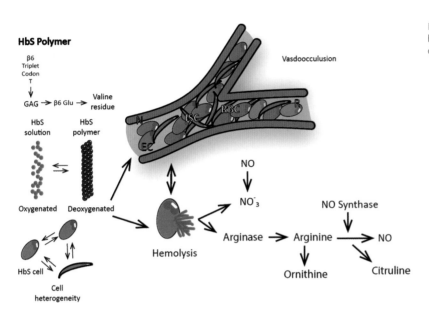

HbS Polymer

β6
Triplet
Codon
T

GAG → β6 Glu → Valine residue

HbS solution   HbS polymer

Oxygenated   Deoxygenated

HbS cell

Cell heterogeneity

Vasdoocculusion

Hemolysis

NO
↓
NO⁻₃

Arginase → Arginine

NO Synthase
↓
→ NO

Ornithine   Citruline

Figure 17.1 Pathophysiology of hemolysis and vaso-occlusion in sickle cell anemia.

Table 17.3 Interpretation of Newborn Screen Results

Newborn screen result: hemoglobins present	Interpretation
Hb F and Hb A	Normal newborn
Hb F, Hb A, and Hb S	Sickle cell trait
Hb F and Hb S	HbSS, HbSβ0, S-HPFH
Hb F, Hb S, and Hb C	HbSC
Hb F, Hb S, and Hb A	HbSβ+

Genetic Modifiers of Severity of Sickle Cell Disease

There is considerable heterogeneity in the clinical severity of sickle cell disease that is seen in homozygous disease. Co-inheritance of sickle mutation with other genes may be responsible for the variable phenotype. There is a protective effect of co-inheritance with alpha-thalassemia that modulates intracellular Hb S. Similarly co-inheritance with HPFH is a milder disease because the percentage of fetal hemoglobin reduces the concentration of Hb S. Non-globin-gene mutations such as glucose-6-phosphate dehydrogenase (G6PD) deficiency also can result in a milder phenotype.

Diagnosis/Newborn Screening

Diagnosis is established by hemoglobin electrophoresis or chromatography. Universal newborn screening programs are established in the United States and many other areas worldwide. Early diagnosis via newborn screening and initiation of penicillin prophylaxis are keys to decreasing morbidity and mortality in the first 2 years of life in sickle cell disease. Even earlier detection via chorionic villus sampling or amniocentesis is possible (Table 17.3).

Complications of Sickle Cell Disease in Children and Adults

There is an overlap in complications in both children and adults, including infections, pain episodes, acute chest syndrome, and stroke. However, in general, these tend to be more severe in adults than in children (Table 17.4).

Infants/Children

Dactilitis and *infection* are the two most frequent complications in this age group. Dactylitis refers to a syndrome of pain, swelling, tenderness, and increased temperature in the hands or feet or both secondary to sickling within the small bones. The child may become systemically unwell with leukocytosis. Symptoms begin as early as 6 months of age, but episodes prior to 1 year of age are usually a marker of the

Table 17.4 Complication in Infants, Children, and Adults

Infants	Children	Adults
Dactylitis	Veno-occlusive crisis	Cardiomegaly/heart failure
Anemia	Acute chest syndrome	Pulmonary hypertension
Enlarged spleen	Splenic sequestration	Retinopathy
Infections	Aplastic crises	Hepatic sequestration
–	Anemia	Liver failure
–	Stroke	Kidney failure
–	Priapism	Nephropathy
–	Retinopathy	Frequent urinary tract infections (UTIs)
–	Cholelithiasis	Bone necrosis
–	Avascular necrosis	–
–	Renal impairment	–
–	Isosthenuria/proteinuria	–
–	Left ventricular hypertrophy (LVH)/cardiomyopathy	–
–	Delayed sexual development	–

overall severity of the phenotype and confer a poorer prognosis. Early recognition, adequate hydration, and analgesia for control of pain symptoms are important.

Infection remains one of the major causes of mortality in young sickle cell patients and probably relates to the early onset of functional asplenia. Prophylactic penicillin administration has been shown to dramatically reduce the risk of sepsis and should be started on diagnosis. Aggressive management of fever in a child with sickle cell anemia before the age of 5 years is recommended, with investigation for bacterial sepsis and early antibiotic therapy. The exact antibiotic regimen varies based on local sensitivities, and most hospitals that manage children with sickle cell disease have a clear protocol that should be followed.

Splenic sequestration occurs in a third of children with a first episode occurring before the age of 2 years. Children who have not yet undergone autosplenectomy can have sudden and rapid splenic enlargement with trapping of a large component of their RBC mass. This leads to rapid anemia (with reticulocytosis), shock, and cardiac decompensation associated with thrombocytopenia. In the past, this was a frequent cause of death, but education of family members and daily spleen palpation have increased detection and reduced morality. Management of an acute episode requires supportive care and usually transfusion to restore oxygen-carrying capacity. However, as the episode resolves, the patients can autotransfuse RBCs from the spleen back into the circulation, so initial transfusions should be modest to avoid polycythemic complications in the recovery phase. Antibiotics to cover possible concomitant sepsis and chest physiotherapy to prevent secondary chest crisis are also important. About half the children with splenic sequestration will have a recurrence. Splenectomy is frequently performed with the second episode, although some centers will wait until the child is over 2 years old and can be vaccinated with the 23-valent pneumococcal vaccine (Table 17.5).

Vaso-occlusive crises (VOCs) occur at all age groups as severe episodic pain requiring opiod analgesia. Unlike dactylitis, there are often no physical signs on examination. The frequency peaks in teenagers and young adults. Known triggers are infection, exposure to cold, asthma exacerbation, and stress. The pain arises because of bone marrow ischemia and infarction. Increasing age, higher baseline hematocrit, and lower fetal hemoglobin are risk factors for VOC. Some centers in the hospital setting use teams specialized in management of pain because both under- and overtreatment of these episodes can have deleterious effects. In the acute setting, front-line management usually includes IV fluids, analgesia

Table 17.5 Differential Diagnosis of Acute Splenic Sequestration versus Parvovirus-induced Aplastic Crises

Features	Acute splenic sequestration	Parvovirus-induced aplastic crises
Spleen	Enlarged	Not enlarged
Reticulocyte count	Increased	Decreased
Nucleated RBCs	Present	Absent
Platelet count	Low	Normal
Transfusion	As soon as possible, quickly	Slowly
Risk of recurrence	Yes	No

(usually opiate), and hospitalization. IV fluids are usually given at maintenance rates because fluid overload increases the risk of secondary lung complications. Antibiotics are required if infection is suspected. Chest physiotherapy as prophylaxis against secondary chest crisis during hospitalization is relevant, especially if the site of vaso-occlusive crisis is the ribs, spine, or abdomen and the child is reluctant to breathe deeply because of pain. Severe episodes may require transfusion therapy aimed at reducing the proportion of Hb SS in the blood.

The management of vaso-occlusive crisis is a major part of sickle cell management, and hospitals responsible for the care of children with sickle cell disease should have well-established protocols that focus on

1. Education of patients and families for early recognition of symptoms and beginning of increased oral fluids and simple analgesia at home to try to abort early crisis.
2. Rapid recognition and treatment of these children in the emergency department. The lack of physical signs can often be a deterrent for inexperienced junior medical staff for giving adequate analgesia, so a clear and unambiguous policy and protocol are required.
3. Specialist pain management input to maximize effective pain management but minimize unnecessary exposure to opiate analgesia and the longer-term risks of dependence. However, the primary premise should be that these children have pain that requires treatment rather than assuming inappropriate drug-seeking behavior. Infusions of patient-controlled analgesia have been shown to be most effective.
4. Ability to escalate prophylactic therapy, either hydroxyurea or transfusions, for children having frequent and severe episodes.
5. Psychosocial support for children and families to facilitate schooling and also the consequences of dealing with severe, frequent painful crises.

Many countries have very well-established national guidelines for the management of sickle cell disease, and these are most useful for the pragmatic details of therapy.

Acute chest syndrome (ACS) is a potentially life-threatening complication of sickle cell disease and the most common cause of complications of hospital admission after vaso-occlusive crises. It is defined as a combination of fever, hypoxia, and new infiltrate on a chest x-ray. It is important to remember that there may be a delay in radiographic features, so fever and hypoxia in a patient with VOC should prompt an urgent chest x-ray and blood counts. Acute chest syndrome is the leading cause of morbidity and mortality in sickle cell patients and, when suspected, should be treated as a medical emergency. Many affected patients will require intensive care admission. Oxygen support, simple transfusion that may need to progress to exchange transfusion, and antibiotics to manage any potential infection are all important and should be started without delay. Analgesia is often required, but the risk of suppressing ventilation is real, and experience and expertise are critical in the successful management of chest crises. Once again, centers that manage sickle cell patients should have clear protocols and clinical care pathways to ensure optimal management.

Stroke and silent cerebral infarcts are an important cause of morbidity and mortality. The incidence of stroke is reported to be 11 percent by age 20 years. Annual transcranial Doppler screening (TCD) is part of routine management of children between 2 and 16 years of age with sickle cell anemia. It assesses blood flow velocity in the distal internal carotid artery (ICA), proximal middle cerebral artery (MCA), and anterior cerebral artery (ACA). An abnormal scan is a time-averaged velocity of 200 cm/s measured on two occasions, and between 170 and 200 cm/s is conditional. Up to a third of children with abnormal scans can have an ischemic stroke within 4 years. The Stroke Prevention Trial in Sickle Cell Anemia (STOP trial) demonstrated that regular blood transfusion reduces the risk of ischemic stroke by 90 percent. TCDs are limited by a lack of availability outside specialist centers.

Silent cerebral infarcts (SCIs) are more common and can occur in up to 37 percent of children with sickle cell anemia. Silent cerebral infarct is defined as an infarction on MRI without focal neurologic deficits on examination lasting longer than 24 hours. They can present with headaches or brief disturbances of vision or speech. These have the potential to develop into overt stroke and can cause a decline in cognitive abilities and academic performance. Optimal treatment is unknown, and the results of the recent Silent Cerebral Infarct Multicenter Clinical Trial (SIT) indicate that blood transfusion therapy reduces the incidence of cerebral infarct recurrence.

Adults

Adults have worsening of the complications just described and experience additional complications that can cause mortality. These include pulmonary hypertension, cardiac failure, transfusional iron overload, sickle cell retinopathy, nephropathy, leg ulcers, and thromboembolism. Death can result from infections, heart failure, pulmonary emboli, ACS, and stroke.

Components of Age-Based Approach to Care via Regular Comprehensive Clinic Visits

Health maintenance and comprehensive clinics are very important in the management of sickle cell disease and have greatly improved outcomes with early diagnosis, education, and regular care. Children should be seen at diagnosis and every 2 to 3 months until the age of 3 years and every 6 months thereafter. Many centers have developed clinical care guidelines based on best available evidence to allow a systematic approach to evaluation. Important age-based aspects of care in children with sickle cell disease are highlighted next:

Newborn

- Identification via newborn screening program and early referral to a specialized center
- Confirming diagnosis and parental testing
- Measuring growth parameters (height and weight)
- Initiation of penicillin prophylaxis
- Emphasizing importance of routine immunizations
- Parental education regarding disease, fever guidelines, and providing genetic counseling

Infancy

- Monitoring growth
- Education regarding fever, spleen size, measurement
- Emphasizing importance of compliance to penicillin prophylaxis
- Management of pain crises including dactylitis

Toddler

- TCD screening commencing regularly at age 2.
- 27-Valent pneumococcal vaccine.

Childhood

- Recording oxygen saturations and blood pressure and blood counts
- Monitoring adherence to penicillin (recommended until 5 years of age)
- Monitoring frequency of acute complications
- Assessment of school performance
- Early detection/prevention of chronic complications – sickle cell retinopathy, nephropathy, avascular necrosis of femur, and sleep apnea
- Consider an echocardiogram to measure tricuspid regurgitation jet velocity (TRJV) and pulmonary function testing (PFT)

Adolescence

- Counseling on transition to adult centers
- Adherence to chronic medications (e.g., hydroxyurea)
- Psychological support

Disease-Altering Agents/Treatment

Hydroxyurea

Hydroxyurea therapy substantially reduces the frequency of painful episodes and ACS events and the need for erythrocyte transfusions and hospitalizations.

Long-term hydroxyurea administration results in a reduction in mortality. Hydroxyurea is a ribonucleotide reductase inhibitor that has been in use since the 1970s to treat persons with myeloproliferative neoplasms. In the 1980s, hydroxyurea was identified as a promising drug candidate for SCD because it increases fetal hemoglobin levels. Subsequent research has shown that there are other beneficial effects as well. Hydroxyurea is rapidly absorbed, has near-complete bioavailability, and is therapeutic with once-daily oral dosing. The predominant short-term side effect is dose-dependent myelosuppression. There are concerns about some long-term side effects of malignancy, effects on male sterility, and teratogenic effects on the fetus if conceived while on therapy, but these have not been substantiated with evidence. There is now emerging data to suggest that it may be of benefit even to those children who do not have a severe clinical course, with recent recommendations that it should be offered to all children with sickle cell disease at 9 months of age regardless of clinical course. Whether hydroxyurea reduces stroke in all children, or those with elevated TCD's is still under investigation. The principles of hydroxyurea therapy are to start with a relatively low dose (20 mg/kg per day) until there is mild myelosuppression or to a maximum of 35 mg/kg per day. Monthly monitoring with full blood counts and in general dose escalations occur 8 weekly. If myelosuppression occurs, then temporary dose reduction and then re-escalation are appropriate, although in some children side effects will require permanent cessation. There are well-established protocols for this process.

Blood Transfusion and Iron Overload/Chelation

Blood transfusion is used to mitigate both acute and chronic complications of sickle cell disease with the goal of reducing the percentage of sickle cells to less than 30 percent. It is used in acute complications including ACS, splenic sequestration, aplastic crises, stroke, recurrent painful episodes, and preoperative correction of anemia. Indications for its use in chronic complications are primarily in secondary stroke prevention.

Blood transfusion corrects anemia, reduces the percentage of sickle cells, and reduces hemolysis. This can be given as a simple transfusion or via erythrocytapheresis (or red cell exchange transfusion), with the latter used if the hemoglobin concentration is high. A simple transfusion is time efficient in a sick patient, whereas the erythrocytapheresis depends on intravenous access placement and availability of personnel to perform it. While most centers have automated erythrocytapheresis machine, some centers do still employ manual exchange.

Surgical procedures in persons with SCD are associated with significant risk for SCD and non-SCD-associated morbidity as well as an increased risk of death. Transfusions are commonly used during the perioperative period to prevent postoperative vaso-occlusive crises, stroke, or ACS. Studies have shown a lowered risk of postoperative complications in persons with SCD undergoing medium-risk surgery when their preoperative hemoglobin level was increased to 100 g/liter; thus elective transfusion prior to surgery is often required. Anesthesia should ensure adequate oxygenation and attention to fluid status, and postoperative pain management to ensure maximal chest recovery without atelectasis is also important. Unless driven by clinical emergency, surgery should be planned and conducted in major sickle cell treatment centers.

The most important complications of recurrent blood transfusion are alloimmunization and iron overload. Extended cross-match including typing for Kell blood group in addition to ABO and Rhesus (Cc/D/Ee) and matching ethnic origin of donor and recipient have reduced the frequency of alloantibodies. Iron chelation is an important aspect of care in sickle cell patients requiring regular transfusion. The pattern of iron deposition in sickle cell disease is different from thalassemia and occurs predominantly in the liver. Desferrioxamine is effective, although parenteral administration limits its use for some patients. Deferasirox, an oral iron chelator, is increasingly being used and has proved to be effective.

Hematopoietic Stem Cell Transplantation (HSCT)

This is the only curative treatment for sickle cell disease. Not everyone has a family donor, and unrelated donor identification is often difficult because of the relatively low representation of specific ethnic groups on unrelated donor panels. There has been recent interest in haploidentical stem cell transplantation in hemoglobinopathy. This is transplant using a parent as a donor for the child. This means that everyone has a donor. There are specific risks of fraft versus host sisease and particular strategies are employed to reduce these risks. All transplant decisions are risk based. It is employed for those with severe complications like cerebrovascular disease and those on a red cell transfusion programme.

Future Therapy

HSCT from unrelated and halloidentical donors with reduced-intensity conditioning as well as gene therapy are future promising cellular therapies aimed at cure. There are other additional targets of sickle cell aimed at increasing fetal hemoglobin (decitabine, butyrate), increasing levels of nitric acid (inhaled nitric oxide, sildenafil, arginine), reduce erythrocyte dehydration (magnesium), and reduce tissue damage (glutamine). Gene therapy trials using lentiviral gene transfer are just beginning.

Thalassemia

1. The thalassemias are a heterogeneous group of inherited red blood cell (RBC) disorders causing a quantitative decrease in globin chain production leading to ineffective erythropoiesis and hemolysis.

2. Seven percent of the world's population are thalassemia carriers (270 million people).

3. The phenotype is variable, ranging from an asymptomatic state with no anemia to severe microcytic anemia with transfusion dependence.

4. The key to management of homozygous thalassemia is regular, comprehensive clinics directed toward appropriate transfusion therapy while addressing iron overload with chelation and managing the multisystem complications.

5. The causes of mortality in thalassemia have changed over the years with the introduction of improved therapies.

6. Thalassemia syndromes are broadly classified as transfusion dependent (TDT) and non–transfusion dependent (NTDT).

7. Stem cell transplantation can cure transfusion dependence in thalassemia major, but its availability is limited by donor availability. Gene therapy using autologous human stem cells (HSCs) holds promise as corrective therapy in those without a suitable donor.

Introduction

The thalassemias are inherited as autosomal recessive disorders primarily conferring a survival advantage as protection against *Plasmodium falciparum* in malaria-endemic areas. Approximately 7 percent of the world's population have some form of thalassemia trait, although this varies by country, with the highest rate being up to 18 percent in the Maldives. About 1.5 percent of the global population is a carrier of the beta-thalassemia gene, with the highest carrier frequency in Cyprus, Sardinia, and Southeast Asia.

Adult hemoglobin is composed of a tetramer of two alpha- and two beta-globin chains (Figure 18.1). The alpha-globin genes are on chromosome 16, and the beta-globin genes are on chromosome 11 (Figure 18.2). In thalassemia, the production of alpha or beta chains is decreased. This results in excess unmatched globin chains that accumulate in RBCs causing ineffective erythropoiesis leading to their in-marrow destruction and in the clinical feature of hemolysis.

Some important details about the pathophysiology of thalassemias are as follows:

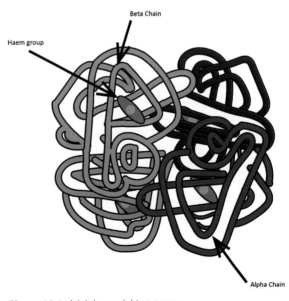

Figure 18.1 Adult hemoglobin tetramer.

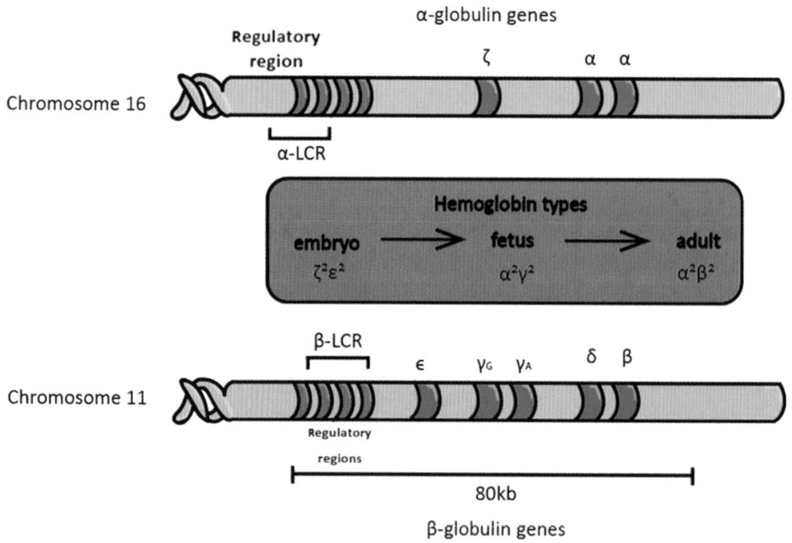

Figure 18.2 Genes for thalassemia.

1. In beta-thalassemia, it is the excess alpha chains that causes RBC death, and in alpha-thalassemia, it is the excess beta-chain production.

2. Thalassemia is characterized by ineffective erythropoiesis. The marrow will hypertrophy to compensate, leading to extramedullary hematopoiesis. This is responsible for some of the features of thalassemia major with splenomegaly and bone thinning.

3. Beta-thalassemia is more commonly a clinical problem than alpha-thalassemia because there are four alpha-globin genes on chromosome 16, whereas there are only two beta-globin genes on chromosome 11. Therefore, a greater genetic lesion is required to cause a quantitatively abnormal alpha-globin chain production sufficient to cause RBC death – because the remaining genes can compensate

4. Beta-thalassemia is not a clinical problem until the switch from gamma- to beta-globin chain production occurs from 3 to 6 months of age. There is no globin chain imbalance until this switch occurs.

5. The genetics of thalassemia are varied, but in a given population, there are common genotypes. There are many genes that cause beta-thalassemia but relatively few likely genes potentially responsible for beta-thalassemia in a child from a single region (e.g. Cyprus). This is important in genetic screening.

6. Most alpha-thalassemia is caused by gene deletion, and most beta-thalassemia is caused by mutation.

There is a genotype–phenotype correlation. Mutations that allow some globin chain output will cause a milder phenotype than mutations that allow no globin chain output.

7. Milder mutations in the beta-globin gene that change quantitative production include splice-site mutations and mutations in the promoter region, whereas more severe mutations might be those that generate a premature stop codon or generate a frame shift (by inserting or deleting one or two nucleotides).

Classifications of Different Forms of Thalassemia

Alpha-Thalassemia

Alpha-thalassemia is caused by reduced or absent production from the four alpha-globin chain genes. The clinical severity of the alpha-thalassemias is based on the number of affected alleles and whether there are deletional or nondeletional mutations. The deletional mutations cause complete or partial deletion of alpha-globin chains, whereas the non-deletional mutations cause reduced production of alpha-globin or structurally aberrant alpha-globins such as hemoglobin Constant Spring (see later).

- Loss of one of the four alleles, written as ($-\alpha$/ $\alpha\alpha$), has no clinical implications or phenotype.

There may be laboratory evidence with a mild microcytic anemia and an increased RBC count but normal RBC distribution width (RDW). The importance of diagnosis is avoiding mislabeling of the child as iron deficient based on the reduced mean corpuscular volume (MCV) and to enable appropriate genetic counseling.

- Loss of two alleles can either occur in *trans*-(-α/-α) or in *cis*-(--/αα). The former is more common in the US populations and the latter in Southeast Asian populations. The two are clinically the same – microcytic mild anemia with normal hemoglobin electrophoresis (in contrast to beta-thalassemia trait). Note that Southeast Asian alpha-thalassemia trait individuals are at risk of having a child with severe hemoglobin Bart syndrome (i.e. hydrops fetalis – four-gene deletion) if they have children with a similar genotype carrier. This is not the case where the alpha-thalassemia gene loss is inherited in *trans*.

- Loss of three alleles gives rise to hemoglobin H (HbH) disease, which gives a mild to moderate to severe hemolytic anemia with splenomegaly. Growth failure can occur, and sometimes transfusions are required, although most commonly this is intermittent and associated with intercurrent illness. There is β^4-hemoglobin (hemoglobin H) on Hb electophoresis.

- Hemoglobin Constant Spring is a variant in which a mutation in the alpha-globin gene produces an alpha-globin chain that is abnormally long (α^{CS}). The quantity of hemoglobin in the cells is low for two reasons. First, the mRNA for hemoglobin Constant Spring is unstable. Some is degraded prior to protein synthesis. Second, the Constant Spring alpha-globin chain protein is itself unstable. The carrier state is undetectable (αα/αα^{CS}). When inherited with α^0-thalassamia (αα^{CS}/--), a more severe HbH disease occurs.

- Loss of all four alleles (--/--) causes *in utero* anemia and hydrops secondary to severe fetal anemia. This is usually not compatible with postnatal life. Screening and early detection are important because women who are pregnant with an affected child have significantly increased risks of maternal complications, and early termination is usually advocated.

Table 18.1 shows the number of affected alpha alleles with their clinical severity.

Beta-Thalassemia

Beta-globin gene mutations causing beta-thalassemia involve both coding and noncoding sequences. Thalassemia major is homozygous or compound heterozygous for β^0 or β^+ genes (beta-globin mutations allowing no [0] or some [+] global chain production), whereas thalassemia minor represents heterozygous disease. Table 18.2 summarizes the beta-thalasssemia syndromes.

Thalassemia major usually presents by 6 months of life when the fetal hemoglobin declines or later in infancy with symptoms of severe anemia, hepatosplenomegaly, and other evidence of extramedullary hematopoiesis manifest. Beta-thalassemia major and intermedia are defined based on RBC transfusion requirements. Those with major disease require more than eight transfusions per year (usually every 3 to 4 weeks), whereas those with intermedia require fewer than eight transfusions per year. The indications for transfusion therapy include severe anemia and prevention of subsequent complications, growth failure, and significant extramedullary hemopoiesis, which should be prevented for a variety of reasons.

Beta-thalassemia intermedia occurs when two beta-globin gene mutations have been inherited, but there is reduced transfusion dependence. It is best understood by considering that the severity of disease reflects the degree of globin chain imbalance that leads to RBC precursor death.

- The beta-globin chain mutation itself allows some beta-globin chain (a β^+ mutation), so there is less of an excess of alpha-globin chains.
- There is co-inherited alpha-thalassemia trait, so there are reduced amounts of alpha-globin chain and so reduced alpha-globin chain excess.
- There is co-inherited hereditary persistence of gamma-globin chain production which as Hb F will reduce the alpha-globin chain excess.

Hemoglobin E

Hemoglobin E disease presenting in either heterozygous or homozygous form is usually a mild disease. However, when co-inherited with heterozygous beta-thalassemia, it can cause a variable phenotype from mild hemolysis to severe hemolysis requiring regular RBC transfusions.

Table 18.1 Alpha-Thalassemia

Genotype	Nomenclature	Phenotype/clinical implication	Blood counts	Newborn screen positive on Hb electrophoresis
αα/αα	Normal	–	–	–
–α/αα	Silent carrier	No clinical disease; important to differentiate from iron deficiency	Mild microcytic anemia, elevated RBC count, normal RDW	No
–α/– α	Alpha-thalassemia trait in *trans*	No clinical disease; important to differentiate from iron deficiency; usually in African ancestry	Moderate microcytosis	No
––/αα	Alpha-thalassemia trait in *cis*	No clinical disease; important clinical implications for reproduction; usually occurs in Southeast Asian ancestry	Moderate microcytosis	No
––/–α	Hemoglobin H disease	Mild to moderate to severe hemolysis ± transfusion/splenomegaly/growth failure	Moderate to severe microcytosis and variable degree of anemia	Yes. Hemoglobin Barts in small amounts
––/ α^{CS}α	Hb Constant Spring	Severe hemolysis and transfusion dependence	Severe microcytosis and anemia and usually transfusion dependent	Yes. Hemoglobin Bart
––/––	Hemoglobin Bart syndrome	Severe anemia/hydrops fetalis	–	Yes. Hemoglobin Bart

Hemoglobin E–beta-thalassemia (Hb E–β-thalassemia) is the genotype responsible for approximately half of all severe beta-thalassemia worldwide. The disorder is characterized by marked clinical variability ranging from mild and asymptomatic anemia to a life-threatening disorder requiring transfusions from infancy, similar to beta-thalassemia. The phenotype is influenced (see thalassemia intermedia discussed earlier) by the co-inheritance of alpha-thalassemia and polymorphisms associated with increased production of fetal hemoglobin. Other factors, including a variable increase in serum erythropoietin in response to anemia, previous or ongoing infection with malaria, previous splenectomy, and other environmental influences, may be involved. The remarkable variation – and the instability – of the clinical phenotype of Hb E–β-thalassemia suggests that careful tailoring of treatment is required for each patient and that therapeutic approaches should be reassessed over time.

Delta-Beta-Thalassemia and Hereditary Persistence of Fetal Hemoglobin (HPFH)

Delta-beta-thalassemia is a form of beta-thalassemia characterized by decreased or absent synthesis of the delta- and beta-globin chains (usually by a large deletion mutation – they are adjacent genes; see Figure 18.2). There is a compensatory increase in expression of fetal gamma-chain synthesis. The condition is found in many ethnic groups.

The heterozygous form of the condition is clinically asymptomatic with mild microcytosis and no elevation of Hb A2 (because the delta gene is also deleted), whereas the few homozygous patients have a mild clinical presentation. When this is inherited with heterozygous classic beta-thalassemia, patients usually have the thalassemia intermedia phenotype.

Hereditary persistence of fetal hemoglobin (HPFH) is a benign condition in which significant fetal hemoglobin (hemoglobin F) production continues well into adulthood. It has no clinical

Table 18.2 Beta-Thalassemia and Hemoglobin E

Genotype	Nomenclature	Phenotype/clinical implication	Blood counts	Hb electrophoresis
β/β	Normal	–	–	–
β/β^{0a} β/β^{+a}	Beta-thalassemia trait	No clinical disease; important to differentiate from iron deficiency; requires genetic counseling prior to reproductive age	Mild microcytic anemia	Elevated Hb A2
β^+/β^+ β^+/β^0	Beta-thalassemia intermedia	Moderate hemolysis	Moderate microcytic anemia; requires intermittent RBC transfusions	Elevated Hb A2
β^E/β^+ β^E/β^0	Beta-thalassemia intermedia/major	Moderate to severe hemolysis	Moderate to severe microcytic anemia; requires intermittent to regular transfusions	Absent Hb A; elevated Hb F, Hb E
β^0/β^0	Beta-thalassemia major	Severe hemolysis	Severe microcytic anemia; requires regular RBC transfusion support	Absent Hb A; elevated Hb F

^{a} β^+/β^0 reduced production of beta-globin chains/absent beta-globin chain production.

significance except to ameliorate beta-thalassemia. It is usually caused by mutation in the beta-global gene cluster.

Beta-Thalassemia Major

Clinical Features

Beta-thalassemia major is clinically suspected in a child with severe microcytic anemia starting at approximately 6 months of age with hepatosplenomegaly and other evidence of extramedullary hematopoiesis. The blood film shows marked RBC anisopoikilocytosis, severe microcytic hypochromic RBCs, and many nucleated RBC forms. Hemoglobin electrophoresis in homozygous β^0 disease shows absence of hemoglobin A. Hb F is present. In β^+-thalassemia, homozygotes show Hb A level between 10 and 30 percent.

Thalassemia is an iron-loading anemia characterized by ineffective RBC production and massive marrow compensatory expansion. Treatment principles are simple:

- Turn off the marrow expansion and ineffective erythropoiesis with red cell transfusion If blood is given – to anyone, not just a thalassemic patient – then the drive for red cell production is suppressed

- Manage the iron overload that is part of the disease and is a complication of a red cell transfusion program.

Complications

Complications are disease related or from therapy directed toward management of anemia or iron overload and are listed below and summarized in Figure 18.3.

1. *Bone marrow expansion and extramedullary hematopoiesis.* Bone expansion thins adjacent cortical bone and causes the typical facial features – 'thalassemia facies' – and the 'bone on end' appearance on skull x-rays. Splenomegaly results from extramedullary hematopoiesis and can cause hypersplenism. Splenectomy can ameriolate transfusion requirements in thalassemia intermedia and in some with beta-thalassemia major whose transfusion requirements are higher than expected. Splenectomy is currently indicated in three clinical scenarios: increased blood requirement that prevents adequate iron control, hypersplenism, and symptomatic splenomegaly. However, splenectomy increases the risk of infection with encapsulated organism, thromboembolic disease, and pulmonary hypertension.

107

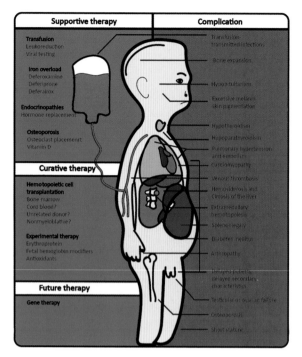

Supportive therapy | Complication

Transfusion
Leukoreduction
Viral testing

Iron overload
Deferoxamine
Deferiprone
Deferatrox

Endocrinopathies
Hormone replacement

Osteoporosis
Osteoclast placement
Vitamin D

Curative therapy

Hemotopoietic cell
transplantation
Bone marrow
Cord blood?
Unrelated donor?
Nonmyeloblative?

Experimental therapy
Erythroprotein
Fetal hemoglobin modifiers
Antioxidants

Future therapy

Gene therapy

Transfusion-transmitted infections

Bone expansion

Hypopituitarism

Excessive melanin skin pigmentation

Hypothyroidism

Hypoparathyroidism

Pulmonary hypertension and embolism

Cardiomyopathy

Venous thrombosis

Hemosiderosis and Cirrosis of the liver

Extramedullary hemotopoiesis

Splenomegaly

Diabetes mellitus

Arthropathy

Delayed puberty delayed secondary characteristics

Testicular or ovarian failure

Osteoporosis

Short stature

Figure 18.3 The multiorgan complications of thalassemia major that are due to the primary disease or as a result of therapy are listed on the right side of the diagram. The potential therapies used to overcome specific problems are listed on the left side of the diagram.

2. *Endocrinopathies.* This is secondary to iron overload. Hypopituitarism, hypothyroidism, hypoparathyroidism, adrenal failure, and diabetes mellitus are all well recognized. These are more common in older patients as a result of iron overload or in whom chelation therapy has not been optimal. Hormone replacement is needed in a few patients.

3. *Pulmonary hypertension.* Risk of increased pulmonary pressure occurs at an older age and in those who have undergone splenectomy. Inflammation and activation of the coagulation system are contributory.

4. *Hypercoagulability.* There is increased risk especially after splenectomy, with a relative risk increase for clinical thrombosis of over six times.

5. *Cardiomyopathy.* This is the most serious life-threatening complication of chronic iron overload and the major cause of morbidity and mortality in patients with inadequate chelation therapy.

6. *Liver iron overload.* This frequently causes cirrhosis of the liver.

7. *Fertility.* Delayed puberty and testicular/ovarian failure can occur in up to 50 percent of adults with thalassemia as a result of hypogonadotropic hypogonadism. This can be corrected with hormone replacement. Women of childbearing age have been able to become pregnancy spontaneously or with assisted reproductive methods.

8. *Osteoporosis.* Bone marrow expansion secondary to ineffective erythropoiesis, endocrinopathies including impaired calcium metabolism, and iron-chelating drugs all contribute to the development of osteopenia/osteoporosis. Optimal chelation, dietary adjustments to increase calcium intake, and vitamin D therapy are effective bone disease management strategies. Bisphosphonates can reduce bone resorption by inhibiting osteoclasts, but they require further study.

9. *Growth failure/short stature.* Chronic anemia and endocrinopathies contribute to growth failure in thalassemia. Growth hormone therapy has had variable success.

10. *Transfusion-related infections.* Infections, particularly hepatitis B and C and HIV, were more common in the older population and are less frequent now because of vaccinations and screening of blood donors. Hemolytic and nonhemolytic reactions can be seen in the immediate post-transfusion period.

11. *Psychosocial.* The thalassemia team must remember that the patient they care for has a chronic illness with an enormous impact on family life, on schooling, and on psychological well-being. The patient's life is fundamentally different from that of his or her neighbor, however well the disease is managed.

The major causes of mortality in thalassemia have changed over the years. Originally, severe anemia was the leading cause of death, but with adequate transfusion therapy, long-term complications of iron overload, predominantly cardiac failure, became the major cause of mortality. With the advent of better chelation therapies, infection is now the most important cause of disease-related death. Across this evolution of care, the life expectancy for patients with thalassemia has improved dramatically. Untreated, patients with thalassemia major would rarely survive late childhood, but now the life expectancy with appropriate transfusion and chelation therapy – as

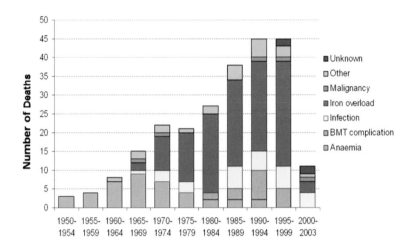

Figure 18.4 Changing cause of death in transfusion-dependent thalassemia (TDT)

well as supportive care as provided within a specific thalassemia treatment center – is approaching that of the normal community (Figure 18.4).

Management of Anemia

Regular blood transfusions are the cornerstone of management of beta-thalassemia major. The goals of transfusion are

- Correction of anemia
- Suppression of extramedullary hematopoiesis
- Prevention of endocrinopathies
- Promoting optimal growth and development

Most patients require regular transfusions before 1 year of age and are initiated based on the presence of clinical symptoms of severe anaemia, including fatigue and poor growth. The frequency of transfusion varies with each individual, but the widely accepted aim is to keep the pretransfusion hemoglobin level between 90 and 100 g/liter. In addition to the risk of infection and hemolytic and nonhemolytic complications, there is a risk of alloimmunization with frequent transfusions, and these patients need extended RBC typing before starting on a regular transfusion program. Some centers routinely use extended antigen-matched blood to reduce alloimmunization.

Iron Overload and Management

The most common complication of transfusions and cause of morbidity and mortality in beta-thalassemia major is transfusional iron overload. Hepcidin, which inhibits iron absorption in the gut when iron stores are elevated, is inappropriately low in patients with thalassemia major. Most patients needs iron chelation after about 10 to 12 RBC transfusions.

There are several measures of iron overload in the patient:

- Ferritin is an unreliable but simple indicator of tissue iron overload, particularly in patients with liver disease. It is frequently used to serially measure iron stores and monitor chelation therapy.
- Some centers perform liver biopsy, but this has fallen out of favor because of its invasive nature, inaccuracy in the face of hepatic fibrosis, and heterogeneous distribution of iron deposition. Furthermore, hepatic iron overload does not always correlate with cardiac iron overload. There may be a role for liver biopsy prior to hematopoietic stem cell transplantation (HSCT).
- The availability of noninvasive means of measuring iron overload by magnetic resonance imaging (MRI) methodology $R2^*$ in the liver and $T2^*$ in the heart has revolutionized monitoring of tissue iron burden.

Iron Chelators

The goal of iron chelation is to keep ferritin below 1,000 ng/ml or liver iron below 7 mg/g of liver tissue. The drug used historically is desferrioxamine with a starting dose of 20 to 30 mg/kg per day to a maximum of 50 mg/kg per day for 12 h as a continuous infusion for 5 to 7 days of the week. The drug has its problems – it is given by subcutaneous administration, and this leads to noncompliance; it has auditory and ocular toxicity; and it has an increased risk of infection (classically with *Yersinia*), which has made it a less favorable option.

Deferiprone and deferasirox are two oral agents that are in clinical use. Deferiprone at doses of 75 to 100 mg/kg per day has proven to be effective, safe, and not associated with liver damage. Side effects are primarily hematologic (neutropenia) and gastrointestinal but reversible. A particular advantage of deferiprone is its combined use with desferrioxamine in reducing cardiac iron overload when more intense chelation is needed. Deferasirox is another oral chelator used in the dose of 20 to 30 mg/kg per day. Side effects include gastrointestinal symptoms, skin rashes, and renal toxicity but are reversible and rarely require discontinuation of the drug.

Components of an Age-Based Approach to Care via Regular Comprehensive Clinic Visits

Visits to a center equipped with the laboratory and imaging capability of monitoring patients with severe hemoglobinopathies are an essential component of care of these patients. Monitoring is particularly essential to gauge the effectiveness of the transfusion regimen and chelation therapy and its side effects, to evaluate endocrine function, and if noninvasive methods are available, to assess for iron burden.

Recommended monthly assessments are as follows:

- Physical examination during visits for blood transfusion
- Laboratory evaluation including CBC, comprehensive metabolic panel (CMP), serum ferritin determination, and urinalysis

Recommended yearly assessments via annual clinic visits are as follows:

- Annual transfusion need. As this rises above 200 ml/kg per year, splenectomy might be considered.
- Ophthalmic and auditory examinations
- Bone densitometry (DEXA scan)
- MRI of heart and liver (T2*/R2*)
- Laboratory evaluation for endocrinopathies – thyroid and parathyroid hormone studies, luteinizing hormone (LH), follicle-stimulating

hormone (FSH), estradiol, testosterone, ionized calcium, vitamin D, serum glucose, and screening for hepatitis B and C

Genetic Modifiers of Homozygous Beta-Thalassemia

These are discussed in the preceding text, but it is important to note that there are some genetic variants that reduce globin chain imbalance resulting in milder phenotypes in beta-thalassemia:

- Co-inheritance of alpha-thalassemia
- Deletion or nondeletional delta-beta-thalassemia
- Genetic determinants that are able to sustain a continuous production of gamma-globin chains (Hb F) in adult life
- Other mutations increasing Hb F productions (Those associated with deletional and nondeletional HPFH are linked to the beta-globin gene cluster.)

Prenatal Diagnosis/Newborn Screening/ Carrier Detection

Carrier Detection

Most carriers are detected by low MCV/mean corpuscular hemoglobin (MCH) and, for beta-thalassemia, elevated Hb A2 by hemoglobin chromatography (HPLC). Other conditions that result in microcytosis and hypochromia with normal/borderline Hb A2 and normal Hb F are iron deficiency anemia, alpha-thalassemia trait, the thalassemia traits that also delete the delta gene (delta-beta-thalassemia, beta+delta-thalassemia), and mild beta-thalassemia trait.

Iron deficiency anemia can be ruled out by appropriate tests. The other thalassemia determinants can be differentiated based on globin gene synthesis (alpha, beta, or gamma). The following are pitfalls to carrier identification:

- Co-inheritance of heterozygous beta-thalassemia and alpha-thalassemia that can raise MCV (but will have high Hb A2)
- Presence of mild beta-thalassemia mutation (e.g. β^+ IVS-I nt 6 mutation) (Co-inheritance of heterozygous beta-thalassemia and delta-thalassemia and gamma-delta-beta carriers may have normal HbA2 [but low MCV]).

- Silent beta-thalassemia, where MCV/MCH and Hb A2 are borderline
- Concurrent iron deficiency (This may falsely elevate the Hb A2, so correction of iron deficiency is required before beta-thalassemia can be excluded by Hb electrophoresis

Prenatal Diagnosis

This is performed via chorionic villus sampling or amniocentesis using polymerase chain reaction (PCR) technology to detect point mutations or deletions. Preimplantation genetic diagnosis is available for families in which the disease-causing mutation has been identified and offers diagnostic testing before implantation. Preimplantation also has been extended to HLA typing on embryonic biopsy, which can allow selection of an embryo that is not affected by thalassemia.

Newborn Screening

Beta thalassemia major is picked up on newborn high-pressure liquid chromatographic (HPLC) screen by the presence of predominantly Hb F and low or absent Hb A. Hb E also may be detected in individuals with Hb E–β-thalassemia. HPLC can also detect hemoglobin Barts at birth, indicating hemoglobin H disease or hemoglobin Constant Spring variants. Newborn screen results should be confirmed by DNA testing.

Hematopoietic Stem Cell Transplantation (HSCT)

Allogeneic HSCT remains the definitive curative treatment in beta-thalassemia. Risk-stratification systems (Lucarelli Classification) classify pretransplant factors such as hepatomegaly, hepatic fibrosis, and effectiveness of iron chelation into groups that can predict post-transplant outcome. One of the limitations of HSCT is the lack of availability of HLA-matched sibling donors. The use of matched unrelated donors (MUDs), cord blood, and haploidentical transplants makes the transplant more difficult and increases the risks, albeit having expanded donor source availability.

There are particular issues in thalassemia transplantation:

- There is an increased risk of graft rejection because of the expanded recipient hemopoiesis. There is no space for donor cells. This might be reduced by pretransplant hypertransfusion regimens.
- There is an increased risk of hepatic vena-occlusive disease (VOD) in the iron-loaded patient. This risk might be reduced by pharmacokinetically targeting the busulfan into a reduced range by adding defibrotide as VOD prophylaxis and by using safer regimens such as those that replace busulfan with treosulfan.

Gene Therapy

Gene therapy is another emerging curative option with ongoing clinical trials that have shown promising results in early stages. The principle of such trials is to collect blood stem cells from the patient that are modified in a laboratory using a lentiviral vector encoding a single-codon variant of the beta-globin gene and then returned to the patient's body after myelobaltive conditioning, where they grow and produce new cells that contain a functioning copy of the gene. The risks of myelobalative bone marrow transplantation (BMT) persist: infertility, transplant-associated morbidity, and mortality. There are no graft-versus-host disease (GvHD) risks. Infection risks are reduced. There may be a risk of insertional mutagenesis, but this seems to be safe with lentivirus.

Neutropenia

Neutropenia is a common problem for the pediatric hematologist, and the thorough assessment of a child with neutropenia should distinguish the following causes:

1. Neutropenia that is *significant* and likely to increase the risk of bacterial and other infection and that which is benign and less likely to be associated with infection (Such clinical significance importantly does not rest on the absolute value of the neutrophil count.)

2. Neutropenia that is caused by *marrow production failure* and neutropenia that is caused by *peripheral consumption* (In general, the former is more likely to result in significant infection than the latter.)

3. *Congenital* neutropenia and *acquired* neutropenia (There are several genetic conditions that are associated with either isolated neutropenia or neutropenia that is part of a more generalized marrow failure.)

4. Conditions in which neutropenia is a likely presenting feature or where it is not the sole presenting feature and appears variably in the course of that condition (For example, neutropenia is common in Fanconi anemia, but it is rare that a child in the clinic who is referred with isolated neutropenia will have Fanconi anemia.)

Introduction

Neutropenia is defined as a decrease in absolute neutrophil count (ANC) that includes both segmented forms and bands. In general, an ANC $< 1.5 \times 10^9/$liter is the lower limit of normal in children, but African and Middle Eastern groups have a lower ANC by about $0.5 \times 10^9/$liter. *Mild* neutropenia refers

to an ANC of 1 to $1.5 \times 10^9/$liter, and *severe* neutropenia refers to an ANC of $<0.5 \times 10^9/$liter. *Chronic* neutropenia refers to neutropenia lasting more than 3 months. The diagnostic approach and useful laboratory tests in the evaluation of neutropenia are listed in Table 19.1.

Distinguishing Benign from Severe Neutropenia

This distinction is mandatory when seeing any child with neutropenia on the wards or in the clinics. *Benign* and *severe* indicate the clinical significance of the neutropenia – that is, how likely is the affected child likely to become ill with infection from the neutropenia. The distinction cannot be made on the ANC alone because it may be very low in both. The indicators of a severe or constitutional neutropenia include

- *History of severe infection ± hospitalization* (e.g. lymphadenitis, cellulitis, omphalitis, pneumonia [abnormal chest x-ray], sinusitis, and sepsis [especially gram-negative sepsis]) (These features should be specifically sought during the initial assessment of the neutropenic child.)

- *Cyclical pattern of infections* (It may be helpful to suggest that families keep a symptom diary.)

- *Clinical features* (These include short stature and dysmorphology that might suggest that the neutropenia is part of a wider illness. Make sure that each neutropenic child is examined for such features and that the child's growth is plotted.)

- *Some laboratory features* (Some laboratory help to make the diagnosis of the illness causing neutropenia and therefore also help to distinguish severe from benign causes. These may be specific to the cause, such as molecular genetic studies in severe congenital neutropenia or bone marrow morphology to distinguish marrow failure from peripheral consumption.)

Table 19.1 Diagnostic Approach and Useful Laboratory Tests in the Evaluation of Neutropenia

Suspected etiology	Tests to consider
Transient myelosuppression	Repeat counts
Chronic/autoimmune benign neutropenia	Anti-neutrophil antibodies (ANAs)
Viral serologies	Epstein-Barr virus (EBV), cytomegalovirus (CMV)
Quantitative immunoglobulins/lymphocyte subsets	Neutropenia associated with immune disorders
Drug-induced neutropenia	Possible dose reduction/alternative agent
Nutritional deficiencies	Serum vitamin B_{12} and folate levels
Cyclic neutropenia	Serial blood counts/genetic test for cyclic neutropenia
Shwachman-Diamond Syndrome	Pancreatic function test, skeletal radiographs
Severe *congenital neutropenia* (SCN), dyskeratosis congenita, other congenital neutropenia	Bone marrow examination with cytogenetics

Benign Neutropenias of Childhood

Chronic Benign Neutropenia/ Autoimmune Neutropenia

This condition is common with a prevalence of 1 in 100,000 children. Both familial and nonfamilial forms have been described. In both forms, the mechanism of neutropenia is similar and secondary to antibodies against the neutrophil-specific antigen (NA), especially FCγRIII. This can present as early as infancy, and the neutropenia can last until age 4. There is no significant predisposition to infections. When stressed with infection, patients are able to increase their peripheral neutrophil counts. ANC can be variable and is usually mild to moderate, but severe neutropenia can occur. There may be a compensatory monocytosis. Anti-neutrophil antibody may or may not be detected and is not necessary for diagnosis. Bone marrow examination may not be necessary unless there are no other worrying features, as described earlier. There is no significant history of infection. There are no findings on physical examination.

Supportive care during infections is the mainstay of management, but infections are few. Parents should have access to immediate medical help during fever. Broad-spectrum antibiotics are indicated if fever and neutropenia are present on admission. Granulocyte colony-stimulating factor (G-CSF) is usually not required but will increase neutrophil counts. The natural history of the condition is spontaneous resolution, although this may be protracted.

Neonatal Alloimmune Neutropenia

This is the neutrophil equivalent of Rh hemolytic disease of the newborn and alloimmune thrombocytopenia. It has a reported incidence of 1 in 500 live births but rarely comes to clinical attention because babies are usually well. The mother is sensitized to antigens on the fetal neutrophils that are paternally derived and not shared by the mother. There is production of immunoglobulin G (IgG) that crosses the placenta and causes destruction of fetal neutrophils.

Newborns have severe neutropenia that can present with skin infections, pneumonias, or sepsis but more commonly is simply an incidental finding on a full blood count (FBC) taken for another reason. Infections are with organisms that are common in the neonatal age group and include gram-negative organisms, *Staphylococcus aureus*, and Group B streptococcus. The average duration of neutropenia is 7 weeks (range 2 to 17 weeks).

The treatment of alloimmune neutropenia is supportive with aggressive management of infections with antibiotics against the specific pathogen. In life-threatening infections, intravenous immunoglobulin (IVIG) or G-CSF may be considered.

Infection-Induced Neutropenia

This is the most common cause of neutropenia. Severe and clinically significant neutropenia can be associated with viral, bacterial, fungal, protozoal, and rickettsial infections. Common mechanisms include redistribution of neutrophils from the circulating to the marginating pool, antibody-mediated destruction, and direct marrow suppression. Neutropenia can be variable and rarely causes an ANC < 500/liter. Treatment is usually supportive, and G-CSF is rarely required.

Hypersplenism

Splenomegaly secondary to infections or portal hypertension can have associated neutropenia because of pooling of neutrophils in the enlarged spleen. These patients have other cytopenias. Cytopenias correct after treatment of the underlying condition or with splenectomy and rarely need specific treatment.

Drug-Induced Neutropenia

The mechanisms of drug-induced neutropenia are both immune and nonimmune. There may be a marrow effect – agranulocytosis, which might be serious. In immune-mediated neutropenia, the drug acts as a hapten to induce antibody formation, complement fixation, and neutrophil destruction or by formation of immune complexes in response to the drug that bind to neutrophils and cause neutrophil destruction within hours to days of drug exposure. Diagnosis is based on neutropenia seen during or after drug exposure. Marrow examination might be indicated to distinguish agranulocytosis from peripheral consumption.

Treatment is usually supportive if the neutropenia is mild to moderate. If the neutropenia is severe, the offending drug should be changed. G-CSF might be helpful.

Severe Neutropenia

Severe Congenital Neutropenia (SCN)

This disorder was initially described by Kostmann. The clinical, blood, and marrow features of severe neutropenia, as detailed earlier, are typically present.

This is a rare condition with a prevalence of 1 to 2 cases per 1 million people. It is characterized by accelerated apoptosis of myeloid precursors. Presentation is in the first few days or weeks of life with severe recurrent infections, including skin and soft tissue infections,

omphalitis, pneumonias, and urinary tract infections (UTIs), which are the hallmark of this disease. Most cases are apparent within the first year of life. The most common organisms are *Staphylococcus aureus*, *Escherichia coli*, and *Pseudomonas*. ANC is usually < 200/liter and often 0.

The blood count and smear show severe neutropenia, often with monocytosis and eosinophilia. Bone marrow shows maturation arrest at the promyelocyte stage. Further investigation should include genetic analysis. The illness as originally described was due to mutation in the *ELANE* (*ELAstase Neutrophil Expressed*) gene, and this remains the most common single-gene mutation identified.

In SCN, the following points are important to note:

- If an *ELANE* mutation is absent, then mutations in other genes should be sought, including *HAX1*, *WAS*, *GF1*, *AK2*, and *G6PC3*. *G6PC3* mutation is a recently described cause of CSN, although the presentation is usually later than in classic SCN and with chronic or recurrent pyogenic infection.
- Management is with G-CSF.
- This is a stem cell disorder, and the natural history includes transformation to myelodysplastic syndrome (MDS) and acute myeloid leukemia (AML). The relationship of G-CSF therapy to development of MDS/AML is uncertain, with a cumulative described incidence of 21 percent by 10 years and 36 percent by 12 years of follow-up in the SCN International Registry (SCNIR). In general, this risk is highest in individuals who require a high dose of G-CSF to achieve an adequate neutrophil count. Some individuals with a mutation in the G-CSF receptor will not respond to G-CSF.
- Allogeneic HSCT from an unaffected HLA-matched donor will correct SCN but is reserved for those who do not respond to G-CSF or those who have evidence of a clonal hematologic disorder or are at high risk of such a disorder (generally those who require more than 8 µg/kg per day of G-CSF).
- Another complication of chronic G-CSF therapy is osteoporosis, which may develop in up to 50 percent of patients. Yearly bone marrow evaluations for morphology and cytogenetics for malignant transformation and bone density study while on G-CSF are therefore recommended as part of ongoing therapy of children with SCN.

- G-CSF use may be associated with extramedullary hematopoiesis, which most often will be in the spleen with clinically apparent splenomegaly. There may then be an association with other cytopenias.

Cyclic Neutropenia

This is a rare cause of neutropenia with an estimated prevalence of 0.6 per 1 million people. It is an autosomal dominant disorder secondary to mutation in the *ELANE/ELA2* gene, and it occurs in a sporadic form. These mutations are distinct from those causing SCN. There is apoptosis of the myeloid precursors, and neutropenia is classically seen in a cyclic manner occurring every 21 ± 3 days and lasts 3 to 10 days. This is a stem cell disorder, and there may be concurrent cycling of platelets, the reticulocyte count, and monocytes.

The history in these patients is often impressive, with predictable, repeating episodes of fever, malaise, oral ulcers, and skin infections. Occasionally, more serious infections can occur, including mastoiditis, pneumonias, intraabdominal infections, and septicemia. Diagnosis is established by serial differential counts twice weekly for 6 to 8 weeks to demonstrate a cyclic pattern. Continuous G-CSF administration will abolish the symptoms of cyclic neutropenia. Typically, a lower dose is required than in SCN; median dose required is 2 μg/kg per day. Malignant transformation is *not* part of the natural history of cyclic neutropenia.

Drug-Related Agranulocytosis

In this condition, there is a reduction in granulocyte production from the bone marrow, secondary to a drug. The effect may be dose dependent and even desired, as in chemotherapy administration. It may be well described but idiosyncratic – such as with carbimazole and certain psychiatric and antonconvulsant drugs. The diagnosis is made following the finding of reduced myeloid progenitors in the marrow examination with reduced myeloid precursors. Neutropenia may be severe and may be associated with significant infection. Therapy usually involves stopping the offending drug and using G-CSF while the blood counts recover.

Shwachman-Diamond Syndrome (SDS)

This is a rare autosomal recessive disorder secondary to mutation of the *SBDS* gene on chromosome 7 (7q11). It is one of the bone marrow failure syndromes

and is discussed in Chapter 10. This disorder is characterized by apoptosis of marrow precursors (hypoplasia) that causes neutropenia. Pancreatic exocrine insufficiency, metaphyseal chondrodysplasia, and short stature are other hallmarks of this disorder. Most patients present in early infancy with growth failure, diarrhea, eczema, recurrent bacterial infections, otitis media, and moderate to severe neutropenia. Diagnosis is established by the classic clinical presentation of neutropenia, growth failure, and pancreatic insufficiency. Bone marrow evaluation is variable, and different findings are reported, including a cellular marrow with a paucity of mature granulocytes and hypocellular marrow. Most patients (>90 percent) have mutations in the *SBDS* gene. G-CSF administration is the mainstay of management of neutropenia because it ameliorates the increased frequency of infection. Generally lesser doses of G-CSF are required than in SCN. Pancreatic insufficiency is managed by enzyme replacement and dietary modification to address the fat malabsorption. This does not correct the growth failure or neutropenia, however. Infections are managed with antibiotics and supportive care. These children are at increased risk of MDS/AML, which occurs at a frequency similar to that noted in children with SCN. HSCT with reduced-intensity conditioning corrects the genetic abnormality but is only indicated in selected patients.

Myelokathexis/WHIM

This is a rare autosomal dominant disorder with mutations in the *CXCR4* gene. It is characterized by myeloid hyperplasia and destruction of precursors and granulocytes in the bone marrow. Myelokathexis is associated with warts (*W*), hypogammaglobulinemia (*H*), and infections (*I*) as part of *WHIM syndrome*. These infants present in infancy with severe neutropenia and recurrent infections. Diagnosis is established by features of neutropenia and related findings as part of WHIM syndrome. The bone marrow shows degenerating granulocytes. Mature neutrophils have cytoplasmic vacuolization, pyknotic nuclei, hypersegmentation, and nuclear strands connecting the nuclear lobes. Management relies on treatment of infection with antibiotics and supportive care. G-CSF is administered to correct the neutropenia during infectious episodes. Correction of hypogammaglobulinemia with IVIG should be considered.

Neutropenia with Other Illnesses

Neutropenia may be part of the presenting features of another underlying condition. This contrasts with the conditions already described, in which neutropenia might be the dominant finding. Neutropenia occasionally might be important in making the diagnosis in the first place, or neutropenia may be a feature of the condition that needs appropriate and separate management.

Neutropenia as part of Constitutional Hypoplastic Anemias and Other Marrow Disorders

Neutropenia is part of the presenting features and natural history of the inherited disorders of stem cell number including Fanconi anemia (FA) and dyskeratosis congenita (DKC), and it may be present in the hypoplastic stage of Diamond-Blackfan anemia (DBA) and amegakaryocytic thrombocytopenia (AMT). Neutropenia is also part of the presentation of any bone marrow disorder presenting with cytopenia, including leukemias.

Neutropenia Associated with Nutritional Deficiency

This is considered more fully in Chapter 14, and neutropenia is rarely the presenting feature but is often present.

Neutropenia Associated with Immune Defects

The overlap between immunologic and hematologic illness is considered in more detail in Chapter 23. Patients with X-linked agammaglobulinemia, hyper-IgM, IgA deficiency, cartilage-hair hyperplasia, common variable immunodeficiency, and reticular dysgenesis can have associated neutropenia. A combined immune-function defect and neutropenia can present a significant risk of infection. IVIG, G-CSF, and HSCT may be used in the management of these conditions.

Neutropenia and Barth Syndrome

Barth syndrome is an X-linked inborn error of metabolism that affects cardiolipin, a lipid that is essential in the mitochondrial respiratory chain. It is characterized by cardiomyopathy, skeletal muscle abnormalities, short stature, and variable neutropenia ranging from mild to severe. In the neonatal period, this can run a fatal course with an overwhelming bacterial infection. Bone marrow examination shows a maturational arrest. G-CSF is used in the presence of severe infection.

Neutropenia Associated with Metabolic Diseases (GSD1B)

Several metabolic disorders can have associated neutropenia. In glycogen storage disease type 1b (GSD1B), there is abnormal myeloid maturation causing neutropenia. The neutropenia may be severe. There may be significant recurrent infection and an associated colitis. G-CSF is used in the treatment of infection and corrects the neutropenia, although there may be associated splenomegaly with extramedullary hematopoiesis. Occasionally, HSCT can be used to correct this condition.

Neutrophil Function Disorders

1. There are primary inherited disorders of neutrophil function and this chapter will deal with such disorders. However, neutrophils may also be dysfunctional in other primary immune deficiencies, including antibody and complement disorders.

2. In order for neutrophils to be functional, they must be able to adhere to the endothelium and leave the circulation, migrate (chemotaxis) to inflammatory areas, ingest (phagocytose) microbes, etc., and then kill ingested infectious material within the phagosome. Inherited disorders can occur in any aspect of neutrophil function.

3. The cardinal evidence of neutrophil dysfunction is infection. There may be unusual organisms or infections in unusual sites, or infections may be more frequent or occur at unusual ages. There may be colitis in chronic granulomatous disease (CGD) and neutrophil-specific granule deficiency, and there may be delayed cord separation classically in leukocyte adhesion deficiency (LAD).

4. Diagnosis of such disorders is usually by flow cytometric techniques and molecular genetics.

5. Treatment may be supportive or via bone marrow transplantation.

Normal Neutrophil Function

Neutrophils must adhere to the endothelium as a first step in their migration from blood vessels to sites of infection. There are several steps in this migration process, and illness can occur from defects in each of the steps:

1. E-selectins expressed on endothelial cells bind to fucosylated proteins on the neutrophil. The best known of these fucosylated proteins is the sialyl-Lewis X antigen (CD15s).

2. Such binding triggers beta-integrin expression on the neutrophil, and these integrins mediate tight adhesion to endothelial cell–expressed intercellular adhesion molecule 1 (ICAM-1) which is itself upregulated in infection. There are three different integrins on the neutrophil, but they all share a common chain – CD18 – which combines with CD11b (CD11b/CD18 complex is known as MAC-1), CD11a (LFA-1), and CD11c.

3. Activated neutrophils detect small changes in the chemoattractant gradient, which causes them to move toward the site of infection.

4. Neutrophils phagocytose bacteria opsonized by antibody and complement. Following phagocytosis, neutrophil granules fuse with phagosomal membranes and release proteases, enzymes, and antibacterial proteins into the phagosomal lumen.

5. Reactive oxygen species (ROS) play an important role in killing microbial pathogens. The major source of ROS is the phagocyte respiratory burst pathway. The initial reaction in this pathway is catalyzed by an nicotinamide adenine dinucleotide phosphate (NADPH) oxidase, which is found in the phagosome membranes of neutrophils. NADPH oxidase produces superoxide free radicals by catalyzing the transfer of electrons from NADPH to molecular oxygen. Superoxide is converted to hydrogen peroxide and, in the presence of neutrophil myeloperoxidase, hypochlorous acid (HOCl), in addition to numerous other microbicidal oxidants that synergize with granule proteins to kill microbes in neutrophil phagosomes (Figure 20.1).

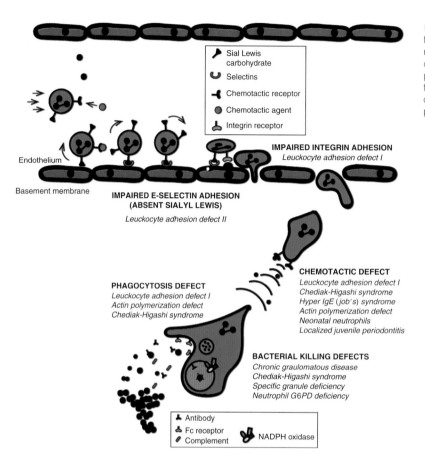

Figure 20.1 Normal neutrophil function. The components of normal neutrophil function are adhesion, chemotaxis, phagocytosis and killing of phagocytosed material. Neutrophil function disorders arise from defects or deficiencies at different points in this pathway.

Leukocyte Adhesion Defect Types I and II

Defective integrin adhesion is responsible for leukocyte adhesion defect type I (LAD I). LAD I is an autosomal recessive disorder characterized by a defect in CD18 and therefore reduced or absent expression of all the beta-integrins. It presents with omphalitis and peridontal disease. Classically, there is delayed cord separation and this history should be specifically sought where the diagnosis is suspected. Moreover, there will be neutrophilia – the patient is stimulated to make neutrophils, but they just cannot get to where they are needed (the differential diagnosis might include a chronic leukemia). Diagnosis is with flow cytometric demonstration of absent integrin expression (usually macrophage-1 [MAC-1] absence). Clinical management is with antibiotics and antifungals, but usually the child is referred for bone marrow transplant.

Note that MAC-1 has other functions in neutrophils. It is the principal neutrophil receptor for the complement fragment C3bi, which coats and opsonizes microbes, so there is also defective phagocytosis

in LAD I. MAC-1 binding is also an important costimulatory signal for the pathways that are important for adhesion, degranulation, and activation of reactive oxidant production.

In LAD II, there is a mutation in the membrane transporter for fucose with associated loss of the fucosylated glycans, including the sialyl-Lewis X (CD15s). LAD II patients have less severe infection than LAD I patients, significant developmental delay and learning difficulties, and the Bombay (hh) phenotype due to the absence of fucoslylated proteins (including the H antigen) on red blood cell (RBC) surfaces. Diagnosis is flow cytometric demonstration of reduced CD15s expression on leukocytes. Management is usually supportive.

Hyper-IgE Syndrome (HIES)

HIES is often considered a disorder of neutrophil chemotaxis, although it has more general immunologic and clinical manifestations and is diagnosed on the basis of certain clinical features and demonstration of a *DOCK8* mutation in the autosomal recessive (AR) inherited condition and a *STAT3* mutation in the autosomal dominant (AD) condition.

The clinical features of this syndrome on which the scoring system depends include

- Eczema that often occurs in the newborn period in AD HIES
- Staphyloccocal skin infections, often without inflammatory features such as erythema and pain
- Virus skin infection – molluscum, herpes virus in AR HIES
- Chronic candidal infection of the skin and nails
- Recurrent lung infection, particularly in AD HIES (There may be bacterial or fungal infection, and there may again be fewer symptoms than in patients with an intact immune system. Pneumatoceles are also particularly prevalent in AD HIES. Patients may appear much better than their x-ray suggests.)
- Involvement of both the connective and skeletal tissues in AD HIES with *STAT3* mutations (An asymmetrical facial appearance with prominent forehead and chin, deep-set eyes, broad nose, thickened facial skin, and a high arched palate are typical of this disease. These features evolve during childhood and become more established by adolescence. Patients with AD HIES exhibit hyperextensibility of the joints. They frequently suffer bone fractures from seemingly insignificant trauma, and bone density may be reduced. Scoliosis is common and typically emerges during adolescence or later in life.)
- Abnormalities affecting dentition in AD HIES with *STAT3* mutations (In contrast to AD HIES patients, those with AR HIES due to *DOCK8* deficiency do not manifest abnormalities in their dentition.)
- Increased risk for malignancies, especially lymphomas, in both AD and AR HIES patients (Other cancers described in STAT3 deficiency include leukemia and cancers of the vulva, liver, and lung. Patients with DOCK8 deficiency are susceptible to papilloma virus-induced squamous cell carcinoma and lymphomas. Autoimmune diseases also have been associated with both types of HIES, but they are most often seen in DOCK8 deficiency.)
- DOCK8-deficient patients have more symptomatic neurologic disease than those with

STAT3 deficiency. Neurologic manifestations may range from limited involvement such as facial paralysis to more severe manifestations such as hemiplegia (one side of the body paralyzed) and encephalitis. The causes of the neurologic complications are not clear, but fungal and viral agents and vasculitis may be responsible. Central nervous system involvement is responsible for a significant number of fatalities in this disorder.

Diagnosis is made on the basis of clinical features and elevated immunoglobulin E (IgE). Absence of DOCK8 protein and mutation analysis of *DOCK8* and *STAT3* are important in making the diagnosis. There are other immunologic abnormalities in AR HIES, including T-cell lymphocytopenia and IgM deficiency. Treatment is supportive or with transplant in more severe cases. Transplant is also used where there is malignant disease.

Chediak-Higashi Syndrome (CHS)

This is a rare autosomally inherited condition. CHS is a disease causing impaired bacterial killing due to failure of phagolysosome formation. There is impaired lysosome degranulation within phagosomes, so phagocytosed bacteria are not destroyed by the lysosome's enzymes. Neutrophils from patients with Chédiak-Higashi syndrome have giant granules that appear to be a coalescence of azurophilic and specific granules. The giant granules are often more prominent in bone marrow neutrophils than in peripheral blood neutrophils. Giant granules are also seen in lymphocytes and natural killer cells from patients with CHS. These patients also have partial albinism. There is recurrent infection and an accelerated phase of the illness in older children that is hemophagocytic lymphohistiocytosis (HLH)-like and triggered by Epstein-Barr virus (EBV) infection.

Diagnosis should be obvious from the blood or marrow smear in a patient with suggestive features. The affected gene is *CHS1* (also known as *LYST*). Usually patients are treated with bone marrow transplantation.

Neutrophil-Specific Granule Deficiency

Neutrophil-specific granule deficiency (SGD) is a very rare disorder characterized by the absence of specific or secondary granules in developing neutrophils. Neutrophils from SGD patients also typically have morphologically abnormal bilobed nuclei. SGD neutrophils are markedly deficient in many important microbicidal granule proteins, including lactoferrin and the defensins. The diagnosis of SGD is made if microscopic examination of neutrophils reveals the absence of specific granules. The diagnosis can be confirmed by assessing expression of granule-specific proteins (e.g. lactoferrin and gelatinase) by staining or other direct assays of the proteins. The disease is caused by inactivating mutations of the *CCAAT/ enhancer binding protein-ε* (*C/EBP-ε*) gene.

Chronic Granulomatous Disease (CGD)

CGD is the most common significant neutrophil function disorder, with an incidence of about 1 in 200,000 individuals. It arises from a genetic mutation in one of the four polypeptide subunits that are critical for NADPH oxidase function. Approximately 70 percent of CGD cases result from defects in the X-linked gene encoding the gp91^{phox} subunit of flavocytochrome b558, a membrane heterodimer that is the redox center of NADPH oxidase. An uncommon autosomal recessive form of CGD (5 percent of cases) is associated with mutations in the gene encoding p22^{phox}, which mediates translocation of two regulatory subunits of NADPH oxidase, p47^{phox} and p67^{phox}. Mutations in genes encoding p47^{phox} (20 percent) and p67^{phox} (5 percent) are affected in two other autosomal recessive subgroups of CGD.

Diagnosis is usually by flow cytometric assay of the oxidation of dihydrorhodamine 123 (DHR) by activated neutrophils. Female carriers of X-linked disease can be demonstrated to have two distinct neutrophil populations – one without and one with the ability to oxidize DHR.

Infection is the cardinal feature of CGD. It usually occurs in skin or lung and draining lymph nodes. *Staphylococcus* is the most common organism, but opportunistic pathogens including *Aspergillus*, *Nocardia*, and *Serratia* are also seen. Abscesses are seen in liver and lung and the nodes and are classically granulomatous. There is no caseation. Children with CGD also have colitis, and this can be a prominent and difficult-to-manage complication of the disease.

Management of the infection should include an attempt to identify the specific causative agent so that antimicrobial therapy can be specific. Most children receive prophylactic cotrimoxazole and prophylactic antifungal treatment. The colitis is managed somewhat similarly to Crohn disease, but immune suppression may increase the risk of infection. Bone marrow transplantation should be considered, especially before the patient has very serious complications of the disease.

Myeloperoxidase (MPO) Deficiency

MPO deficiency is the most common inherited disorder of phagocytes, with complete deficiency occurring in approximately 1 in 4,000 individuals. However, MPO deficiency is rarely associated with clinical symptoms. MPO is inherited in an autosomal recessive manner and is caused by mutations in the *MPO* gene on chromosome 17. Deficiency in MPO inhibits formation of hypochlorous acid from chloride and hydrogen peroxide. There is a remarkable lack of clinical symptoms in most individuals with MPO deficiency despite in vitro defects in the ability to kill *Candida albicans* and *Aspergillus fumigatus*.

The Child with Newly Presenting Acute Leukemia

The newly presenting child with leukemia is a common scenario for all practicing hematologists. It is imperative to get this situation right for the child and the family. Much trust is engendered for the following treatment with good medicine and good communication in these first days.

In this scenario, the approach to the newly diagnosed leukemia is separated into four related areas:

1. Are there emergency situations to be recognized and dealt with?

2. What are the routine treatments for the newly presenting child?

3. What are the routine diagnostic tests for such a child?

4. What should be said to the family, and how should consent be taken, including consent to the local clinical trial?

For the newly presenting child with acute leukemia, then, there are several separate questions to address on the first day in the hematology ward, and these are summarized in Table CS1.1:

- Are there emergency situations to be dealt with?
- What are the routine treatments for a child with acute leukemia? This will include blood products, hydration, tumor lysis prophylaxis, transfusion, etc.
- What tests are necessary to make an exact diagnosis?
- What should the family be told? What should the patient be told? This might include consent to enrollment in a national clinical trial.

Emergency Situations in Acute Leukemia Presentation

Hyperleukocytosis

This is dealt with in Clinical Scenario 2.

The Mediastinal Mass

Management of a child with a mediastinal mass is dealt with in Clinical Scenario 3. Here it should be noted that all children with newly presenting acute leukemia must have a chest x-ray as a matter of routine and certainly prior to any general anesthetic for diagnostic procedures.

Abnormal Renal Function and Tumor Lysis in Newly Presenting Leukemia

Abnormal renal function is most commonly due to tumor lysis. The biochemical hallmarks are given in Table CS1.2. There may also be contributions from direct renal infiltration with leukemia, and this might be more commonly seen in T-cell acute lymphoblastic leukemia (T-ALL) and monoblastic acute myelogenous leukemia (AML). Sepsis and drugs such as aminoglycosides might contribute to renal dysfunction and should be managed appropriately with fluid support/antibiotics and judicious use, respectively.

The clinician should do the following:

- Give rasburicase.
- Involve the renal team early.
- Avoid the use of nephrotoxic medications.
- Institute a rigorous fluid balance.
- Provide hydration as above, but make sure that the urine output is sufficient. The hydration fluid must not contain added K^+.

Table CS1.1 Questions to Address for Newly Presenting Child with Leukemia

Area of focus	Things to consider
Are there emergency situations?	1. Is there hyperleukocytosis? Remember that symptomatic hyperleukocytosis will occur at a lower white blood cell (WBC) level in acute myelogenous leukemia (AML) than in acute lymphoblastic leukemia (ALL). 2. Is there already evidence of tumor lysis syndrome? 3. Is there a mediastinal mass? 4. Is there disseminated intravascular coagulation (DIC) or is there evidence of significant bleeding? 5. Is central nervous system (CNS) function normal? 6. Is renal function normal? What are the causes of such dysfunction? What tests should be performed?
What are the routine treatments for the newly presenting child with acute leukemia?	1. What transfusion support should be given? What are the target hemoglobin and platelets? Are there any inhibitors to transfusion (e.g., where there is hyperleukocytosis)? 2. What fluids should be prescribed? 3. What infection prophylaxis should be given? 4. What tumor lysis prophylaxis should be given?
How can a diagnosis be made?	1. Can a diagnosis be made from the peripheral blood counts? This is especially important when the child is not fit for anesthesia and bone marrow aspiration. In general the diagnosis of acute leukemia is from a bone marrow examination. 2. What tests should be done on the aspirate bone marrow – morphology, immunophenotyping, cytogenetics, and molecular genetics? 3. Should a lumbar puncture be performed routinely? Should intrathecal therapy always be given? Are there risks to a lumbar puncture at diagnosis?
Keep the family and patient informed.	1. The child is in the right place 2. A certain diagnosis will be made. 3. With the diagnosis will follow treatment, which is there to cure the child. 4. There will be many conversations over the next days; too much information about what the diagnosis and treatment *might* be is likely to be more confusing than a later conversation about what the diagnosis and treatment actually are. 5. Reassure the family that as more information becomes available after diagnostic procedures, they will be told everything. No information will be kept from them. 6. Informed consent is needed to participate in a national clinical trial.

- Check the electrolytes regularly and often depending on the extent of abnormality. Remember that potassium may leak from blast cells and that measured K^+ may not be in vivo K^+ (see Table CS1.2).
- Basic clinical management of hyperkalemia includes nebulized salbutamol, insulin/glucose, etc.

- Furosemide might help the urine output in tumor lysis syndrome. Dialysis might be necessary for electrolyte disturbance unresponsive to these simpler measures or for oliguric renal failure associated with fluid overload causing clinical dysfunction (e.g. pulmonary edema). Note that if dialysis is required during these early days, then the prognosis for eventual renal function remains good.

Table CS1.2 The Biochemical Indices of Tumor Lysis Syndrome

Increased phosphate

Reduced calcium

High potassium. Note that K^+ can be high *in vitro* and not *in vivo* because it leaks from the blast cells. To distinguish them, take the sample quickly to the laboratory (or do near to bedside on a blood gas analyzer), and avoid pneumatic sample transport tubes. Do an electrocardiogram (ECG), and look for evidence of the peaked T waves of hyperkalemia.

High creatinine

Reduced urine output and edema, including pulmonary edema.

Raised uric acid. (Once rasburicase has been given, the uric acid is usually measured as below the lower limit of detection because the drug also works *in vitro*.)

Table CS1.3 Causes of Depressed CNS Function in Children with Newly Presenting Leukemia

CNS disease. Parenchymal or leptomeningeal leukemic infiltration.

CNS bleeding

Hyperviscosity with reduced tissue perfusion accompanying sluggish blood flow of hyperleukocytosis.

CNS thrombosis. For example, sagittal sinus thrombosis.

Drug-related. For example, related to intrathecal chemotherapy.

Raised intracranial pressure. May be seen in hyperleukocytosis or obstructive hydrocephalus after CNS bleed, for example.

Abnormal CNS Function

Children with depressed consciousness level during leukemia presentation require urgent CNS imaging. They may need anesthesia with intensive care in order to carry out such imaging. If such anesthesia is required, then central venous access for leukemia treatment should be secured under the same anesthetic. Platelets should be given immediately on presentation. Fluid administration must be cautious prior to imaging in case there is cerebral edema. Management of the cause of the CNS depression is critical. Lumbar puncture with intrathecal therapy can be deferred, of course, while CNS imaging takes place and while hyperleukocytosis, coagulopathy, and so on are managed and resolved.

Routine Management and Investigation of the Newly Presenting Child with Acute Leukemia

Many of these investigations will be part of a national leukemia treatment protocol. There may be central molecular analysis of ALL patients for minimal residual disease (MRD) quantification. There may be national cell banking of viable cells for future research. Blood, marrow and spinal fluid are taken.

Unless the emergency situations noted earlier apply, the new patient receives adequate hydration therapy (usually 2.5- 3 liter/m^2 per day), and K^+ is not added in this fluid. Blood and platelets are given, if necessary. Antibiotics are given to the febrile child after blood cultures have been taken. Consults with anesthesia and surgery are made because diagnostic procedures in children will be routinely performed under general anesthesia, and central venous access might need to be secured. There will be institutional practices concerning such access in new leukemia patients but a line will always be needed in AML and in 'risk' ALL, where anthracyclines are routinely employed in induction. For 'low risk' ALL, a line might be avoided if there is good peripheral venous access, for only vincristine is needed, and there will be a reduced risk of central line–associated thrombosis.

Routine investigations of blood, marrow, and cerebrospinal fluid (CSF) are done, as shown in Table CS1.4.

Keep the Family and Patient Informed

All clinicians will have their own ways of talking to families of newly presenting children. These notes are not prescriptive, but merely suggestive of one approach.

Table CS1.4 Routine Investigation of the Newly Presenting Child with Acute Leukemia

Blood:
- Morphology of blast cells
- Does the child require platelet transfusion? There will be an institutional transfusion threshold, so platelets might be given when the count is fewer than 10 or 20×10^9/liter. Platelets should be given to keep the circulating count higher when the patient has a high presenting WBC count.
- Does the child require red cell transfusion? There will be an institutional transfusion threshold. Caution should be exercised where there is hyperviscosity, as discussed earlier.
- What is the blood group and antibody screen of the patient?
- What is the renal function?

Marrow:
- What is the marrow blast cell morphology and therefore the FAB classification of the leukemia?
- What is the immunophenotype? Is there a blast cell immunophenotype that can define the population for MRD testing?
- Marrow should be sent for cytogenetic analysis.
- Marrow should be sent for molecular studies.

CSF:
- Are there cells on cytospin? What is the morphology of those cells? It is not usual to perform immunophenotyping of the cells in the CSF?
- What is the cell count of the CSF?
- Is the protein elevated in the CSF, and what is the CSF/blood glucose ratio?

Families need to be able to trust their hematologist. We think that it is helpful to have some simple objectives to give to families at the first meeting and not to become immersed in a conversation about causes of leukemia and prognosis when families are at their most anxious. We therefore state that there are three things that matter:

- That the child has reached the right place. (The road to diagnosis might have been a long one with several fruitless contacts with family doctors or pediatricians.)
- That a certain and exact diagnosis will be made. (How this diagnosis will be reached is a practical question for families to deal with. The clinician can say that there are lots of different types of leukemias and that these tests will exactly distinguish these.)
- With exact diagnosis comes exact treatment. That treatment will be of curative intent. There is reason for a family to have hope for their child.

When we go back to families after this conversation and once diagnostic procedures have yielded a diagnosis, they are usually in a totally different place. The preceding conversation can be had again and more information given as it becomes available.

Box CS1.1

Leukemia cells are analogous to weeds in a flower bed, and normal blood cells are the flowers in that flower bed. At presentation, the gardener can only see the weeds. After treatment, there are only flowers to see, but there might still be weeds within the flower bed that would grow back if treatment were stopped. The difference between cure and remission is that in cure there are no weeds left to grow back. MRD technology is a special test the gardener has developed for telling how many weeds are left behind even when he or she cannot see them.

At each conversation, then, the preceding information can be given again and consolidated.

There is the weeds and flowers analogy, which is a framework that doctors and families can go back to as treatment continues (see Box CS1.1).

Consent to treat will often include consent to a clinical trial. Clinical trials have allowed children to be cured of leukemia. Forty years ago, all such children died from the disease. Now most such children are cured. There are three components to consent to a phase III randomized, controlled leukemia treatment for a child, and these are given in Table CS1.5.

Table CS1.5 The Elements of Consent to Participation in a National or Collaborative Group Phase III Clinical Trial

1. That the child will receive evidence-based treatment	<ul><li>The family should know that this is a national trial and that wherever they are in the country the newly presenting child will be offered this treatment.</li><li>That many leukemia experts have formulated this treatment.</li><li>That the trial has been through a rigorous national ethics process in which the family and child's interests are specifically and independently represented.</li><li>That if they decline to participate, then the child will be treated with the previous best treatment, which is also an arm of the trial.</li></ul>
2. That we ask permission to record some information about the child anonymously and for the purposes of research	This is so that we can know just how well children in this country (or collaborative group) are doing with leukemia and make sure that the results are as good as elsewhere in the world
3. That participation in randomized elements of the trial where children receive previous best treatment or previous best treatment modified in a small way (The modification is made because there is evidence to suggest that it might be even better treatment.)	Randomization is difficult, especially on the first day of presentation as treatment is just beginning. The researcher must distinguish experimental treatment ('a drug that worked well in the guinea pig') from the clinical trial question that is addressed. <ul><li>The backbone of therapy is the same.</li><li>The changes in treatment are small.</li><li>Most of these increments have improved outcomes over the years.</li><li>There is ongoing statistical analysis of one arm against the other, and the trial would stop if differences were shown.</li><li>One arm of the trial is the previous best published therapy.</li></ul>

Families must know that the responsibility of the treating clinician is to their child: that the physician will always treat the child first for his or her needs regardless of the trial protocol. Such a statement is perfectly consistent with enrollment of the patient in the trial. The physician knows that trials are good in general but that sometimes patient-specific management is needed.

Hyperleukocytosis

1. Hyperleukocytosis is a raised WBC count in a newly presenting child with acute leukemia.

2. It may occur in acute myeloid leukemia (AML) or acute lymphoid leukemia (ALL). In ALL, it is more typically found in T-ALL. A high WBC count is a risk feature of newly presenting ALL.

3. Hyperleukocytosis may present as a medical emergency for the hematologist. Specifically, hyperleukocytosis is associated with:
   . Increased blood viscosity, and the sluggish circulation impairs oxygen delivery to the tissue
   . Increased risk of tumor lysis
   . Increased risk of bleeding

The clinician should

1. Make a diagnosis of leukemia type from the blood, and defer invasive procedures.

2. Limit RBC transfusion so as to prevent further viscosity rise.

3. Get the WBC count down with either treatment of the leukemia or exchange transfusion.

In hyperleukocytosis there is a markedly elevated WBC count in the peripheral blood. This is more common in T-ALL than in precursor B-ALL and might be seen in AML. There are several clinical problems associated with such a high disease burden:

1. There might be hyperviscosity of the blood because the WBCs impair blood flow. This is more likely seen in AML than in ALL because the cells are bigger and have that much more impact on blood flow. There might be confusion or decreased conscious level with increased viscosity because tissue oxygenation is impaired by sluggish blood flow.

2. There is an increased risk of tumor lysis. The laboratory features and management are described in Table CS1.2 and related text in Clinical Scenario 1. There might already be evidence of such.

3. There is an increased risk of bleeding including into the CNS. This is partly a consequence of the increased blood viscosity. Retinal hemorrhage might be visible.

The management of hyperviscosity syndrome is focused on

- *Making a diagnosis of the leukemia.* If the WBC count is high, then all important diagnostic tests that usually might be used on a marrow can be done on the blood. A diagnosis of the leukemia can be made after microscopy of the blood smear, immunophenotyping of the blood blasts, and samples can be sent for cytogenetics and molecular genetics.

- *Checking renal function.* If it is normal, then prevent tumor lysis with rasburicase and hydration.

- If renal dysfunction is present, then ask for a renal ultrasound (see later), and ask for involvement of the renal team. It is better that this team is involved early rather than late. Commence rasburicase and hydration, but meticulously record the fluid balance of the child. The hydration fluid must not contain added K^+.

- *Keeping the platelet count high because the risk of bleeding is increased.* Correct any associated significant coagulopathy.

- Transfusion of packed RBCs might increase the viscosity further and so should be performed cautiously. Hydration is continued, and RBCs are given 'little and often' to prevent rapid change in hematocrit.

It is important to get the WBC count down. This can be done in one of two ways:

- The best way to do this is to make a diagnosis and treat the leukemia. If the diagnosis is ALL, then it is easy enough to start treatment with steroids alone without securing central venous access. In AML, it might be necessary to secure venous access with a central line so that AML treatment can be started. The assistance of an experienced pediatric anesthesia team and surgical team is required, and these teams should be consulted early.

- Exchange transfusion or partial exchange transfusion will reduce the circulating WBCs. This does not treat the leukemia at all but might temporarily reduce the WBC count.

Management of the Child with a Mediastinal Mass

1. The mediastinal mass might cause compression of the airway and hypoxia and compression of venous return in superior vena cava (SVC) obstruction.

2. The most likely diagnosis is T-cell lymphoblastic non-Hodgkin lymphoma (NHL).

3. There are three questions: (a) What is the clinical condition of the child? (b) What is the diagnosis? And (c) can a diagnosis be made without surgical intervention?

4. Careful assessment is needed, including clinical examination and imaging, to decide whether the child is fit for surgical biopsy if the diagnosis cannot be reached by simple blood tests.

5. If the child is not fit for surgery, then steroids and sometimes other drugs are given to shrink the mass sufficiently to allow safe anesthesia. Tumor lysis prevention should be given. The anesthetist, surgeon and hematologist should be involved in this decision.

6. In a critically ill child who is poorly oxygenated, emergency measures including intensive care are necessary.

A mediastinal mass is a hematologic oncologic emergency. The immediate management is focused on three questions that are linked. *A child who has clinically compromised respiration is not fit for surgical intervention, including biopsy.* During such anesthetic, there may be irreversible airway obstruction as the child lies flat and voluntary muscle tone is lost. Note that the mass is likely to extend below an endotracheal tube, so it may not be possible to intubate the child during general anesthesia. *In such cases, steroid therapy may be necessary in the absence of a proven*

diagnosis to stabilize the patient and shrink the mass to a point where surgery is possible.

1. *How is the mediastinal mass affecting the immediate welfare of the patient?*
   It might be compressing the airway, causing stridor. It might be compressing the great veins, obstructing venous return from the head and upper limbs in SVC obstruction.

2. *What is the histologic diagnosis?*
   A correct diagnosis is needed for the appropriate treatment to be given. The most likely diagnosis is T-cell lymphoblastic lymphoma when there is airway compression or SVC obstruction. Other lymphomas might present in this way, including Hodgkin lymphoma and primary mediastinal B-cell lymphoma.

3. *Can the diagnosis be made without surgical intervention?*
   In T-cell lymphoblastic NHL, there may be blast cells in the blood. This is often obvious, but sometimes it is less so. If there are blasts in the blood, then all diagnostic tests including immunophenotyping, cytogenetics, and molecular testing for subsequent minimal residual disease (MRD) can be done on those blasts. Sometimes there are few blasts in the blood but other evidence on the blood film examination that there is marrow involvement (e.g. a leukoerythroblastic appearance). In this instance, a bone marrow aspirate is likely to yield diagnostic information and can be carried out under local anesthetic on the cooperative child by an experienced hematologist. Note that if the child is not fit for a general anesthetic, the child must be cooperative during these tests or the condition may be worsened by anxiety.

Assessing the Child

The patient's respiratory status can be assessed clinically. The child might be breathless at rest or cyanosed. There might be stridor. There also may be difficulty lying flat because in this position the airway compression is exaggerated compared to when the child is sitting up. The oxygen saturation should be determined or a blood gas taken. There may be associated cervical lymphadenopathy. There may be signs of SVC obstruction with conjunctival suffusion, visible venous distension, or limb edema.

The child should have the following simple tests:

- Plain posteroanterior (PA) x-ray and a CT scan of the chest. The airway should be specifically imaged. There is a poor correlation between patient symptoms and the size of the mass on imaging. The presence and degree of tracheal compression and associated carinal or bronchial compression should be specifically recorded. The likelihood of surgical complications related to the mass is increased with increased tracheal compression and the presence of additional bronchial compression.
- An echocardiograph.
- Older patients should have erect and supine peak-flow measurements as a baseline. Improvement in these measurements with steroid therapy may be useful to the anesthesia team.

Management of the Child with a Mediastinal Mass

This is a multidisciplinary management decision. The hematology, anesthetic, and surgical teams at least are involved. Sometimes the teams from pediatric intensive care and ear, nose, and throat (ENT) are involved. Several situations are possible:

1. The diagnosis can be reached from the blood tests (circulating lymphoblasts) or from a marrow aspirate performed without sedation under local anesthetic. Definitive treatment can be started, and the only surgical question is when a Hickman line can be inserted.
2. The diagnosis can only be reached from biopsy of the medistinal mass or cervical lymph nodes,

but only when the clinical picture and CT imaging demonstrate that anesthesia is safe. The anesthesia team should be experienced, and fiberoptic and rigid bronchoscopy equipment must be available. The use of a muscle relaxant may be delayed until adequate ventilation is demonstrated. Induction of anesthesia may be started in the sitting position.

3. Anesthesia is unsafe but needed for a diagnosis. In this instance, the likely diagnosis – T-cell non-Hodgkin lymphoma (T-NHL) – is treated with steroids (e.g. prednisolone 60 mg/m^2 per day or dexamethasone 10 mg/m^2 per day), and the anesthetic assessment is repeated on a daily basis. The mass will shrink with steroids alone or with other agents such as cyclophosphamide (100 to 200 mg/m^2 per day). The daily assessment by the MDT determines the right time to biopsy (when there is still tumor to biopsy) because the tumor may disappear quickly. Tumor lysis prevention will be necessary with such treatment, including hydration and rasburicase.

4. In the critically compromised child, the immediate need to oxygenate the patient is the priority. There might no be time in this exceptional case to wait for steroids, even with other chemotherapy added in, to shrink the mass. The options are threefold. They carry the risk of failure, but these risks are taken when the child is critically ill:

- The experienced ENT and anesthesia teams may ventilate one lung after intubating through the mass.
- Extracorporeal membrane oxygenation (ECMO) is used in certain centers. There is direct oxygenation of the blood in an extracorporeal ('bypass') circuit.
- There may be surgical (cardiothoracic) debunking of the mediastinal mass.

The Approach to the Neutropenic Child with Fever

Key Messages

1. The likely most common referral for the hematology/oncology junior medical staff is to see a child with cancer and neutropenia who is newly febrile.

2. Prompt administration of antibiotics is essential in such cases and indeed is lifesaving.

3. The choice of antibiotics should be according to the institution's protocol. Antibiotics are chosen to be effective in institutional blood culture isolates and are reviewed frequently.

4. The time to antibiotic administration should be audited so that the delay is minimal. The different components of the time to administration include time to complete blood count (CBC) being taken, time to CBC result, time to physician seeing the child, time to prescription of antibiotics and time to subsequent administration.

5. In prolonged fever in a child who is receiving antibiotics, certain possibilities should be sought:
   a. An organism that is resistant to first-line ('institutional') antibiotics (Note that such resistant organisms will be expected to grow in blood cultures.)
   b. Line infection (This involves repeatedly positive line blood cultures despite the use of antibiotics to which the isolated organism is sensitive.)
   c. Fungal infection (The risk of such infection is principally related to the depth and duration of neutropenia. Imaging is the principal investigation where fungal infection is suspected.)
   d. Other causes of focal infection (There should be focal [i.e. localizing] symptoms.)
   e. Virus infection (There might be focal symptoms.)

Introduction

A fever consult is common for the junior hematology medical staff and a common scenario for patients. It is suggested that the student should approach this topic in three related ways:

1. Immediate management of the neutropenic patient – doing the simple things well
2. Governance aspects of neutropenic fever management for the pediatric hematology treatment center
3. Management of the pediatric patient with persistent neutropenic fever – this will include the investigation of such fever without cause and management of specific situations, including line-related fever, fungal infection, and viral infection.

Immediate and Immediately Subsequent Management of the Neutropenic Child with Fever

This is largely about good, basic pediatric medical assessment – doing the correct blood tests and making sure that broad-spectrum intravenous antibiotics are given promptly. The former requires a timely assessment of each child with neutropenic fever – whether on the in-patient ward or in the emergency room – by a pediatric physician or experienced nurse-practitioner. The questions are simple, and this is basic pediatric medicine.

What Are the Important Physical Signs?

These include heart rate, blood pressure, respiratory rate, and oxygen saturation. Many institutions will have used such basic physiologic parameters to develop scoring systems (*early-warning scores*) that aid in identification of the potentially sick child.

What Blood Draws Should Be Taken and from Where?

Blood draws should be taken through the indwelling central venous catheter, if present. There is no need to take blood from a peripheral vein. This will only likely delay testing and inflict unnecessary discomfort on the child. If the line is not working or 'giving blood' – because it sometimes is not in the 'real world'! – then antibiotic administration should not be delayed in a neutropenic child. A chest x-ray (CXR) may be performed, especially if there are respiratory signs or hypoxia.

- Complete blood count (CBC) (This can be done from a capillary sample in advance of line access because the result may determine the need for further intervention.)
- Blood culture
- Blood to transfusion so that if transfusion is indicated on the CBC, the sample is already in the appropriate laboratory
- Renal function and liver function
- Blood clotting, including fibrinogen

What Antibiotics Should Be Given?

Empirical broad-spectrum antibiotics should be given that should be effective against organisms – gram-negative infection and *Staphylococcus aureus* infection – that can cause rapid demise. The choice of antibiotics should be determined by institutional practice (see below). The physician should not have to think! Empirical antibiotic therapy may include a penicillin, in which case the empirical choice must include an alternative for patients who are allergic to penicillin. Even if there are focal symptoms, these empirical antibiotics can be prescribed and are the safest first-line choice. Even in an afebrile but sick neutropenic child, it is appropriate to give these antibiotics so that infection is covered. Administration of first-line antibiotics is never wrong.

What Happens to the Patient Next?

Antibiotics are given after the blood cultures are drawn and after a clinical assessment has been made. Several subsequent scenarios can be seen:

- *The fever settles and the blood cultures become negative.* As long as the child remains clinically well, the antibiotics can be stopped at 48 hours, and the child can be allowed to go home.
- *The fever continues and the child is considered to be 'high risk.'* See Figure CS4.1 for risk criteria. The antibiotics should be continued and management should be that of prolonged febrile neutropenia (see below).
- *The fever continues and the blood cultures are negative at 48 hours, but the child might be considered 'low risk.'* This child might be discharged at 48 hours on oral antibiotics.
- *The blood culture is positive.* The child should receive appropriate antibiotic therapy based on the sensitivity of the organism isolated. Note that while fever continues, the antibiotics should include both empirical neutropenic antibiotics and those directed at the isolated organism. Once the fever has settled, the only antibiotics required are those directed at the organism. Repeat blood cultures should be taken to confirm that the infection has cleared.

Anticipated neutropenia <7 days
  Defined as patients NOT having
    Acute myelogenous leukemia
    Burkitt lymphoma
    Acute lymphoblastic leukemia in the induction phase of
      therapy
    Progressive or relapsed disease with bone marrow
      involvement
No significant comorbidity at presentation
  Hypotension
  Tachypnea or hypoxia (o_2 saturation less than
    94% on room air)
  New infiltrates on CXR
  Altered mental status
  Mucositis requiring intravenous narcotics
  Vomiting or abdominal pain
  Evidence of a significant focal infection defined as tunnel
    infection, perirectal abscess, or cellulitis
  Other reasons beyond febrile neutropenia requiring inpatient
    management

Figure CS4.1 Risk criteria for a neutropenic child with fever.

Governance (Institutional) Aspects of the Management of Febrile Neutropenia

Prompt administration of appropriate antibiotics to neutropenic children saves lives and permits intensive chemotherapy of acute myeloid leukemia (AML) and so on and successful stem cell transplantation. Governance of febrile neutropenia is about making the management of such a common hematogic emergency as safe as possible.

There are several components to such governance of neutropenic fever. All components should be subjected to periodic and regular audit in order to ensure that optimal practice is maintained:

1. Education of families of children who are likely to become or are already neutropenic. Fever should be defined (e.g., two temperatures above 38ºC or one above 38.5ºC). Families should be taught how to take their child's temperature and what to do if the child has a fever.

2. Febrile children who are likely or possibly neutropenic should have direct access to an area of a specialist or local hospital where they can be promptly assessed by trained staff.

3. For inpatients, the temperature of children should be checked regularly and the rules for when to call the on-call physician or nurse specialist should be clearly defined.

4. There should be adequate numbers of trained staff. The time to patient assessment should be as quick as possible, whether the child is an inpatient or in the emergency room. Such patients should not join a queue in their local emergency room.

5. There should be a febrile neutropenia protocol. This protocol must include what investigations are to be performed and what antibiotics are to be prescribed. The time from antibiotic prescription to administration should be minimal.

6. The choice of empirical antibiotic therapy should be regularly audited against the blood culture isolates from local neutropenic children. The empirical antibiotics selected must be appropriate to the local isolates so that empirical therapy is effective. This is likely to become more important as antibiotic resistance grows.

7. Unnecessary antibiotic use should be minimized to reduce the risk of resistance. This is part of the rationale to the management of 'low-risk' febrile neutropenia, as discussed earlier (see earlier and Figure CS4.1).

Persistent Neutropenic Fever

Persistent fever is fever that continues in a neutropenic child despite empirical antibiotic therapy. It may still be a bacterial infection. Such an infection is either resistant to the empirically chosen antibiotic therapy and the antibiotics should be changed based on the sensitivity of the isolate or is in the indwelling line. In the latter case, the line but not peripherally drawn blood cultures are positive. This is more common with certain species, including *Klebsiella*, *Staphylococcus aureus* and *Pseudomonas* species. Fever, rigors, and occasionally collapse with line flushing might be clinical indicators of such infection. Removal of the line may be necessary.

Other infections might be responsible for persistent neutropenic fever:

- Classically fungal infection will present as prolonged fever associated with neutropenia. Such an infection might be better diagnosed with CT scan of the chest and abdomen. Bronchial alveolar lavage (BAL) or biopsy of suspicious lesions may yield the organism. Some units might serially test blood for components of the fungal wall, such as galactomannan, to otherwise diagnose invasive fungal infection. Depending on institutional practice, all children with persistent fever might receive empirical antifungal therapy or only those with abnormal imaging.

- Virus infection might cause persistent fever. This is more common where T-cell numbers are reduced, such as following allogeneic stem cell transplant. Routine testing of blood for cytomegalovirus (CMV), adenovirus and Epstein-Barr virus (EBV0) is usual following transplantation. Testing for other viruses is directed by patient symptoms. For a child with upper respiratory symptoms, the secretions can be tested by polymerase chain reaction (PCR) for respiratory viruses including influenza virus, parainfluenza virus, and respiratory syncytial virus (RSV). For the child with gut symptoms, stool can be tested by PCR for enteric viruses and, similarly, cerbrospinal fluid (CSF) can be tested for infections associated with meningoencephalitis and urine for BK and JC viruses.

- Persistent fever may be caused by other organisms that are not bacterial, fungal, or viral. Usually there will be focal symptoms and abnormal imaging (e.g. *Pneumocystis jirovecii* infection will cause cough and hypoxia, and there will be an abnormal chest x-ray). Diagnosis will follow testing for the organism with PCR of bronchiolar lavage (BAL) fluid or respiratory secretions.

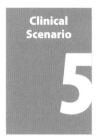
Approach to the Child with Pancytopenia

1. Pancytopenia indicates a reduction of all normal cellular elements – red blood cells (RBCs), neutrophils, and platelets – in the peripheral blood.

2. Understanding the causes of pancytopenia in children and how to distinguish these causes and make a diagnosis is a large part of understanding clinical pediatric hematology.

3. There may be bone marrow causes – production failure – or there may be systemic causes – consumption of formed cells.

4. Some of the causes of pancytopenia are inherited diseases, and some are acquired. The differential diagnosis is different for children of different ages.

5. In making a diagnosis, hematologists do it all, and this is one of the joys of everyday clinical hematology. They take the history from patients and their families. They examine patients. They look at the peripheral blood counts and blood smear. They take and examine the bone marrow aspirate and smear. Once a diagnosis is made and explained, they manage the patients.

Introduction

Pancytopenia indicates a reduction in the normal cellular elements in the blood. It must not be confused with aplastic anemia, which is a particular – and rare – cause of pancytopenia. Pancytopenia may be life threatening, and making a diagnosis as quickly as possible is important.

The hematologist will make a diagnosis from history, examination, blood count with a blood film, and bone marrow examination. All cytopenia – either single lineage or multilineage – is either because of bone marrow failure or because the cells are being used up at a greater rate than normal. This is also true of pancytopenia.

Bone Marrow Failure

The causes of bone marrow failure resulting in pancytopenia are listed in Table CS5.1. The key features in the history, examination, and blood in the presenting child that alert to this diagnosis are given for each diagnosis.

In order for the bone marrow to make blood,

- There must be physical space for bone marrow stem and progenitor cells. Infiltration with malignant cells (leukemia) will reduce this available space. (Note that solid-tumor marrow involvement rarely causes pancytopenia; it might cause anemia or there will commonly be primitive cells on the smear including nucleated RBCs and myelocytes, ie a leukoerythroblastic appearance.) A rarer infiltrative cause is un-remodeled bone in malignant infantile osteopetrosis (MIOP).

- Drugs may affect bone marrow function in either a dose-related or dose-unrelated (idiosyncratic) fashion. The most common cause of bone marrow failure in our hospitals is chemotherapy, and for most chemotherapeutic agents, there will be bone marrow failure if you give enough of the drug.

- There must be adequate nutritional elements for the massive cellular proliferation that gives rise to blood elements. This requires vitamin B_{12} and folate, and deficiency of these elements will give rise to pancytopenia.

- In aplastic anemia, there is a deficiency of hematopoietic stem cells. This may be acquired or due to an inherited bone marrow failure syndrome.

Table CS5.1 Bone Marrow Causes of Pancytopenia

Infiltration with leukemia (most common cause perhaps) (see Chapters 36 and 37)	• Examination might show evidence of infiltration elsewhere, including lymph nodes, skin, and spleen. • Blast cells may be present in the blood film. • Diagnosis is made on bone marrow aspirate.
Infiltration with trabecular bone (malignant infantile osteopetrosis) (see Chapter 25)	• There might be a family history, and the illness is more common in a consanguineous family. • There are features of extramedullary hematopoiesis on examination – including splenomegaly. • There is evidence of bone compression elsewhere beyond the marrow. There will frequently be clinical blindness or roving-eye movements (compression of the optic nerve by excess bone as the nerve passes through the optic foramen). • There may be associated developmental delay. • The blood film is leukoerythroblastic and without blast cells. This reflects disruption of the bone marrow–blood architecture and the extramedullary hemopoiesis. • The abnormal cortical bone is visible on plain x-ray of the long bones or ribs.
Nutritional deficiency (vitamin B$_{12}$ and folate) (see Chapter 14)	• There might be an appropriate dietary history. • In infants, there will be associated developmental delay (TCII deficiency or infant of a deficient mother). • There will be blood features with macrocytes, circulating megaloblastic RBC precursors, and hypersegmented neutrophils. • The bone marrow aspirate is cellular and megaloblastic with giant metamyelocytes. • The exact diagnosis will follow appropriate testing.
Drug-related causes: a. Dose related – chemotherapy b. Dose unrelated – idiosyncratic	• The cause is clearly evident on the history. • Note that whole-body radiotherapy will also cause dose-related pancytopenia, and this is also used with high-dose chemotherapy in bone-marrow transplantation. • Remember that some drugs that might cause bone marrow failure are used beyond the hematology ward (e.g. azathioprine in autoimmune or transplant medicine). • Altered renal or liver function or inherited polymorphisms affecting drug metabolism may sensitize patients to hematologic toxicity from these drugs. • A drug history should be taken in all patients admitted with pancytopenia. Chloramphenicol is the best-known idiosyncratic drug cause of bone marrow failure and pancytopenia.
Acquired aplastic anemia (see Chapter 11)	• There is no evidence of extramedullary hematopoiesis – no spleen or nodes, etc. • There is frequently macrocytosis on the full blood count (FBC) and smear. • There are no primitive cells in the blood smear. • Definitive diagnosis is made by marrow aspirate and trephine biopsy.
Inherited bone marrow failure syndrome (see Chapter 10)	• There might be a family history, and most of these disorders are autosomal recessive and therefore more common where there is consanguinity. • There might be associated features of disease such as short stature, skin abnormalities (DKC and FA), and skeletal abnormalities (FA and SDS). • There might be macrocytosis in the blood. • There are no primitive RBCs in the blood smear. • The marrow might not be as hypoplastic as in acquired aplastic anemias (there is an element of ineffective blood cell production). • There may be dysplastic features in the bone marrow aspirate. • Definitive diagnosis will test for the specific condition (e.g. chromosome fragility testing for FA). • Pearson's anemia is an important but rare cause of inherited bone marrow failure (see Chapter 12)

Table CS5.1 (cont.)

Immune causes (e.g. HLH) (see Chapter 24)	• HLH is an important cause of pancytopenia in infancy.
	• This is often a genetic illness, and this is more common where there is parental consanguinity, and there may be a family history of HLH or death in infancy.
	• The affected child is often ill, and there is usually fever (one of the diagnostic criteria).
	• There is frequently splenomegaly (another of the diagnostic criteria).
	• The blood film does not show circulating blast cells.
	• A comprehensive, systematic search for the diagnostic criteria should be initiated. The genetic causes should be sought.
	• There may be many contributors to pancytopenia: bone marrow suppression by hypercytokinemia, hemophagocytosis of formed cellular elements, and splenomegaly and hypersplenism.
	• Urgent treatment may be needed in this condition.

Table CS5.2 Consumptive Causes of Pancytopenia

Splenomegaly	• The presence of splenomegaly in itself is neither an adequate cause of pancytopenia nor does it necessarily imply that bone marrow function is normal.
	• Some bone marrow causes of pancytopenia are usually associated with hypersplenism (see Table CS5.1, 'Infiltration with leukemia'). MIOP and HLH are associated with splenomegaly.
	• A cause for splenomegaly must be ascertained. It might be thalassemia or another hematologic condition, a metabolic illness, chronic liver disease with portal hypertension, or an immunologic cause.
	• The pancytopenia of hypersplensim is rarely severe, and splenectomy is rarely indicated.
Immune causes (see Chapter 23)	• Many of the inherited primary immune deficiencies (PIDs) are associated with either humoral or cellular autoimmune cytopenia, which might be pancytopenia.
	• HLH is a PID that is also associated with pancytopenia (see 'bone marrow causes' above).
	• Systemic lupus erythematosus (SLE) may cause pancytopenia.
	• Rheumatologic illness may be associated with pancytopenia that is mutifactorial and includes macrophage activation syndrome (MAS), which is part of the spectrum of HLH.
Infection (see Chapter 16)	• Severe infection may cause pancytopenia.
	• Activation of the coagulation cascade and disseminated intravascular coagulation (DIC) may contribute to the thrombocytopenia of severe infection.
	• The hematologist must distinguish bone marrow failure and pancytopenia as a cause of infection, from pancytopenia as a consequence of infection.

Peripheral Consumption

The peripheral causes of pancytopenia are usually obvious and are given in Table CS5.2. Important comments for each cause are given as well.

Does This Child Have Lymphoma?

1. This is a common referral to pediatric hematologists from primary care clinicians and from pediatric colleagues in other specialties.

2. The clinical hallmark of lymphoma is usually pathologic enlargement of an involved lymph node or group of lymph nodes, and the diagnosis of lymphoma is usually made following histologic examination of an involved lymph node.

3. There are certain clinical features that suggest that lymph node involvement is due to malignant disease. These include site, size, and feel during examination. Imaging with ultrasound or computed tomographic (CT) scan may help to distinguish benign from malignant disease involving the node, but histology is definitive.

4. Presentation of lymphoma with pyrexia of unknown origin (PUO) is unusual but not unknown. There are other more common causes of PUO in pediatric medicine.

5. The bone marrow aspirate and biopsy are more useful in the staging of lymphoma than in the diagnosis of lymphoma. A staging marrow in lymphoma is used to assess how disseminated the lymphoma is and whether there is bone marrow involvement. This is frequently misunderstood by referring clinicians.

6. Lymphoma in pediatric medicine might be non-Hodgkin lymphoma (NHL) or Hodgkin lymphoma (HL). NHL is more often high-grade disease than in adult disease, where indolent low-grade disease is commonly found. This type of disease is less commonly seen in children.

7. NHL and HL each may be associated with primary immunodeficiency and the immunodeficiency associated with HIV infection.

8. Prompt diagnosis of high-grade NHL is important so that definitive therapy can begin.

9. NHL – especially those of a T-cell immunophenotype – may present as an HLH like illness. This is particularly true for anaplastic NHL.

Which Nodes to Worry About?

Hematologists are often involved in the diagnosis of lymphoma. They are referred children either because of the presence of palpable lymph nodes or because the child has other features that are reported to also occur in children with lymphoma such as PUO.

- Palpable lymph nodes in children are common and more likely to be due to causes other than lymphoma.
- Table CS6.1 gives some of the indications to think that a lymph node might be enlarged due to lymphoma. Where this is the case, lymph node biopsy is indicated.
- Few cases of lymphoma present with PUO alone. The bone marrow test is a poor diagnostic test for lymphoma in such a case.

Types of Lymphoma in Children

In general, lymphoma is diagnosed by histologic examination of an involved lymph node. The specific features of the diagnosis are beyond the scope of this book, but the elements of diagnosis are similar to

Table CS6.1 When to Consider Malignancy as a Cause of Lymph Node Enlargement

Where is the enlarged lymph node?	• Neck nodes are common in children. • Nodes that are high in the neck are often benign. • Supraclavicular lymphadenopathy is *always* pathologic (not necessarily malignant). • Inguinal nodes are normally palpable in all children.
How big is the node?	• Big nodes are more likely to be involved with lymphoma than smaller nodes. • Is there enlargement of other lymph node groups or is the spleen enlarged?
What has happened to the node?	• Has the node changed in size and is becoming rapidly bigger? • Has it been there for a long time? Sometimes bigger and sometimes smaller – this is less likely to be due to malignant disease.
Are there other clinical features?	• Is the child unwell? • Has the child lost weight? • Is there fever? • Is there an obvious cause for regional lymph node enlargement other than malignancy? • Is there a significant past medical history suggesting a primary diagnosis that might predispose to malignancy?
Are there laboratory test abnormalities that might indicate malignant lymphoma?	• Lymphoma might be associated with the anemia of chronic illness. • HL is associated sometimes with a blood eosinophilia. • The lactate dehydrogenase (LDH) level is often elevated in lymphoma. A normal LDH does not exclude lymphoma, and a raised LDH is not specific for lymphoma. • Is imaging abnormal? The chest x-ray might show mediastinal lymphadenopathy, which can be better delineated on CT scan. Similarly, abdominal lymphadenopathy can be seen on ultrasound, and the lymph node architechture (normal, reactive, or malignant) also can be assessed by ultrasound.

those employed in leukemia diagnosis (see Chapters 35 and 36), namely, clinical features, morphology, immunophenotyping, cytogenetics, and molecular genetics.

Lymphoma is either HL or NHL. As for leukemia, there is a World Health Organization (WHO) classification. Each is subdivided further, and the important classifications are given below. The student is referred to more comprehensive lymphoma texts for further discussion. Here the key features of HL and several more common NHL types are discussed.

Hodgkin Lymphoma

• Diagnosis rest mainly on the finding of Reed-Sternberg (RS) cells.

• May be related to EBV infection
• May be seen in primary immune deficiency (PID)
• May be associated with HIV infection

WHO classifies HL into two main types – the four classic subtypes and the nodular lymphocyte predominant. The former have more RS cells than the latter. The classic four subtypes are

• Nodular sclerosing (this is the most common)
• Mixed cellularity
• Lymphocyte predominant
• Lymphocyte depleted

The staging of HL is according to the Ann Arbor System and is part of the risk assessment of a child presenting with HL. More advanced disease receives more treatment. Part of the risk assessment includes

Table CS6.2 Staging of HL

I	Single lymph node group
II	Multiple lymph node groups on the same side of the diaphragm
III	Multiple lymph node groups on both sides of the diaphragm
IV	Multiple extranodal sites or lymph nodes and extranodal disease
X	Bulk > 10 cm
E	Extranodal extension or single, isolated site of extranodal disease
A/B	B symptoms: weight loss > 10 percent, fever, drenching night sweats

response to treatment, including by positron emission tomographic (PET) scanning – comparing pretreatment scans and scans after a defined treatment.

Lymphoblastic NHL

- Immunophenotype of the malignant cells is the same as in acute lymphoid leukemia (ALL). This is a lymphomatous (solid lump) presentation of the same disease.
- T-cell lymphoblastic NHL commonly presents as a mediastinal (thymic) mass. This is stage III disease. Management of a child with a large mediastinal mass is dealt with separately in Clinical Scenario 3.
- Precursor B NHL is rarer than T-cell lymphoblastic NHL but likely has an inferior prognosis to ALL and is treated usually more intensively (even though the child may be young and with a low white blood cell count).

The St. Jude System divides NHL in children into four stages. In general, stage I and II lymphomas are considered limited-stage disease and are treated the same way. Stage III and IV lymphomas are usually thought of as advanced-stage disease and are also treated alike.

- Stage I: The lymphoma is in only one place, either as a single tumor not in lymph nodes or in lymph nodes in one part of the body (neck, groin, underarm, etc.). The lymphoma is not in the chest or abdomen (belly).
- Stage II: The lymphoma is not in the chest, and one of the following applies:

  - The lymphoma is a single tumor and is also in nearby lymph nodes in only one part of the body (neck, groin, underarm, etc.).
  - The lymphoma is more than one tumor and/or in more than one set of lymph nodes, all of which are either above or below the diaphragm. For example, this might mean nodes in the underarm and neck area are affected but not the combination of underarm and groin nodes.
  - The lymphoma started in the digestive tract (usually at the end of the small intestine) and can be removed by surgery. It might or might not have reached nearby lymph nodes.

- Stage III: One of the following applies:

  - The lymphoma started in the chest (usually in the thymus or lymph nodes in the center of the chest or the lining of the lung). T-cell lymphoblastic NHL is therefore stage III disease.
  - The lymphoma started in the abdomen and has spread too widely within the abdomen to be completely removed by surgery.
  - The lymphoma is located next to the spine (and may be elsewhere as well).
  - The lymphoma is more than one tumor or in more than one set of lymph nodes that are both above and below the diaphragm. For example, the lymphoma is in both underarm and groin lymph nodes.

- Stage IV: The lymphoma is in the central nervous system (brain or spinal cord) or the bone marrow when it is first found. (If more than 25 percent of the bone marrow is cancer cells, called *blasts*, the cancer is classified as acute lymphoblastic leukemia [ALL] instead of lymphoma.)

Burkitt Non-Hodgkin Lymphoma

- Burkitt lymphoma has particular clinical, morphologic (histopathologic and cytologic), immunophenotypic, cytogenetic, and molecular features.
- Burkitt lymphoma is often extranodal, although nodal and leukemic presentations are not uncommon.

- Morphology of infiltrate is 'starry sky' rather than diffuse. The blackness of the sky is the B-cell infiltrate, and the stars in the sky are the macrophages scattered within the infiltrate.
- Aspirate morphology (cytology) is of L3 lymphoblasts (see Chapter 35).
- The immunophenotype is a mature B cell, distinguishing this disease from precursor B- or precursor T-cell lymphoblastic disease. The pan-B-cell markers CD79a, CD20, and CD22 are positive, and there is surface expression of immunoglobulin that is class restricted – expressing either kappa or lambda – because this is a clonal disease.
- Cytogenetics involves translocation of the *c-myc* oncogene on 8q24 – t(8;14) is the most common, followed by t(2;8) and t(8;22).
- All B-cell lymphomas will have molecular evidence of immunoglobulin gene rearrangement. Where there is doubt about the diagnosis of malignancy, clonal Ig gene rearrangement or light-chain restriction is useful in confirming the infiltrate to be malignant.
- Therapy is by intensive chemotherapy, and conventional ALL-type treatment will fail. Outcome with short intensive therapy, though, is good. Monoclonal antibodies directed at B-cell antigens (rituximab, anti-CD20) may improve response rates when added to chemotherapy schedules.

Diffuse High-Grade B-Cell Lymphoma

- Diffuse large B-cell lymphoma is most commonly nodal disease, and the most common sites of involvement are the mediastinum and abdomen.
- This is the most common lymphoma associated with primary and acquired immunodeficiency states.
- The histology is diffuse replacement of nodal architecture rather than the 'starry sky' of Burkitt lymphoma.
- t(14;18) with involvement of the anti-apoptosis *BCL2* gene is seen in about 30 percent of patients, and the remainder often have complex cytogenetics.
- Treatment is by intensive chemotherapy regimens as for Burkitt lymphoma. Response and cure rates are also good. Sometimes the disease may be primarily mediastinal, and the response rates in this presentation are somewhat inferior.

Anaplastic Large-Cell Lymphoma

- This is a rare T-cell tumor.
- It might present as an HLH illness. HLH in an older child should raise the consideration of this tumor as the primary cause.
- The tumor cells are T cells and express CD30 classically. There is a typical cytogenetic alteration associated with this tumor, which is the t(2;5) translocation and involves the nucleophosmin gene on chromosome 5.
- The product of this fusion gene may be identified by immunohistochemistry using antiserum to ALK protein. Probes are available to identify the translocation by fluorescent *in situ* hybridization (FISH) and are useful diagnostically.

Diamond-Blackfan Anemia, Transient Erythroblastopenia, or Other Cause of Red Cell Aplasia in Children

1. Red blood cell (RBC) aplasia with a reticulocytopenic anemia may be a constitutional disease, Diamond-Blackfan anemia (DBA), or it may be an acquired illness.

2. The most common acquired cause is transient erythroblastopenia of childhood (TEC), but it may be more rarely a feature of autoimmune disease or malignant disease in children.

3. Most, but not all, children with DBA are diagnosed in infancy, and many will have other evidence of disease, including somatic abnormality and short stature. Some will have a family history. There are certain laboratory and genetic tests that help to make the diagnosis of DBA.

4. Parvovirus may cause RBC aplasia in the setting of immune deficiency so that viremia is prolonged or; when there is shortened RBC survival and hence the RBC production failure is more pronounced, for example in chronic hemolytic anemia.

DBA or TEC?

Both these disorders will present in early life with a reticulocytopenic anemia. TEC is a self-limiting disorder of uncertain etiology. The following are the features that help to distinguish these two conditions for the clinician:

- *Age at presentation.* Most DBA is diagnosed in infancy, and most TEC is diagnosed after infancy. However, DBA is heterogeneous, and some will present later in life, even in adult life. Some TEC will present in infancy. Age at presentation does not absolutely distinguish the two.

- DBA is a multisystem disorder. There are associated somatic abnormalities. These are discussed in Chapter 10. Growth may be affected.
- There might be a family history in DBA. No such history is found in TEC. The same genetic lesion may cause very different hematologic disease in different family members.
- The anemia is usually macrocytic in DBA, although this is not the case in TEC until the recovery phase, when there is a reticulocytosis. Other cytopenias are seen more commonly in TEC than in DBA. The RBC *adenosine deaminase* (ADA) level is elevated in DBA. The hemoglobin F level is elevated in DBA but also may be increased during the recovery phase of TEC.
- There are particular genetic mutations associated with DBA that are described in Chapter 10 and should be looked for in a new potential case of DBA.
- TEC patients will recover. DBA patients will not usually recover without treatment. Both patients may require transfusion therapy as supportive care. Usually only one or two transfusions are necessary in TEC patients because there is recovery thereafter. Thus in unclear cases, it is desirable to withhold steroids until failure of recovery is demonstrated, or a positive diagnosis of DBA is made (ADA or genetic). Given that long term steroid therapy is required to maintain remission in DBA, erroneously commencing steroids in a case of TEC is a poor outcome for a child who would have recovered spontaneously.

Other Causes of RBC Aplasia

- Parvovirus B19 is specifically cytopathic to RBC presursors. In anyone with this virus, there is therefore a RBC aplasia associated with infection. Once the virus is cleared by the immune system,

141

the RBC aplasia stops. There are two circumstances where this RBC aplasia is apparent:

- Where the immune system does not clear the virus: such as infection during fetal life; or where there is immune deficiency associated with HIV infection or primary immune deficiency (PID); and during acute lymphoid leukemia (ALL) treatment following hematopoietic stem cell transplantation (HSCT). In such cases, the chronic infection is associated with chronic RBC aplasia.
- Where there is shortened RBC survival so that the drop in Hb during transient infection is more noticeable than when RBC survival is normal. This is the aplastic crisis of chronic hemolytic anemia of hereditary spherocytosis or other inherited hemolytic anemias.

- The parvovirus serology (IgM and IgG) should be positive in acute infection when the immune

system is competent, or parvoviremia should be detectable by PCR when the immune system is incompetent.

- RBC aplasia may be the first or most prominent manifestation of a bone marrow failure syndrome (see Chapter 10). The hematologist must look for other cytopenias and for associated clinical features.
- Refractory anemia is part of the myelodysplastic syndromes and forms part of the differential diagnosis of such a presentation (see Chapter 38).
- Pure RBC aplasia may be associated with malignancy. Thymoma is the classic such malignancy, but this is rare in childhood.
- Pure RBC aplasia may be autoimmune and associated with childhood systemic lupus erythematosus (SLE), and there may be anti-EPO antibodies in renal patients given erythropoietin (EPO) for the anemia of renal disease.

8 Approach to Evaluation for a Bleeding Disorder in a Child with Suspected Inflicted or Nonaccidental Injury

Key Messages

1. The hematologist is involved in two ways in the child with inflicted injury as the cause of bleeding. Children may be referred for evaluation of bruising or bleeding and the haematologist might be the first to suspect inflicted injury as the cause. They may also be consulted as experts where inflicted injury is thought by others to be the cause of bruising or other bleeding but hematological causes must be excluded, including as part of a legal process.

2. The importance of thorough history and examination and a knowledge of safeguarding procedures are imperative where the hematologist is the first to suspect non-accidental injury (NAI) in a child referred for evaluation of bruising and bleeding.

3. There are no proven evidence-based strategies to dictate the hematologic evaluation of children with bleeding and/or bruising in the context of suspicion of NAI, and hence practice varies.

4. No single panel or test rules out a bleeding disorder.

5. Virtually any bleeding disorder can present with bruising/bleeding symptoms that can mimic NAI

6. NAI can occur in a child with an inherited bleeding disorder.

7. Fractures or other injuries are never caused by bleeding disorders.

Introduction

A child with bruising may be referred to the hematologist who is the first to suspect in clinic that inflicted injury or NAI is the cause of the bleeding. The hematologist in such a setting must act as a pediatrician first and a hematologist second. The child's welfare and safety depend on appropriate diagnosis being made and the appropriate procedures being followed. Excluding a bleeding disorder is insufficient.

The history must be consistent with the bruising observed. If excessive bruising is observed for the history given then either the child has a bleeding disorder or that history is incorrect. Other injuries must also be sought. Fractures are never caused by a bleeding disorder and a skeletal survey might be considered routine in such a setting. If shaking is suspected, then an ophthalmological examination for retinal hemorrhage is mandated.

All hospitals will have safeguarding procedures and policies where NAI is suspected and the practicing hematologist must know these procedures and follow them.

More commonly the hematologist is involved in NAI as an 'expert'. They exclude hematologic causes of the observed injuries. They are consulted by pediatric colleagues or social workers, as part of the routine investigation of children with NAI. It is important that this is done thoroughly and completely in such cases since the hematologic investigations might become part of legal proceedings. Moreover, on occasions a child being managed for/ or suspected of NAI, will in fact have a bleeding disorder, and a rapid positive diagnosis stops a family being accused of something they did not do. Finally, some children with bleeding disorders suffer from NAI, and only an experienced hematologist can reasonably separate the usual symptoms of a bleeding disorder from those caused by non accidental mechanisms of injury.

Table CS8.1 Guidance for Categorizing Bruising from Suspected NAI According to Location

Location suspicious for NAI	Location less suspicious for NAI
Face (excluding forehead)	Forehead
Ears	Exposed arms
Neck	Shins/ankles
Upper arms/legs or thighs	Spinous process of back
Trunk	Hips
Hand/wrist	
Genitalia	
Buttocks	

Approach to Evaluating for a Bleeding Disorder in a Child with Bruising Suspicious for NAI

Virtually any bleeding disorder can present with bruising. The number and distribution of bruises can help to discriminate bruising secondary to bleeding disorders or NAI (Table CS8.1). Bruising in an infant who is nonmobile (i.e. not yet crawling or walking) is suspicious for NAI. Pattern of bruising as slap or object marks is not likely to be secondary to a bleeding disorder. There are other medical disorders that can cause bruising, such as connective tissue disorders, and testing should be directed toward identify those as a cause of bruising if the history or physical examination warrants.

The following factors may not exclude the need for a bleeding disorder evaluation, since it is imperative to be thorough and complete, but are clear evidence in their own right of NAI:

- Bruising secondary to witnessed trauma
- Locations or patterns of bruising that are suspicious for NAI (e.g. slap/object or bite marks)

Which Tests for Evaluation of a Bleeding Disorder Should Be Carried Out for Bruising?

Bleeding disorders that can cause bruising include platelet disorders, coagulation factor deficiencies, von Willebrand disease, and, rarely, fibrinogen disorders or disorders of the fibrinolytic pathway. A suggested testing panel to distinguish bruising secondary to bleeding disorders versus NAI is as follows:

- Full blood examination and blood film
- Prothrombin and activated partial thromboplastin time (PT/APTT)
- Von Willebrand panel

- Platelet function screening test (PFA-100)
- Thrombin time (TT)
- Fibrinogen assay/concentration
- FXIII assay

If these tests are all normal, then it is reasonable to state that there is no evidence of a bleeding disorder (in the absence of clear family history that would direct the clinician to further investigation, or a clinical examination that would suggest a collagen-, vascular or other connective tissue disorder). Significant malnutrition may result in bruising or bleeding for example due to scurvy (vitamin c deficiency), without abnormalities in the tests listed.

The PFA-100 level is frequently abnormal due to either sample problems or recent nonsteroidal anti-inflammatory drug (NSAID) intake. PFA-100 is only a screening test and does not prove a platelet function disorder, and if the test is repeatedly and consistently abnormal, then formal platelet function testing is required to confirm any diagnosis. As explained in Chapter 3, no child should be labeled with a diagnosis of a bleeding disorder on the basis of one abnormal test, and careful attention to preanalytic variables is required.

Bleeding Disorder Evaluation in Children Presenting with Intracranial Bleeding

There are associated injuries that strongly direct the clinician to suspect NAI. Retinal bleeding suggests shaking. An examination by a pediatric ophthalmology team is mandatory. A skull fracture implies trauma as the cause of intracranial bleeding.

The coagulation testing for a bleeding disorder in isolated intracranial bleeding should be the same as those in bruising and bleeding as above. Being thorough and complete is important. The investigations and the results that they yield may be subject to cross examination in a legal process. Appropriate age-associated reference ranges become critical in this circumstance (see Chapter 4). The absence of a specific investigation, however rare a cause of bleeding it might be, might lead to an inappropriate conclusion that the child has been injured. Hence the history, family history and examination are paramount to determine if any additional testing is required.

False-positive tests can occur in certain circumstances, especially if sample integrity is compromised. Presence of a lupus anticoagulant or transient factor inhibitor can prolong PT or APTT. Children with ICH can have a transient coagulopathy, and testing

in those circumstances should be repeated after the acute presentation. However, false negative tests can also occur in the setting of sample activation for example. Just as we would never diagnose a bleeding disorder based on one test, if our clinical suspicion is high, then we should not exclude a bleeding disorder based on one test either.

Apart from testing for coagulopathies, careful review of diagnostic imaging to exclude vascular anomalies such as arteriovenous (AV) malformations is important. Children with a bleeding disorder can also suffer NAI. The investigation and diagnosis of such injury can be difficult and require a collaborative approach including a pediatric hematologist and a forensic or safeguarding pediatrician.

The Neonate with Catheter-Related Thrombosis

1. Up to 90 percent of thromboses in neonates are central catheter related.

2. Umbilical venous catheters and percutaneously inserted central catheters (PICCs) are the most common catheters placed in neonates.

3. Birth weight < 1,000 g, infections, and longer catheter days are risk factors.

4. Common sites of catheter-related thrombi are the hepatic vein, the inferior vena cava (IVC), and the right atrium.

5. Most thrombi are detected on imaging as an incidental finding.

6. Complications include infection and occlusion; death is rare.

7. Testing for prothrombotic risk factors for catheter-related thrombosis in the presence of other clinical risk factors is currently not recommended.

8. Management of a neonate with catheter-related thrombosis is primarily based on the clinical context and risk factors present.

Clinical Presentations of Catheter-Related Thrombosis

1. Distal extremity swelling with central catheters in limbs, occasionally bilateral leg swelling with IVC thrombosis

2. Head, neck, or arm edema, superior vena cava (SVC) syndrome, arrhythmias with upper extremity central catheters

3. Thrombocytopenia

4. Catheter malfunction

5. Sepsis

In the neonatal intensive care unit (NICU), about 15 percent of babies and 50 percent of all preterm infants with birth weight (BW) < 1,000 g have an umbilical or peripherally inserted central venous catheter (CVC) placement. CVC placement is one of the most important risk factors for thrombosis and is likely due to large catheter size relative to the vessel diameter and vessel wall damage. Duration of catheterization, BW < 1,000 g, and the number of catheterizations have been investigated as possible risk factors but not conclusively proven. It remains unclear why some infants with indwelling catheters develop thrombotic events, whereas others do not. Prophylactic heparin infusion for umbilical arterial catheters and peripherally inserted arterial catheters prolong the duration of catheter use by preventing occlusion but do not prevent thrombosis.

Management

The treatment of CVC-related thrombosis remains ill defined, but most clinicians would treat a symptomatic thrombus, occlusive thrombus, or one that is propagating. The clinical dilemma of choosing to treat or to watch conservatively arises if the thrombus is detected as an incidental finding on imaging for another clinical indication and the neonate is asymptomatic. In these circumstances, it is reasonable to consider clinically watching the neonate for evolving symptoms and using radiologic surveillance to watch for thrombus propagation. This approach is also appropriate if there is a contraindication to antithrombotic therapy because of clinical instability or bleeding. Spontaneous resolution may occur in some nonocclusive thromboses or in umbilical venous catheter (UVC)–related thromboses.

If the neonate has occlusive thrombosis and is symptomatic, antithrombotic therapy with unfractionated heparin (UFH) or low-molecular-weight heparin (LMWH) is indicated. Antithrombotic therapy

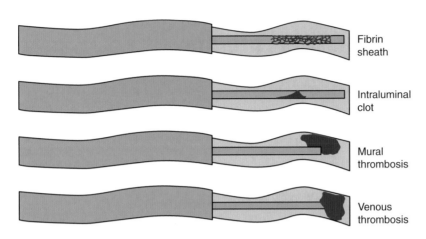

Figure CS9.1 Types of occlusion with CVCs.

is also indicated for central venous catheter (CVC)–related intracardiac thrombi with high-risk features, which include a right atrial thrombus that is >2 cm in diameter, pedunculated, mobile, or snake shaped. The risks and benefits of each therapeutic option should be individualized based on the location of the thrombus, its extent, and the risk of bleeding. There is a relative contraindication to antithrombotic therapy in a neonate who is less than 34 weeks of gestational age and less than 2 weeks postnatal age because of the risk of intracranial hemorrhage (ICH). The decision to treat any neonate with thrombosis should be made by a multidisciplinary team that includes input from the neonatologist and the hematology team. This rationale stems from the fact that there are no randomized, controlled clinical trials that have clearly established the efficacy and safety of existing treatment regimens. LMWH is the treatment of choice for confirmed CVC thromboses that are progressive and in the absence of renal dysfunction. It is important to remember that preterm neonates require increased doses of LMWH to achieve a therapeutic target anti-Xa level compared with term infants.

Thrombolytic therapy is recommended in neonates in whom there is a concern for limb or organ compromise. Tissue plasminogen activator (tPA) is a more preferable option among other thrombolytic agents such as urokinase and streptokinase because of fibrin specificity, poor antigenicity, and short half-life. The treatment of these neonates should preferentially target the use of tPA through the venous catheter with prior administration of fresh frozen plasma (FFP) or plasminogen concentrates for effective thrombolysis. Therapy with tPA needs close clinical monitoring of hematologic parameters and should be guided by radiologic imaging. Recommendations for prevention of catheter-related thrombosis involve the use of catheters only in acute need and prompt removal if malpositioned and when they are no longer needed (see Figure CS9.1).

Neonatal Renal Vein Thrombosis

1. Renal vein thrombosis is the most common spontaneous thrombosis in the neonatal period.

2. Prematurity is frequently associated with renal vein thrombosis.

3. Males are more commonly affected than females.

4. RVT is frequently detected shortly after birth. Some are detected in the antenatal period.

5. At least one of cardinal sign of flank mass, hematuria, or thrombocytopenia is the presenting feature at diagnosis.

6. Adrenal hemorrhage is not uncommon.

7. Thrombophilia testing is not advocated in most circumstances.

8. Decreased renal perfusion and parenchymal hemorrhage are predictors of poor clinical outcome.

The presence of one of the cardinal signs of renal vein thrombosis (RVT) – flank mass, hematuria, or thrombocytopenia – prompts the clinician to get a diagnostic evaluation. Other signs and symptoms that raise suspicion for RVT are the presence of hypertension or oliguria/anuria. Ultrasound Doppler is the most convenient modality for diagnosis of RVT, easily obtained at the bedside and most commonly used. The acute management is a multidisciplinary approach by neonatologists, hematologists, nephrologists, and radiologists. The nephrologist guides fluid and electrolyte management and assesses the need for dialysis and correction of acid–base imbalance. The hematologist is consulted for anticoagulation management.

Acute Management of a Neonate with Renal Vein Thrombosis

The choice of anticoagulation versus conservative management is influenced by the extent of RVT on ultrasound, presence of renal failure, and whether the neonate is premature. The important features for the hematologist to note on ultrasound are

- Is the RVT unilateral or bilateral?
- Is the inferior vena cava involved?
- Is adrenal hemorrhage present?

For unilateral kidney involvement without renal impairment, either supportive therapy or antithrombotic therapies with unfractionated heparin (UFH) or low-molecular-weight heparin (LMWH) are options. Follow-up imaging is important if the decision is made to continue supportive therapy only to assess for further thrombotic extension. If there is unilateral kidney involvement with inferior vena cava (IVC) extension or renal impairment, antithrombotic therapy should be initiated with UFH or LMWH if there are no contra-indications. For bilateral kidney involvement with or without IVC involvement, initial therapy with tissue plasminogen activator followed by UFH or LMWH should be considered. Other things to note are that preterm infants require higher doses of UFH or LMWH for therapeutic anti-Xa effect. Because both agents are eliminated by the kidneys, they need dose reduction and/or more careful monitoring for drug accumulation/bleeding symptoms in the presence of renal insufficiency. It is prudent to get a head ultrasound prior to starting antithrombotic therapy, especially in preterm infants. If the decision is made to start antithrombotic therapy, it is usually continued for 3 months.

About 10 percent of RVT is complicated by the presence of adrenal hemorrhage. Left-sided RVT is more commonly associated with this because the left adrenal vein drains directly into the left renal vein. Presence of adrenal hemorrhage is not considered a contraindication to antithrombotic therapy unless there is an increase noted on follow-up imaging.

Is Thrombophilia Testing Indicated?

Because RVT is most often a spontaneous thrombotic phenomenon, some clinicians suggest thrombophilia testing. Protein C, protein S, and antithrombin levels have to be interpreted in the context of gestational age and day of life reference ranges. Thrombophilic risk factors are found in more than half the neonates with RVT. Similar to other thrombotic disorders, RVT is thought to be multifactorial, and other risk factors in addition to thrombophilia are considered to contribute to its pathogenesis. The results of thrombophilia testing do not change immediate management and are of limited value in predicting recurrence or longer term outcome. Hence the value of thrombophilia testing remains controversial. The risk of recurrence of thrombosis in these infants is unknown.

What Are the Predictors of RVT Outcome?

Whether anticoagulation affects short- or long-term outcome of renal function or risk of thrombosis recurrence is unknonw. Findings on Doppler that are predictors of poor renal function include

- Decreased perfusion of the affected kidney
- Presence of hemorrhagic infarction on the initial Doppler ultrasound
- Enlarged kidneys in the acute phase
- Requirement for dialysis

What Is the Long-Term Renal Outcome?

Regardless of treatment choice in the acute phase, there is a risk of renal scarring and renal atrophy. Hypertension can develop in up to 25 percent of infants with either unilateral or bilateral renal involvement. A small percentage of infants with bilateral renal involvement can develop end-stage renal disease.

Inherited Thrombocytopenia

1. Inherited thrombocytopenia may present at any age.

2. Bleeding manifestations can be variable and not dependent on platelet number.

3. Mutation in one gene can cause different phenotypic expression (e.g. *MYH-9 mutations*)

4. Some inherited thrombocytopenias are associated with characteristic identifying features or are part of a constellation of findings specific to a syndrome.

5. Inherited thrombocytopenia may be associated with platelet dysfunction.

6. Despite identification of novel mutations, more than half of children with inherited thrombocytopenia have a disorder that has not been characterized.

7. Management will include the prevention of bleeding episodes. The use of platelet transfusion will be associated with a risk of sensitization (to HLA proteins or to other platelet proteins), and such sensitization will reduce the efficacy of future platelet transfusions. The decision to use platelets should be carefully considered, and the future risks weighed against the risk posed by the current bleeding episode.

Introduction

Inherited thrombocytopenias are a heterogeneous group of disorders that are variable in their clinical presentation, bleeding manifestations, course, and prognosis. Identification of novel mutations has helped in diagnosing the cause of thrombocytopenia in those cases where the cause of the thrombocytopenia was thought to be 'unknown or idiopathic' or erroneously diagnosed as immune thrombocytopenia (ITP). A correct diagnosis has helped to anticipate clinical course, prognosis, and even management of these disorders and avoided unnecessary therapy with steroids or intravenous immunoglobulin (IVIG) and in some cases even splenectomy. Additionally, better understanding of inherited thrombocytopenia has helped unravel unique aspects of megakaryopoiesis and the biology of platelet production.

Classification of Inherited Thrombocytopenia

Inherited thrombocytopenia can be classified based on platelet size, mode of inheritance, or mechanism of platelet production. Because platelet size can be readily assessed based on mean platelet volume (MPV) on the complete blood count (CBC) and evaluation on a peripheral blood smear, classifying inherited thrombocytopenia based on platelet size is the most practical way to classify these disorders (Table 21.1).

Generic Pointers in the History or Physical Examination in Inherited Thrombocytopenia

Inherited thrombocytopenia can present at any age. Therefore, for a child presenting to the pediatric hematologist for evaluation of thrombocytopenia, for the initial visit, every effort should be made to gather previous counts. History should include inquiries regarding the presence of bleeding symptoms and any history of bleeding during hemostatic challenges. For example, for boys it is important to ask about any history of bleeding after circumcision and so on.

Table 21.1 Inherited Thrombocytopenia Based on Platelet Size

Disorder	Inheritance	Gene	Associated defects
Large platelet size			
MYH-9-related disorders, including May-Hegglin anomaly, Sebastian, Fletchner, Epstein syndromes	Autosomal dominant (AD)	*MYH9*	Leukocyte inclusions, renal failure, deafness
Bernard-Soulier syndrome	AD/ autosomal recessive (AR)	*GP1BA*, *GP1BB*	–
Type 2B von Willebrand disease (vWD)	AD	*GPIBA*	–
Paris-Trousseau and Jacobsen syndromes	AD	*FLI1*	Facial dysmorphology, heart defects, feeding difficulties, developmental delay
Gray platelet syndrome	AD, AR	*NBEAL2*	–
GATA1-related X-linked cytopenia	X-linked	*GATA1*	Hemolytic anemia
FLNA-related disorders	X-linked	*FLNA*	–
TUBB1-related disorders	AD	*TUBB1*	–
Upshaw-Shulman syndrome	AR	*ADAMTS13*	Microangiopathic hemolytic anemia (MAHA)
Single-gene disorders	AD	*ITGB3*, *ITGA2B*	–
Sitosterolemia	AR	*ABCG5*, *ABCG8*	Stomatocytosis, hemolytic anemia
Normal platelet size			
Congenital amegakaryocytic thrombocytopenia (CAMT)	AR	*MPL*	Bone marrow aplasia
Thrombocytopenia absent radius (TAR)	–	*RBM8A*	Absent radii
Familial platelet disorder	AD	*CBFA2*	Myelodysplastic syndrome (MDS), acute myeloid leukemia (AML)
ANKRD26-related thrombocytopenia	AD	*ANKRD26*	Predisposition to leukemia
Congenital thrombocytopenia radioulnar synostosis (CTRUS)	AD	*HOXA11*	Radioulnar synostosis, bone marrow aplasia
CYCS-related disorder	AD	*CYCS*	–
Small platelets			
Wiskott-Aldrich syndrome (WAS)	X-linked	*WASP*	Eczema, immunodeficiency
X-linked disorders	X-linked	*WASP*	Mild or no immunodeficiency

Suspicion of inherited thrombocytopenia on history will be raised if:

- Platelet counts are always low or when an acquired etiology cannot be clearly elicited.

- Other family members have thrombocytopenia. However, absence of family history does not rule inherited thrombocytopenia out.

- A family history of AML or MDS in close relatives (e.g. familial platelet disorder with *RUNX1* or *ANKRD26*).
- A personal history of eczema and repeated infections (WAS).
- An associated finding of developmental delay, feeding difficulties, and cardiac defects (Jacobsen).

Some inherited thrombocytopenias present as syndromic disorders. A careful physical examination is essential to diagnose those groups of disorders.

- There is incomplete arm supination (CTRUS).
- Skeletal survey shows absence of radii (TAR).
- There are facial dysmorphic features (Jacobsen).
- There is presence of deafness or cataracts (*MYH-9*).

Evaluation of Peripheral Blood Smear in Inherited Thrombocytopenia

The peripheral blood smear provides vital pieces of information that can aid diagnosis. First, one must establish that the thrombocytopenia is truly present and is not secondary to platelet clumping (due to ethylenediaminetetraacetic acid [EDTA] effect, and the platelet count is normal when the CBC is repeated and the anticoagulant is changed to citrate). Evaluation of platelet size helps to classify most inherited thrombocytopenias, but a mean platelet volume (MPV) determination may not always be reliable or accurate. Because large platelets are also a feature of immune-mediated thrombocytopenia, it is important to look for abnormalities in other cell lines (e.g. Döhle body inclusions in leukocytes in *MYH-9*-related disorders). Some of the features to note on the peripheral blood smear are as follows:

- Giant platelets (platelet larger than a RBC) in *MYH-9*-related disorders
- Hemolytic anemia/stomatocytes in *GATA1*-related disorder/sitosterolemia
- Microangiopathic hemolytic anemia (congenital deficiency of ADAMSTS13)

Electron microscopy is not readily available from most centers but can be useful in establishing the diagnosis of some rare forms of inherited thrombocytopenia (e.g. absence of alpha granules in gray platelet syndrome). Rarely, platelets with both a decreased number and large alpha granules are seen in Jacobsen syndrome.

Inherited Thrombocytopenia Associated with Disorders of Platelet Structure, Function, and Accelerated Destruction

Inherited thrombocytopenia resulting from bone marrow failure is discussed in detail in Chapter. The following is a brief review of the more common forms of inherited thrombocytopenia associated with disorders of platelet structure, function, and accelerated destruction.

MYH-9-Related Disorders

These are the most common forms of inherited thrombocytopenia. They exemplify the concept that mutations in one gene (in this case, *MYH-9*) can cause different phenotypic expression. May-Hegglin, Sebastian, Epstein and Fechtner syndromes were previously recognized as separate disorders but are all now collectively referred to as the *MYH-9 group of disorders*, since they are caused by mutations in this gene. Mutations can be throughout the gene, but it is now known that when a mutation affects the head domain of myosin-9, patients have lower platelet counts and more bleeding symptoms, and they develop renal disease and deafness later in life, whereas a mutation in the tail region results in higher platelet counts and no associated defects. The diagnosis is suspected in a patient with giant platelets and characteristic Döhle body inclusions in leukocytes that are cytoplasmic aggregates of abnormal myosin protein. Thrombocytopenia is usually not severe, although the FBC may be lower than the actual platelet count because the analyzer may not count the large platelets of this disorder as platelets (rather counting them as red cells). The major morbidity is from the associated renal disease and deafness. Testing for *MYH9* mutation is commercially available at many centers. Active management is required for surgeries and in women with menorrhagia, but overall treatment is supportive.

Bernard-Soulier Syndrome

Bernard Soulier was one of the earliest forms of thrombocytopenia to be described. The disorder has both monoallelic (AD) and biallelic (AR) forms and is caused by mutation in the GP1b/IX/V complex that is involved in adhesion of platelets to exposed subendothelium during vessel wall trauma. In the monoallelic form, bleeding can be severe, and patients often have large platelets and giant forms on the peripheral blood smear. The less-common biallellic form is associated with a mild reduction in the platelet count with absence of any clinically relevant bleeding symptoms. Diagnosis is established by platelet aggregation studies showing absent or markedly reduced response to the agonist ristocetin or by glycoprotein expression (flow cytometry) study that shows reduced GP1b/IX/V glycoprotein expression. Management is primarily controlling the bleeding symptoms, often with platelet transfusions. These patients can develop platelet refractoriness secondary to development of alloantibodies to GP1b similar to that seen in patients with Glanzmann thrombasthenia. Severely affected patients – especially those in whom there is such sensitization – might be offered bone marrow transplantation.

Wiskott-Aldrich Syndrome (WAS) and X-Linked Thrombocytopenia

This syndrome is caused by mutation in the *WASP* gene located on the X chromosome. X-linked thrombocytopenia is a milder form of WAS and should not be confused with thrombocytopenia associated with *GATA1* mutation, which is also frequently referred to as *X-linked thrombocytopenia*. WAS should be suspected in a patient with eczema, immune dysregulation, and recurrent infections. The platelets are moderate to severely reduced in number and are characteristically small in size. Gene sequencing is available as well as flow cytometry for expression of the WAS protein. Patients either succumb to infections, development of lymphoproliferative disease/lymphoma, or severe bleeding and are usually cured with hematopoietic stem cell transplantation (HSCT). Once diagnosis is established and while awaiting HSCT, these children need antibacterial prophylaxis and monthly IVIG. X-linked thrombocytopenia is usually managed with supportive care.

General Principles of Management of Inherited Thrombocytopenia

Prevention and treatment of bleeding episodes is the cornerstone of management of inherited thrombocytopenia.

- Families and general practitioners should be educated regarding avoidance of drugs that impair platelet function (e.g. nonsteroidal anti-inflammatory drugs [NSAIDs]).
- Good dental hygiene should be encouraged to avoid dental procedures and extractions that can result in bleeding.
- It is prudent for patients with severe thrombocytopenia to avoid activities or sports with a high risk of trauma such as contact sports.
- Menorrhagia in young women can be managed with hormonal therapy or by the use of antifibrinolytic agents.
- Platelet transfusions are generally reserved for severe bleeding complications, and their use should be restricted to selected clinical scenarios. Where platelet transfusion is elective, HLA-selected platelets might be chosen to reduce HLA sensitization. Note that alloantibodies against mutated platelet proteins (e.g. glycoprotein Ib in Bernard-Soulier disease) can follow platelet transfusion because this native protein is different. This is a feared complication of platelet transfusion. The decision to use platelet transfusion therapy in these conditions should be made by an experienced pediatric hematologist.

Role of Thrombopoietic Agents in the Management of Inherited Thrombocytopenia

There is limited experience with these agents in pediatrics. Their use has been reported in case series or case reports in patients with severe thrombocytopenia associated with *MYH-9*-related disorders. They have an advantage over platelet transfusions, especially in the group of inherited thrombocytopenic disorders that have a high risk of developing alloimmunization or platelet refractoriness. They are unlikely to be of benefit where there is associated platelet dysfunction or in patients with CAMT, in whom there is lack of thrombopoietin receptor (TPO receptor) expression. Their use should be carefully weighed against potential long-term side effects of therapy.

Chapter 22

Acquired Thrombocytopenia and Immune Thrombocytopenic Purpura (ITP)

1. Nonspecific thrombocytopenia is common in sick children, especially neonates.

2. Spurious thrombocytopenia is very common in pediatrics owing to activation of the sample during collection. Careful inspection of the blood film and repeat testing are often required.

3. There are a number of specific illnesses associated with thrombocytopenia, including hypersplenism, disseminated intravascular coagulation (DIC), and some vascular malformations.

4. Many drugs commonly used in tertiary pediatric hospitals can cause iatrogenic thrombocytopenia.

5. The most common acquired cause of isolated thrombocytopenia in well children is immune thrombocytopenic purpura (ITP).

6. ITP in children follows a different clinical course than ITP in adults.

7. Many children with acute ITP do not require treatment.

Introduction

Thrombocytopenia is arguably the most common abnormality identified on full blood examination (FBE) in children. Spurious thrombocytopenia is especially common, usually due to difficult collection, failure to properly mix the tube (leading to failure of EDTA to effectively stop coagulation), or occasionally EDTA-driven platelet clumping. Careful inspection of the sample and careful blood film examination usually can identify such problems, but occasionally, only a fresh sample from a clean venipuncture (including taking the sample into a citrate tube) can ensure that the child does indeed have a normal numbers of platelets.

Many children with viral or bacterial infections or other inflammatory disorders will develop transient and nonspecific thrombocytopenia that usually resolves as the underlying illness resolves, although there may be a lag time. Often the thrombocytopenia in these children is not so low as to require any intervention but may do so, especially if surgery is required for other indications. Of course, equal numbers of children will develop thrombocytosis in the setting of infection or inflammation, and this almost never requires treatment.

Splenomegaly and hypersplenism can be associated with significant thrombocytopenia, and if liver disease is also present, then the bleeding risk can be increased by the coexistence of coagulopathy. There is no direct correlation between spleen size and platelet count. Spontaneous bleeding is uncommon, but a requirement for platelet transfusion support around diagnostic or surgical procedures is very common. Platelet transfusions often do not lead to sustained, measurable increments in platelet counts but, despite this, are often clinically hemostatic.

Renal vein thrombosis is classically suggested by the clinical findings of flank mass, hematuria, and thrombocytopenia. The thrombocytopenia is usually not a barrier to anticoagulation therapy if it is required and usually resolves over subsequent weeks.

Disseminated intravascular coagulation (DIC) is a global coagulopathy secondary to vascular endothelial dysfunction that, with increasing severity, can also demonstrate thrombocytopenia. Platelet transfusions may be required, although they are usually avoided, if possible. DIC is covered in detail in Chapter 29.

Finally, some vascular anomalies are associated with thrombocytopenia presumably secondary to local destruction within the lesion. This may be an isolated abnormality or associated with microangiopathic hemolytic anemia. Primary therapy of the vascular lesion is the most appropriate therapy. Platelet support is occasionally required at the time of curative therapy, although the platelet count usually recovers quickly once the lesion is removed.

Immune Thrombocytopenic Purpura (ITP)

ITP is a common childhood disease with a reported incidence of 6.4 per 100,000 children. This is almost double the frequency of ITP in adults. The peak age group involved is approximately 2 to 10 years of age, but infants younger than 1 year of age and teenagers are important age groups that require specific consideration.

The classic clinical presentation of ITP is petechial rash with or without mucosal bleeding in an otherwise well child who may give a history of a recent viral illness. The diagnosis is a diagnosis of exclusion, and there are no definitive tests to prove ITP.

1. In the setting of a classic clinical presentation as described previously, the absence of systemic symptoms, including weight loss or fever, suggests the diagnosis.
2. Physical examination should reveal no evidence of lymphadenopathy or hepatosplenomegaly.
3. The FBC and, in particular, the blood film examination should demonstrate an isolated, significant thrombocytopenia with normal RBCs and normal white blood cells (WBCs). Most commonly, the platelet count is less than $20 \times 10^9/$liter. Viral reactive lymphocytes are an acceptable abnormality and still consistent with the diagnosis of ITP.

Should any of these three parameters fail to be met (i.e. history suggestive of systemic symptoms, presence of lymphadenopathy or splenomegaly, or other abnormalities on the FBC and blood film), further investigation, including bone marrow examination, is indicated to exclude other potential diagnoses such as leukemia.

If the history, examination, and blood findings are consistent, then a presumptive diagnosis of ITP is reasonable, and no further investigations are required. In children, ITP is usually an isolated disorder. However, it may be secondary to systemic lupus erythematosus (SLE), anti-phospholipid antibody syndrome, as part of Evans syndrome, common variable immune deficiency (CVID), following transplantation, or secondary to some drugs.

If the amount of bleeding is out of keeping with the observed platelet count (i.e. more bleeding than expected for the platelet count), then checking the coagulation profile and autoimmune workup may be relevant. This is particularly relevant where the platelet count is not particularly low. Occasionally, ITP that presents as part of an anti-phospholipid antibody disease associated with the presence of a prothrombin inhibitor that drives considerable bleeding (due to prothrombin consumption, discussed in Chapter 29) . If the child has had recurrent infections in the past, then consideration of CVID is worthwhile. Unlike adults, there is no association between ITP and *Helicobacter pylori* infection, and tests for *H. pylori* are not useful. ITP as a vaccine side effect will be discussed later.

The majority (~80 percent) of ITP in childhood is of short duration. Table 22.1 shows the current accepted terminology when describing ITP. Chronic ITP occurs in approximately 20 percent of cases, and the identifiable risk factors include age of greater than 10 years at presentation and platelet count of greater than $20 \times 10^9/$liter at presentation. Even so, approximately half of all chronic cases will resolve spontaneously in the subsequent 4 years.

The risk of major spontaneous bleeding in acute ITP is small, and studies to date report overall rates of intracerebral hemorrhage (ICH) of approximately 1 in 1000, although it would seem that for many children the real risk of major bleeding in the absence of trauma is far less. Whether major bleeding events can be prevented with treatment is controversial. However, this is usually the primary indication for treatment (i.e. to further reduce the risk of ICH).

Identification of higher-risk individuals is important. The presence of bleeding or of mucous membrane lesions is thought to be associated with increased risk. Thus, in the physical assessment of any child with ITP, careful examination of the mucous membranes and the fundi is required. The distinction between dry purpura (skin lesions only) and wet purpura (mucous membrane and/or retinal lesions) is important because it often is the deciding factor as to whether treatment is required. The presence of mucosal bleeding, rapidly increasing skin petechiae, or increased menstrual bleeding also should be determined. These features may warrant treatment in their own right or be a marker of increased risk of ICH. Current international recommendations support the idea that children with skin

Table 22.1 Current Terminology for Describing ITP

Term	Definition
Newly presenting ITP	<3 months since diagnosis
Persistent ITP	3 to 12 months since diagnosis
Chronic ITP	>12 months since diagnosis
Severe ITP	Bleeding requiring treatment irrespective of platelet count
Primary ITP	Idiopathic ITP, with no secondary cause
Secondary ITP	Immune thrombocytopenia secondary to drug or other disease
Steroid-dependent ITP	Need for steroids >2 months to maintain platelets >30×10^9/liter or to avoid bleeding
Platelet threshold	100×10^9/liter
Complete response	Platelets >100×10^9/liter or doubling platelets from baseline plus no bleeding
Partial response	Platelets >30×10^9/liter or less than doubling from baseline plus no bleeding
No response	Platelets <30×10^9/liter or less than doubling from baseline or ongoing bleeding
Refractory ITP	No response or loss of response after splenectomy

manifestations only (purpura or petechiae) should be managed with observation alone.

For children who are managed with observation (or those who receive treatment), lifestyle modification to reduce the risk of significant head injury is justified. Avoidance of contact sports where head injury is likely is advised. Helmets must be compulsory when riding bikes, rollerblades, skateboards, horses, and so on and perhaps increased caution shown. Most children and families can tolerate abstinence from some activities in the short term. If the ITP becomes persistent or chronic, then more negotiation may be required. Normal school activities are usually no problem. Aspirin, ibuprofen and other NSAIDS should be avoided.

Occasionally, it is appropriate to offer treatment to children who might not otherwise require therapy based on parental anxiety, social or geographic concerns that likely impair the child's ability to be monitored appropriately, or to enable the child to maintain reasonable lifestyle choices. For example, school, camps, or family holidays often can be made much more palatable for all concerned with a short course of treatment to temporarily stabilize the child's platelet count.

The treatment options for acute ITP are usually either prednisolone or IVIG. There are a number of dosing schedules for prednisolone and no real data to support one regime over another. Many patients respond to a minimal dose of steroid, so 1 mg/kg per day seems a reasonable starting dose. Responses occur in about 70 percent of patients and usually within 3 to 4 days, although some children may not respond for up to 2 weeks. Irrespective of response, it is reasonable to start weaning the prednisolone in 2 to 4 weeks, and even in the absence of response or with loss of response in terms of platelet counts, many children have minimal symptoms and can be safely managed without ongoing treatment. The persistence or recurrence of mucous membrane lesions limits the ability to wean therapy. There is no need for bone marrow examination prior to steroid therapy if the previously stated diagnostic framework has been followed. IVIG is usually given as a single dose at 0.8 or 1 g/kg, and again, approximately 70 percent of children will respond, usually within 48 to 72 hours. Both prednisolone and IVIG usually provide only short-term remission. Intravenous methylprednisolone or dexamethasone can be used as alternatives, but there seems no advantage in terms of response rate, speed of response, or duration of response. Each therapy can be used again, but there can be tachyphylaxis with IVIG. Obviously, minimizing the long-term exposure to steroids is important. Anti-D immunoglobulin is also used as acute therapy in some countries.

For the small percentage of children with persistent or chronic ITP, other therapeutic options may be required. No therapy is required if skin petechiae are the only manifestation. Potential treatments include danazol, azothiaprine, cyclosporine, dapsone, cyclophosphamide, vinblastine, and vincristine, but none has been shown to be particularly effective.

For chronic ITP, the two most common treatment options to date have been splenectomy and rituximab administration. Splenectomy has an approximately 70 percent response rate, which occurs almost immediately postoperatively and usually gives long-term remission. Splenectomy obviously requires surgery, and appropriate presplenectomy vaccination as well as postsplenectomy antibiotics are required. Rituximab is usually given in a dose of 375 mg/m^2 per week for 4 weeks. The response rate is reported to be approximately 80 percent, and there is a secondary immune suppression that is mostly well tolerated. Rituximab response often lasts for 12 months, and repeated courses can be given. Most clinicians defer the use of splenectomy or rituximab until at least 12 months after diagnosis unless there is persistent and problematic bleeding before then.

Eltrombopag and romiplostim are thrombopoietin analogues, and early data suggest that they may revolutionize the treatment of acute and chronic ITP in patients in whom bleeding is a problem. Further data are expected in the coming months and in particular specific pediatric data. While it is unlikely that these drugs will replace prednisolone or IVIG as first-line therapy for acute ITP, they may well replace all other options in chronic or poorly responsive ITP.

Ancillary treatments that may be useful in teenage girls with problematic menstruation include tranexamic acid taken at 0.5 to 1 g qid for the first 5 days of each period. Alternatively, hormonal treatment to render a time of amenorrhea may be appropriate and preferred. Menstrual bleeding or indeed epistaxis can be severe in ITP, and transfusion support may be required. Female patients who are approaching menarche or their first period since diagnosis should be warned of the potential need for hospitalization for transfusion if menstrual bleeding is really heavy. Any child with epistaxis should be given clear instructions on the first aid management of epistaxis and a plan for when to seek medical intervention.

ITP in children younger than 6 to 12 months of age is not common but definitely reported. This age group probably should have further investigation including bone marrow examination to exclude the potential for congenital thrombocytopenia unless there have been clearly documented normal platelet counts prior to presentation. Children of this age often have more problematic bleeding and require treatment, although they rarely develop chronic ITP and usually remit spontaneously.

ITP is a recognized complication of the measles-mumps-rubella (MMR) vaccine, occurring in approximately 1 to 4 per 100,000 children after vaccination. However, primary measles infection induces ITP in 6 to 1,200 per 100, 000 children, so even from an ITP perspective, vaccination is much safer than the native disease. Current recommendations are that even in the presence of a past history of ITP, the first MMR vaccine should be given as per national schedule. In children with either non-vaccine- or vaccine-related ITP who have already received their first dose of MMR vaccine, vaccine titers can be checked. If the child displays full immunity (90 to 95 percent of children), no further MMR vaccine should be given. If the child does not have adequate immunity, then the child should be reimmunized with MMR vaccine at the recommended age.

Approximately 20 percent of children with ITP report significant fatigue as a symptom of their ITP. The pathogenesis of the fatigue is unclear and is not related to the presence of other autoimmune disease. Many children report difficulty in completing the school day or the need for excessive naps after school. The fatigue seems to improve as the platelet count recovers, but whether treatment should be offered purely to resolve this symptom is unknown. Adjusting the child's lifestyle to help manage this tiredness seems appropriate.

Immune Deficiency

1. Primary immune deficiency (PID) is a rapidly changing field with the description of new conditions, as the genetic lesions known to cause PID increase with the application of newer technologies such as genome sequencing to this field.

2. PID is of relevance to the practicing pediatric hematologist for several reasons:

    a. There is an overlap in clinical presentation. Many pediatricians will refer the child with recurrent, unexpected, or refractory infection to a hematologist, and hematologists must be able to recognize PID and know the relevant principles of investigation.

    b. Hematologic cytopenia is a common manifestation of PID and is due to several mechanisms, including antibody or cellular autoimmunity, immune dysregulation such as occurs in hemophagocytic lymphohistiocytosis (HLH) and bone marrow failure associated with PID itself, PID-associated malignancy, or that seen as a side effect of the drugs used to treat viral or other PID-associated infections.

    c. PID is associated with malignancy, including lymphproliferative disease.

    d. Certain PIDs including HLH and disorders of neutrophil function will often be looked after by hematologists, and the treatment of these and other PIDs includes treatment with hematopoietic stem cell transplantation (HSCT).

3. Acquired immune deficiency is common as a consequence of treatment for hematologic illness. Children infected with HIV also may have hematologic cytopenias and may also present to the hematology team.

Primary Immune Deficiency (PID)

This is a rapidly changing and complex field. There are at least 200 genetically defined PIDs, and this number continues to grow rapidly. This is partly as a consequence of greater collaboration between centers, leading to the recognition of new, rare syndromes and partly as a consequence of advances in molecular genetics, including whole-genome sequencing, enabling rapid identification of disease-causing mutations.

There are eight groups of PIDs – listed in Table 23.1 – and these will be dealt with separately. Within each group there are many different conditions, and the key differences between the conditions will be considered. Some of these PIDs are considered in greater detail elsewhere in this book (Chapters 10 [inherited BMF syndromes], 19 [neutropenia], 20 [neutrophil function], and 24 [HLH]).

Combined T- and B-Cell Immunodeficiencies

If there is lymphopenia on the complete blood count (CBC) or there is T-cell lymphocytopenia using immunophenotyping, then this is severe combined immune deficiency (SCID). This is further classified according to the cells that are actually present in the blood: by enumerating B-cells numbers and natural killer (NK) cell numbers

1. T–B–NK– SCID is most commonly caused by adenosine deaminase (ADA) deficiency, which is autosomally recessively (AR) inherited. There is a buildup of deoxyadenosine, which is toxic to

Table 23.1 Groups of PIDs

PID group	Examples of conditions of relevance to the hematologist

Combined T- and B-cell deficiencies	1. Severe combined immunodeficiency (SCID)
	
	   a. T-B-NK1 (ADA deficiency)
	   b. T-B-NK+ (*RAG1/RAG2* mutation)
	   c. T-B+NK– (common gamma chain) X-linked
	   d. T-B+NK+ (DiGeorge)
	
	2. Omen syndrome (hypomorphic mutation of *RAG1/RAG2*)
	3. Hyper-IgM syndromes (CD40 and CD40L deficiency)
	4. Purine nucleoside phosphorylase (PNP) deficiency

Well-defined syndromes associated with immune deficiency	1. Cartilage hair hypoplasia 2. Hyper-IgE syndromes (DOCK8 and STAT3 deficiency); see Chapter 20 3. Dyskeratosis congenita 4. Wiskott-Aldrich syndrome (WAS) (X-linked mutation) 5. Disorders of DNA repair, including Bloom syndrome (*BLM* mutation), ataxia telangiectasia (mutation in *ATM*), and Nijmegen breakage syndrome (mutation in *NBS1*)
Predominantly antibody deficiency	X-linked agammaglobulinemia (mutation in *BTK*)

Disorders of immune regulation	1. Hemophagocytic syndromes, including familial hemophagocytic lymphohistiocytosis
	2. Lymphoproliferative conditions
	
	   a. XLP1 (X-linked mutation in *SH2DIA* and SAP deficiency)
	   b. XLP1 (X-linked mutation in *XIAP*)
	
	3. Syndromes with autoimmunity
	
	   a. Autoimmune lymphoproliferative syndrome (ALPS) (mutation in *FAS* or FAS ligand)
	   b. Immune dysregulation, polyendocrinopathy, enteritis, X-linked – immune dysregulation, polyendocrinopathy, enteropathy, X-linked (IPEX) (mutation in *FOXP3*)

Disorders of neutrophil number or function	1. Severe congenital neutropenias (see Chapter 19) 2. Monocytopenia and mycobacterial infection (MonoMAC) syndrome (AR mutation in *GATA2*) 3. Chronic granulomatous disease 4. Leukocyte adhesion deficiency-1 (LAD1) and LAD2
Defects in innate immunity	1. Isolated congenital asplenia (mutation in *NKX2-5*) 2. Chronic mucocutaneous candidiasis (heterogeneous disorder genetically with several different mutations in different genes responsible for the condition)
Autoinflammatory disorders	1. Early-onset inflammatory bowel disease (AR mutation in *IL10* or *IL10R*) 2. Familial Mediterranean fever (*MEFV* mutation)
Complement deficiencies	1. C1q deficiency (mutation in *C1QA*, *-B*, or *-C*) 2. CD59 deficiency (*MIRL* mutation)

proliferating lymphocytes. It can be treated by pharmacologic administration of enzyme as well by hematopoietic stem cell transplantation (HSCT). There are also lentivirus gene therapy trials for ADA

SCID in which autologous HSCs are corrected by lentivirus-delivered copies of the normal gene.

2. T–B–NK+ SCID might be associated with microcephaly and facial dysmorphism in DNA

ligase IV deficiency or not in defects in the recombination activating genes *RAG1/2*. The protein products of these genes play an important role in recombination of the T-cell receptor and immunoglobulin genes that generate diversity in the T- and B-cell repertoire. They are inherited in an AR manner. Treatment is with HSCT.

3. T–B+NK– is classically caused by mutations in the common gamma chain, also known as the IL2 receptor subunit gamma, which is common to the receptor complexes for many different interleukin receptors. Inheritance is X-linked.

4. T–B+NK+ is caused by a number of different mutations, some of which are associated with other clinically evident manifestations, including complete DiGeorge syndrome. In this syndrome caused most commonly by 22q11.2 deletions, there is lymphoproliferation, autoimmunity, impaired T-cell proliferation, and dysmorphic features. The deletion can be demonstrated by fluorescence *in situ* hybridization (FISH).

If T-cell lymphocytopenia or whole-blood lymphopenia is not present, then the diagnosis is combined immune deficiency (CID). A number of mutations and conditions are described. Some are important to the hematologist.

1. Hypomorphic mutations in *RAG1/2* cause Omenn syndrome, in which there is chronic inflammation of the skin, including erythroderma, that is graft-versus-host disease (GvHD) and is mediated by autologous autoreactive T cells. Other clinical features include diarrhea, hepatosplenogaly, and alopecia. There is eosinophilia, elevated IgE, depressed IgM, and no circulating B cells.

2. In hyper-IgM syndrome there is most commonly deficiency of a protein – CD40 ligand – that binds with CD40 expressed on B cells and instructs them to switch their class of immunoglobulin from IgM to either IgG or IgA. CD40 ligand inheritance is X-linked, but the illness is indistinguishable from CD40 deficiency, which is inherited in an AR manner. Affected patients suffer from infection. *Pneumocystis jiroveci* pneumonia and chronic diarrhea with *Cryptosporidium* are classic infections in this syndrome, and there are often neutropenia and other autoimmune cytopenias, including thrombocytopenia and hemolytic anemia.

Diagnosis is from genetic investigation of a child suspected on the basis of clinical features and a high IgM level.

3. Purine nucleoside phophorylase (PNP) is a key enzyme in the purine salvage pathway that catalyses the conversion of inosine and guanosine to hypoxanthine. PNP deficiency leads to a buildup of deoxyguanosine triphoshphate, which is toxic to developing T cells.

Well-Defined Syndromes Associated with Immune Deficiency

Such syndromes include

1. *Cartilage hair hypoplasia* . There is short-limbed dwarfism arising from metaphyseal dysostosis, sparse hair, and predisposition to malignancy, but there is also bone marrow failure and autoimmunity. Inheritance is AR, and the gene defect is *RMRP*.

2. *The hyper-IgE syndromes.* These are either AR (DOCK8 deficiency) or X-linked (STAT3 deficiency) and are dealt with in Chapter 20.

3. *Dyskeratosis congenita and DiGeorge syndrome.* DiGeorge syndrome is discussed above and Dyskeratosis Congenita was discussed in Chapter 10.

4. *Wiskott-Aldrich syndrome (WAS).* This is an X-linked inheritance of a mutation in the *WAS* gene. Reduced or absent WAS protein expression can be identified using flow cytometry. There is thrombocytopenia, and the platelets are small and dysfunctional. Milder mutations might cause thrombocytopenia alone (X-linked thrombocytopenia), and indeed, mutations in *WAS* also may be responsible for X-linked neutropenia. Other clinical features include splenomegaly, eczema, autoimmunity, and predisposition to infection. There is an increased incidence of malignancy, including leukemia and lymphoma. Therapy is with HSCT or gene therapy.

5. *AR inherited disorders of DNA repair.* There are several such disorders, including

   a. *Bloom syndrome.* There are characteristic ('birdlike') facies with marrow failure, photosensitivity, and predisposition to leukemia and lymphoma. There is mutation in the *BLM* gene.

   b. *Njmegen breakage syndrome.* There is microcephaly, characteristic facies, chromosomal instability, and predisposition to lymphoma. There is mutation in the *NBS1* gene.

c. *Ataxia telangiectasia syndrome* . There is ataxia, elevated alpha-fetoprotein (AFP) and chromosomal instability with an increased incidence of T-cell leukemia. There is mutation in the *ATM* gene.

Predominantly Antibody Deficiencies

These disorders are diagnosed after quantification of serum levels of IgM, IgG, and IgA. Several syndromes are recognized:

1. IgG, IgA, and/or IgM deficiency with absent B cells is most commonly X-linked agammaglobulinemia with mutation in the *BTK* gene. The protein product of this gene is a tyrosine kinase whose deficiency leads to a block in B-cell development at the pro-B to pre-B stage. Affected boys present in early childhood with recurrent, severe bacterial infection, particularly of the respiratory tract, and are treated with replacement immunoglobulin. This is usually given at home by weekly subcutaneous infusion.

2. IgA and IgG reduced with raised IgM is characteristic of CD40 ligand or CD40 deficiency, discussed earlier.

Disorders of Immune Dysregulation

The hemophagocytic lymphohistiocytosis (HLH) syndromes including familial HLH, those familial HLH syndromes associated with hypopigmentation (Chediak Higashi, Griscelli), and with Epstein-Barr virus (EBV)–associated hyperproliferation (XLP-1 and XLP-2) are dealt with more fully in Chapter 24.

There are several syndromes where the genetic defect of immune dysregulation manifests primarily as autoimmunity, but the clinical hematologist is likely to commonly encounter only two such syndromes:

1. Autoimmune lymphoproliferative syndrome (ALPS) is a rare genetic disorder of abnormal lymphocyte survival caused by defective Fas-mediated apoptosis. Normally, the immune system downregulates by increasing Fas expression on activated B- and T-lymphocytes and Fas ligand on activated T-lymphocytes. Fas and Fas ligand interact to trigger the caspase cascade, leading to cell apoptosis. Patients with ALPS have a defect in this apoptotic pathway leading to chronic nonmalignant lymphoproliferation including lymph node enlargement and splenomegaly, autoimmune disease including autoimmune hematologic cytopenia, and secondary cancers. There are increased numbers of CD3$^+$ T cells that are doubly negative for CD4 and CD8, and defective Fas-mediated apoptosis can be demonstrated *in vitro*. Therapy is mainly directed toward control of autoimmunity with steroids, immune globulin treatment, and other drugs including mycophenolate mofetil (MMF), methotrexate, and sirolimus. Inheritance might be autosomal dominant (AD) or AR.

2. Immune dysregulation, polyendocrinopathy, enteropathy, X-linked (IPEX) is a syndrome caused by X-linked mutations in *FOXP3* that lead to a deficiency in circulating CD3$^+$ CD25$^+$ FOXP3$^+$ regulatory T cells, and there is early presentation with autoimmune enteritis, diabetes, and thyroiditis and autoimmune hemolytic anemia and thrombocytopenia. Treatment is with HSCT in a center experienced in such transplantation.

Disorders of Neutrophil Number, Function, or Both

These inherited disorders of neutrophil number (severe congenital neutropenia) and function (including LAD, CGD, and GATA2) are dealt with more fully in Chapters 19 and 20.

Defects in Innate Immunity

These disorders include isolated congenital asplenia caused by AR inheritance of NKX2-5 deficiency and chronic mucocutaneous candidiasis, which is a heterogeneous group of disorders characterized by recurrent or persistent superficial infections of the skin, mucous membranes, and nails with *Candida* organisms, usually *C. albicans*. These disorders are confined to the cutaneous surfaces, with little propensity for systemic dissemination. AD (gain-of-function *STAT1* and *IL17F* mutations) and AR (*IL17RA*) inheritance are recognized.

Autoinflammatory Disorders

These include IL10 or IL10 receptor deficiency early-onset inflammatory bowel disorder (EOIBD), which is treated with HSCT, and familial Mediterranean fever (FMF), which is caused by mutation in the *MEFV* gene and includes recurrent fever episodes with polyserositis and abdominal pain. Inheritance is AR, and it is complicated by amyloidosis. Management is with colchicine, which is effective in most cases. Anakinra (IL1 inhibitor) is also effective in this disorder.

Complement Disorders

The proteins and glycoproteins that constitute the complement system are synthesized by hepatocytes, but significant amounts are also produced by macrophages, including C1q. There are three pathways of activation, and each generates homologous variants of the protease C3-convertase. The classic complement pathway typically requires antigen–antibody complexes (immune complexes) for activation (specific immune response), whereas the alternative pathway can be activated by C3 hydrolysis or antigens without the presence of antibodies. In both pathways, C3-convertase cleaves and activates component C3, creating C3a and C3b and causing a cascade of further cleavage and activation events.

- C3b binds to the surfaces of pathogens, leading to greater internalization by phagocytic cells by opsonization.
- C5a is an important chemotactic protein, helping to recruit inflammatory cells.
- Both C3a and C5a directly trigger degranulation of mast cells.
- C5b initiates the membrane attack pathway, which results in the membrane attack complex (MAC), consisting of C5b, C6, C7, C8, and polymeric C9. MAC is the cytolytic end product of the complement cascade.

Several complement disorders are relevant to the hematologist:

- C1q deficiency is caused by AR inherited mutations in the *C1QA*, *C1QB*, or *C1QC* gene and leads to a familial systemic lupus erythematosus (SLE) syndrome. Because C1q is produced by cells of the hematopoietic system, this syndrome is manageable by HSCT.
- In paroxysmal nocturnal hemoglobinuria (PNH), there is an acquired mutation in the *PIGA* gene. *PIGA* encodes a glycosyl-phosphatidylinositol (GPI) biosynthesis protein, and GPI-linked proteins protect the red blood cell (RBC) from

complement lysis. One of these proteins is CD59, and AR-inherited CD59 deficiency (*MIRL* gene) is described to cause similar problems as seen in PNH, namely, chronic hemolytic anemia and thrombosis.

Who and How to Investigate for PID

PID is principally suspected in children with unusual infections:

- Infection may be with unusual organisms – opportunistic infections – and sometimes the organism identified is itself suggestive of a particular PID diagnosis. CGD is characterized by infection with *Staphylococcus*, but infection with *Aspergillus* and *Burkholderia cepacia* is very suggestive of this diagnosis. Infection with *Pneumocystis* is indicative of a PID with SCID or CD40 or CD40 ligand deficiency
- There may be recurrent infection, or the infection may be difficult to eradicate. The infection may occur at an unusual age.

The National Institutes of Health (NIH) published 10 warning signs that should trigger investigation for a primary PID (Table 23.2). The first three of these are the most important.

There may be other features that suggest a PID diagnosis. There may be the typical dysmorphic appearances seen, for example, in Nijmegen breakage syndrome. There may the erythroderma of Omenn syndrome. PID also may present to the hematologist with cytopenia, and this is considered separately.

The screening investigations for PID should include

- A CBC with differential including the total lymphocyte count
- An exact enumeration of circulating T, B, and NK cells
- The total serum IgG, IgE, IgA, and IgM
- Measurement of the specific antibody to the organisms against which the child has been vaccinated. The ability to generate specific antibody is a good test of the functioning of the immune system.

Further more specific investigations will be toward a suspected diagnosis. Such investigations will include assessment of WAS protein expression in WAS or the nitroblue tetrazolium (NBT) test in CGD.

Table 23.2 Warning Signs for a Primary PID

Failure of an infant to thrive and gain weight normally

Need for intravenous antibiotics to clear infection

Family history of PID or unexplained infant death

Eight or more new ear infections in 1 year

Two or more serious infections in 1 year

Two or more episodes of pneumonia within 1 year

Recurrent deep skin or organ abscesses

Two or more deep-seated infections such as sepsis or meningitis

Persistent thrush in mouth or fungal infection of the skin

Greater than 2 months on oral antibiotics without effect

Cytopenia in PID

From the preceding discussion, it is clear that hematologic cytopenias are frequently encountered in the PID conditions and that several mechanisms underpin such cytopenias.

- Autoimmunity that may be humeral (antibody-mediated), as seen in ALPS and CD40 or CD40L deficiency or cellular (T-cell mediated) as in WAS
- There may be immune dysregulation such as in HLH, XLP, and the IPEX-like syndromes
- There may be bone marrow failure such as in cartilage hair hypoplasia or the monoMAC syndrome associated with *GATA2* mutation
- Cytopenia may accompany significant infection or the drugs used to treat that infection (e.g. the neutropenia that accompanies cytomegalovirus [CMV] infection and its treatment with ganciclovir)

Malignancy in PID

PID is associated with an increased risk in malignancy. This may be lymphoproliferative, such as the B-lineage lymphomas and leukemia seen in XLP-1 or the T-lineage disease seen in ataxia telangiectasia. Myeloid malignancy is seen in GATA2. Other cancers might arise as a consequence of defects in immune surveillance.

HIV Infection

The structure of HIV is relevant to its infection of CD4 lymphocytes. The HIV virus membrane is crossed by a protein p41, which is associated with an extracellular protein p120. The latter binds the CD4 receptor and the chemokine receptor CCR5, inducing a conformational change that allows p41 to find the lymphocyte cell membrane and initiate fusion of virus and cell membrane. Such fusion delivers the virus capsid into the cytoplasm of the lymphocyte. The following processes occur:

- The single-chain viral RNA is transcribed into single-strand (ss) DNA by viral *reverse transcriptase*. Drugs used to treat HIV include nucleoside and non-nucleoside inhibitors of reverse transcriptase.
- The ssDNA is replicated to doubled-stranded (ds) DNA by viral *RNA polymerase*.
- dsDNA migrates to the CD4 lymphocyte nucleus.
- Viral *integrase* incorporates this dsDNA into host genomic DNA at random sites.
- The virus-incorporated DNA is transcribed by host RNA polymerase, and this mRNA is translated by the host, and production of virus RNA copies ensues.
- Viral proteins and RNA are assembled by viral *protease* enzyme. Some drugs for HIV inhibit this viral protease.

Hematologic Complications of HIV Infection

Anemia

Anemia is common in HIV infection, and several factors contribute:

- *Anemia of chronic disease.* This anemia is likely related to HIV infection of monocytes, and the resulting cytokines – tumor necrosis factor (TNF) and interleukin 1 (IL1) – will suppress erythropoiesis.
- *Anti-HIV drug therapy.* Zidovudine inhibits *in vitro* erythroid colony development in a dose-dependent manner.
- *Other drug therapy.* This includes ganciclovir therapy of CMV infection.
- *Parvovirus infection.* An intact immune system is required to clear parvovirus, so chronic parvovirus infection will lead to reticulocytopenic anemia as in similar infection in children receiving maintenance therapy for ALL and in

children whose immune system is not yet recovered following HSCT. Diagnosis will be made with parvovirus polymerase chain reaction (PCR) of the blood.

- *Other opportunistic infections.* These also may have marrow involvement that contributes to anemia, including histoplasmosis, leishmaniasis, and atypical mycobacterial infection. Diagnosis will be with marrow aspiration and appropriate culture and PCR techniques.
- Autoimmune hemolytic anemia might occur in a patient with a dysfunctional immune system. Note that a positive direct antiglobulin test (DAT) is more common than actual hemolytic anemia in HIV infection.
- HIV itself, the infections that are opportunistic in HIV (CMV, tuberculosis, EBV), and the tumors associated (NHL, Hodgkin lymphoma) with HIV all may be causes of HLH. Exclusion of infectious and malignant causes must be carefully undertaken before management of the HLH with the usual therapy can be undertaken.

Thrombocytopenia

Some of the causes of thrombocytopenia including drug therapy for HIV and its associated infections and as well as direct marrow involvement with infection suppress marrow platelet production. However, immune thrombocytopenic purpura (ITP) is common in HIV infection and may occur early. Indeed, it may be a presenting manifestation. Other consumptive thrombocytopenias occur in HIV, and thrombotic thrombocytopenic purpura (TTP) and hemolytic-uremic syndrome (HUS) are both more common in HIV-infected individuals.

Neutropenia

Infections themselves, drugs to treat infections and opportunistic infections, and autoimmune causes are the principal causes of neutropenia in HIV-infected individuals.

HIV-Related Hematologic Malignancy

Lymphomas are increased in incidence in individuals infected with HIV. The risk of such disease is related to the extent of immune suppression and the CD4 lymphocyte count. In this era of highly active antiretroviral therapy (HAART), the incidence of such malignancy in the developed world is reduced. The histology of such illness includes classical Hodgkin lymphoma, Burkitt lymphoma, and diffuse large B-cell lymphoma, including primary CNS lymphoma. There is a smaller increase in the risk of other hematologic malignancies, including acute leukemia. In general, treatment of the lymphoma includes effective anti-HIV treatment and is based on protocols for similar diseases in the absence of HIV. Prognosis is similar to that in the non-HIV population.

Chapter 24

Hemophagocytic Lymphohistiocytosis (HLH) and Other Nonmalignant Histiocytic Disorders

Key Messages

1. Hemophagocytic lymphohistiocytosis (HLH) is a life-threatening disorder of immune dysregulation with hyperstimulation and inflammation.

2. HLH may be found in familial (FHLH) disease, where there is mutation in one of several genes affecting granule-mediated cytotoxic T-lymphocyte (CTL) function and in a number of other genetic diseases including the X-linked disorders X-linked lymphoproliferative disease (XLP) and X-linked inhibitor of apoptosis (XIAP) deficiency.

3. HLH is also found in acquired diseases, including malignant, autoimmune, metabolic, and infectious diseases.

4. Diagnosis may be difficult. The clinician must consider the possibility of HLH. Immune system activation must be demonstrated and defined dialgnostic criteria evaluated. These diagnostic criteria reflect hypercytokinemia in the patient. Genetic disease must be excluded through specific evaluation of certain protein expressions by flow cytometry (perforin, SAP) and the demonstration of effective cytotoxic T-lymphocyte (CTL) function through the granule release assay. In both genetic and acquired illness, a trigger to the HLH process should be sought.

5. Treatment of acquired HLH is sometimes treatment of the trigger. However, in some acquired illness and in all genetic disease, HLH is treated by powerful immune suppression, and genetic disease will usually also require hematopoietic stem cell transplantation (HSCT).

6. Where response to therapy is limited, or where patients relapse during therapy, the diagnosis should be re-evaluated, including a repeated assessment for a disease trigger. Additional immune suppression including with the pan-lymphocyte-depleting antibody alemtuzumab might be indicated.

Hyperinflammation and HLH

When properly regulated, the immune system should turn on when stimulated, deal with the stimulus – clear antigen, etc. – and then turn off again. In HLH, the immune system is dysregulated so that is turned on and then further on and on. This occurs either because the immune system is intrinsically (primarily) flawed and unable to clear infection so that antigen presentation and immune activation continue, or because in acquired disease the nature of stimulation is such that it continues to stimulate the immune system.

Diagnosis of HLH

HLH looks like infection. The manifestations of HLH are those of infection because they are those of a stimulated immune system. In HLH, however, this immune response is both disproportionate and progressive. Many infants will have died of 'culture-negative' sepsis when the diagnosis actually should have been HLH. The first step in the diagnosis of HLH therefore is the recognition by the attending clinician that the child *might* have HLH. In order to make the diagnosis, it must first be even considered. One of the duties of the practicing pediatric hematologist is to raise the profile of this diagnosis within his or her institution so that the diagnosis is considered in a timely manner.

There are diagnostic criteria for HLH, and they may appear to be a somewhat arbitrary collection, but in reality, they reflect the hypercytokinemia of the activated, dysregulated immune system. There are eight criteria, and five of them must be reached in order to allow a diagnosis of HLH to be made. Before these eight criteria are considered, five points should be made to the clinician:

1. A child with a genetic lesion that confers HLH might be asymptomatic and diagnosed because of an affected sibling. This child might be offered HSCT if there is an appropriate donor or at the very least kept under close surveillance.

2. Familial HLH may present with inflammatory brain disease and should form part of the differential diagnosis of such disease of uncertain etiology in young children. There may be seizures, altered mental state, brain stem signs, and ataxia.

3. A ferritin level of >500 μg/liter is consistent with a diagnosis of HLH and allows a diagnosis to be made. However, in practice, the ferritin level may be very much higher, and a level of $>10,000$ or $20,000$ μg/liter is very suggestive of HLH indeed because there are few other illnesses that so raise the serum ferritin.

4. Abnormal liver function tests do not form part of the HLH diagnostic criteria, but it is the exception to see a child who has HLH and normal liver function. Liver disease and jaundice with lactic acidosis are a well-recognized presentation, so inborn errors of metabolism might form part of the differential diagnosis.

5. The disorder is progressive. If the diagnostic criteria cannot be reached on Monday, they may all be present by the Thursday or the following Monday. Children with stuttering disease are recognized but are unusual. In some cases, the patient may be gravely ill without all the criteria being reached, and in these circumstances, treatment of HLH may need to be started after appropriate multidisciplinary team meetings involving different medical specialists, including immunology, intensive care, metabolic diseases, infectious diseases, and so on. In such circumstances, waiting for all criteria to be met may result in a dead child.

Diagnostic Criteria of HLH

The eight diagnostic criteria reflect organ infiltration by activated immune cells, hypercytokinemia, and the downstream effects of hypercytokinemia or the intrinsic immune defect itself:

- Fever – induced by interleukin 1 (IL1) and IL6
- Splenomegaly
- Cytopenia affecting two-thirds of the lineages, including hemoglobin (Hb) < 90 g/liter, platelets $< 100 \times 10^9$/liter, and neutrophils $< 1.0 \times 10^9$/liter (Cytopenia is the consequence of the inhibitory effects of high levels of tumor necrosis factor α [TNF-α] and interferon-γ on hematopoiesis rather than hemophagocytosis.)
- Hypertriglyceridemia (fasting triglycerides > 3 mmol/liter) and/or hypofibrinogenemia (fibrinogen < 1.5 g/liter) (The former arises from TNF-α inhibition of lipoprotein lipase and the latter from the secretion from activated macrophages of plasminogen activator and induction of fibrinolysis. There are also elevated levels of D-dimers or fibrin degradation products [FDPs].)
- Ferritin > 500 μg/liter (This is secreted by activated macrophages.)
- Hemophagocytosis in bone marrow, liver, spleen, or lymph nodes (The hemophagocytosis is often performed by small, activated histiocytes. It may be easier to see in trephine biopsies than in aspirates.)
- Soluble CD25 > 2400 IU/ml (This is the IL2 receptor and derives from activated lymphocytes.

Table 24.1 Diagnostic Criteria for Familial HLH

1. Familial disease/known genetic defect
2. Clinical and laboratory criteria (five of eight)

- Fever
- Splenomegaly
- Cytopenia

  - Hb < 9 g/liter
  - Platelets $< 100 \times 10^9$/liter
  - Neutrophils $< 1.0 \times 10^9$/liter

- Hypertriglyceridemia and/or hypofibrinogenemia

  - Fasting triglycerides > 3mmol/liter
  - Fibrinogen < 1.5 g/liter

- Ferritin > 500 μg/liter
- cCD25 $> 2,400$ U/ml
- Decreased or absent NK cell activity
- Hemophagocytosis in bone marrow, cerebrospinal fluid (CSF), spleen or lymph nodes.

Other cytokines are elevated and may be directly measurable but do not form part of these criteria.)

- Low or absent natural killer (NK) cell activity (This assay is often not performed because it is not widely available and not relevant in very young infants.)

The diagnostic criteria for familial HLH are listed in Table 24.1.

Etiology of HLH

HLH may be primary or acquired. In general, primary disease affects infants and young children, whereas acquired disease affects older children and adults and an initiating illness or infection can be identified. These distinctions are not absolute: An infectious cause can sometimes be identified in genetic disease, and primary disease may present in older subjects, including adults.

There are four subtypes of HLH that should be specifically looked for by additional investigation in children who have HLH:

- *Familial HLH (FHLH).* In FHLH there is genetic mutation in the lymphocyte granule–mediated cytotoxic pathway (Figure 24.1). In this pathway, CTL activation is accompanied by the mobilization of intracellular cytotoxic granules containing perforin and granzyme to the cell surface, where they fuse with the cell membrane, thereby releasing their contents. Based on genetic etiology, FHLH has been subclassified – in

FHLH1, the gene is not known but has been localized to chromosome 9q21.3; in FHLH2, there is mutation in the gene encoding perforin (*PRF-1*); in FHLHL3, there is mutation in the gene encoding Munc 13–4 (*UNC13D*); and in FHLH4 and FHLH5, there is mutation in the gene encoding syntaxin 11 (*STX11*) and syntaxin-binding protein 2, Munc 18-2 (*STXBP2*), respectively.

- HLH is described in three genetic disorders of more widespread intracellular granule trafficking and therefore has pigmentary abnormalities and defective cytotoxicity. The clinician should be alerted to the possibility of these conditions when the patient has pigmentary abnormalities including albinism. These are Griscelli syndrome (mutation in *RAB27A*), Chediak-Higashi syndrome (*LYST*), and Hermansky-Pudlak syndrome type II (*AP3B1*).

- There are two X-linked disorders that do not affect the cytotoxic pathway directly but are associated with Epstein-Barr virus (EBV)–associated HLH. These are X-linked lymphoproliferative disease (XLP) with mutation in the *SHDIA* gene (signaling lymphocyte-activating molecule-associated protein [SAP]) and the more recently described X-linked inhibitor of apoptosis (XIAP) deficiency.

Secondary HLH follows a clearly demonstrable cause in the absence of a demonstrable genetic mutation. Secondary causes include

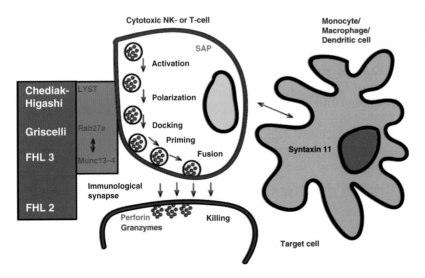

Figure 24.1 The genetic mutations in the lymphocyte granule–mediated cytotoxic pathway found in familial HLH.

- *Infection.* Herpes family viruses including EBV and cytomegalovirus (CMV) are the most common triggers. Neonates may have herpes simplex virus (HSV)–associated HLH. *Leishmania* species may cause HLH, and the parasite may be difficult to see in marrow smears. This is a presentation of leishmaniasis in the very young.
- *Rheumatologic illness* may trigger HLH and is more commonly referred to as the *macrophage activation syndrome* (MAS). This is seen especially in systemic-onset juvenile rheumatoid arthritis. In contrast to genetic HLH, the cytopenia may be less pronounced but the ferritin level may be very high and the hemophagocytosis very pronounced. Granulopoiesis is often increased, the C-reactive protein (CRP) level may be very high, and the IL-1β level also may be very high.
- *Metabolic illness.* HLH is described in several metabolic illnesses, including lysinuric protein intolerance and Wolman syndrome.
- *Malignancy.* HLH is seen in anaplastic large cell lymphoma (ALCL) and Hodgkin lymphoma. It is also described in other malignancies at presentation and in the course of treatment of malignancy, presumably then associated with infection.

Investigation of HLH

Following from the preceding sections, it is logical that there are three aims in the investigation of a child with suspected HLH. These will usually be conducted in parallel. The first is an evaluation of the diagnostic criteria for HLH; the second is an assessment of the possible genetic causes of HLH; the third is an evaluation of the trigger of the HLH episode.

1. *Is this HLH?* The diagnostic criteria should be evaluated and reevaluated in the suspected case. Remember that HLH is a progressive disorder, and if the diagnostic criteria cannot be reached today, then they may be reached tomorrow.
2. *Is there a genetic cause of HLH?* A specific and planned examination of the known genetic causes of HLH should be undertaken. The investigation

of the cause of HLH should not hinder treatment of a critically ill child. There may be a family history or certain clinical features (e.g. albinism) that might direct investigation toward a particular disorder immediately. Usually there will be a regional or national reference laboratory where these will be undertaken. These tests will include

a. Blood film to specifically examine the neutrophil granules that are seen in Chediak-Higashi syndrome
b. Flow cytometry to determine cell expression of perforin (FHLH2), SAP (XLP-1), and XIAP (XLP-2/XIAP)
c. The granule release assay (GRA). This is a test of the granule-mediated cytotoxicity of CTL and NK cells. During the granule release that accompanies competent T-cell activation, the membrane of the cytotoxic vacuole fuses with the cell membrane, and vacuole membrane protein CD107a becomes expressed on the cell surface [Figure 24.2]. The GRA is abnormal, when there is a defect in the pathways that control cytotoxic vacuole movement and with the genetic defects of FHLH3 [*UNC13D* gene, Munc13–4 protein], FHLH4 [*STX11* gene, syntaxin-11 protein], FHLH5 [*STXBP2* gene, syntaxin-binding protein, Munc 18-2], Griscelli syndrome [*RAB27A* gene], Chediak-Higashi syndrome [*LYST* gene], and Hermansky-Pudlak type II syndrome [*AP3B1* gene].)
d. There can be direct (Western blot) determination of protein expression and direct sequencing of a suspected gene. These confirmatory tests often follow abnormal flow cytometry or abnormal GRA assays.

3. *What is the trigger to this HLH episode?* This will be directed by clinical features. In general, viral polymerase chain reaction (PCR) determination for EBV, CMV, and so on will always be undertaken. If there is a history of travel, then *Leishmania* investigation (bone marrow, trephine, serology, and PCR) will be included, and in a neonate, a specific search for HSV, including by PCR, should be undertaken. Tumor will be diagnosed by biopsy. Rheumatologic illness will be diagnosed by clinical features and may be aided by autoantibodies.

(A)

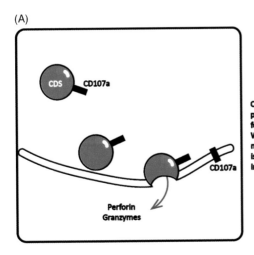

CD107a (LAMP-1) is a lysosome associated protein found in the membrane protein found in the membrane of cytotoxic granules. When the granules fuse with the cell surface membrane to release their contents, C107a is present on the cell surface and is then internalised.

Figure 24.2 (A) During granule release that accompanies competent T-cell activation, the membrane of the cytotoxic vacuole fuses with the cell membrane, and vacuole membrane protein CD107a becomes expressed on the cell surface. (B) Flow cytometric detection of membrane CD107a. (B) Flow cytometric detection of membrane CD107a. There is reduced expression in FHL4, syntaxin deficiency but there is epxression in XLP-1

(B)

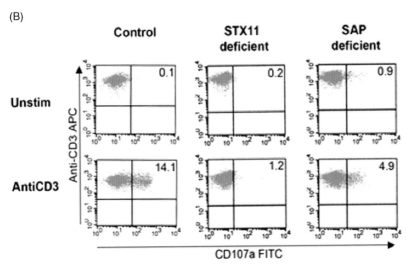

Treatment of HLH, Including Considerations in Refractory Disease

Treatment of HLH will include several or all of the following components:

- Treatment of the primary condition
- Supportive care of the cytopenia (requiring blood products, antibiotics, etc.) and often very sick child (many children with HLH will require intensive care and organ support)
- Treatment of the hyperinflammatory state
- Definitive correction of any underlying genetic defect
- Separate consideration of refractory disease
- Treatment of the primary condition is usually sufficient in malignancy-associated HLH and is

sufficient in leishmaniasis-associated HLH. Rituximab therapy is used for EBV-associated HLH, but in this and other infection-associated HLH, specific therapy of the hyperinflammatory state with immune-suppressant treatment such as employed in the genetic HLH conditions is often required. Once stimulated, the HLH immune system rather has a life of its own even once the initial trigger is turned off.

- In rheumatologic-disease associated MAS, pulsed high-dose steroids and cyclophosphamide have benefit. Other therapies including monoclonal antibodies – etanercept and infliximab block TNF-α, for example – have some role in management of both MAS and the primary disorder. Once full-blown HLH has developed, the

169

management might be that of the HLH as in the management of the genetic disease.

- Immune-suppressant therapies include those of the Histiocyte Society's clinical trials HLH-94 and HLH-2004. The backbone of both is an 8-week regimen with tapering dexamethasone (10 mg/m^2 for 2 weeks and then 5, 2.5, and 1.25 mg/m^2 each for 2 weeks during the ensuing 6 weeks) and etoposide (150 mg/m^2 twice weekly for 2 weeks and then weekly for 6 weeks). In HLH-2004, ciclosporin is added from the initiation of treatment, whereas in HLH-94, its introduction was delayed somewhat. Another regimen has employed anti-thymocyte globulin (ATG), and, more recently, hybrid regimens that include ATG, steroids, and chemotherapy are in clinical trial. Fever resolution is usually prompt, but cytopenia remains for several weeks and often may deepen with the chemotherapy. Correction of coagulopathy is usually between correction of fever and correction of cytopenia. Serial bone marrow aspirates are not helpful. Response rates in excess of 70 to 80 percent may be expected with such protocols.

- Transplant will cure genetic disease by replacing the incompetent patient's immune system with the competent immune system of the donor. Results are better when the hyperinflammation of HLH is controlled before conditioning therapy of HSCT is undertaken. Increasingly reduced-intensity conditioning protocols are used in the transplantation of children with HLH. Such protocols are particularly important in the transplant management of children with XIAP deficiency because results of transplantation in this condition with myeloablative conditioning are particularly poor. Results are improving all the time, and most children with genetic HLH may expect to be cured with appropriate supportive care, management, and control of the hyperinflammatory state and correction of the underlying defect with transplantation.

Children who are failing standard treatment should have both their diagnosis and their treatment reassessed early. The search for a primary trigger should be undertaken afresh. Specifically infection and malignancy should be excluded. Leishmaniasis and Hodgkin lymphoma may both cause HLH and yet themselves be relatively inconspicuous and not be responsible for most of the presenting symptoms. Persistent hyperinflammation in HLH might be managed with alemtuzumab, which is often used to control HLH to allow transplantation – as a 'bridge' to transplantation. Filtration of the plasma may aid control of HLH in the severe setting because the cytokines that are responsible for disease manifestations are removed in this process.

Osteopetrosis

Key Messages

1. Osteopetrosis is a condition characterized by increased bone density due to defective osteoclast-mediated bone remodeling.

2. Severe forms present in infancy with cytopenia and hepatosplenomegaly and are often first recognized by hematologists.

3. The pathologic defect usually resides in the osteoclast, which is a specialized tissue macrophage and is therefore derived from the hematopoietic stem cell.

4. Hematopoietic stem cell transplantation (HSCT) might correct the condition because stem cells from an unaffected donor will provide the tissues with unaffected, competent osteoclasts.

5. The decision to transplant is time-critical if vision and hearing are to be saved before loss of these senses due to bony overgrowth of the cranial foramina is irreversible.

6. The genetic pathogenesis of osteopetrosis is largely now known. Those forms of severe, recessively inherited osteopetrosis where the defect is intrinsic to the osteoclasts should respond to transplantation. Where there is associated neurodegenerative disorder, transplantation should be avoided. There are specific transplant-related complications and management issues in these diseases.

Pathology of Osteopetrosis: The Central Role of the Osteoclast

Osteopetrosis is a genetic condition characterized by increased bone density due to the absence of, or defects in, osteoclast-mediated bone resorption. Bone in the human body is constantly being remodeled. The remodeling process involves the resorption of bone by osteoclasts, which is matched by the formation of new bone by osteoblasts.

Osteoclasts begin the process of remodeling by binding to the surface of the bone. Following attachment, osteoclasts undergo polarization and use exocytosis to insert proton pumps into the plasma membrane facing the bone surface. This plasma membrane is now called the *ruffled border*. The osteoclast is tightly sealed to the surface of the bone, and the space between the bone and osteoclast is referred to as the *resorption lacunae* (Figure 25.1). Acid and proteases are delivered across the ruffled border into the resorption lacunae by exocytosis and direct transport. The enzymes attack the bone and dissolve the organic portion of the bone. Acid is secreted to dissolve the inorganic salts of the bone matrix. Chloride ion (Cl^-) channels are fused into the ruffled border to ensure the electroneutrality of the acid secretion by the V-type H^+-ATPase pump into the resorption lacunae. Bone proteins and minerals then enter the osteoclast and are excreted into the extracellular space. The next step of bone remodeling involves the migration of osteoblasts, which begin to lay down the components of new bone.

Osteopetrosis has varying degrees of severity and can be classified due to the mode of inheritance as either autosomal recessive or autosomal dominant. Autosomal dominant osteopetrosis is less severe than the autosomal recessive form, which is also called *malignant infantile osteopetrosis* (MIOP). MIOP is relatively rare, with an incidence of 1 in 200,000 individuals in the general population. Incidence is significantly increased in regions such as Costa Rica, the Middle East, the Chuvash Republic of Russia, and the province of Västerbotten in northern Sweden due to a combination of founder effect, geographic isolation, and a higher rate of parental consanguinity. It is this severe form that presents in early life to pediatric hematologists.

(A)

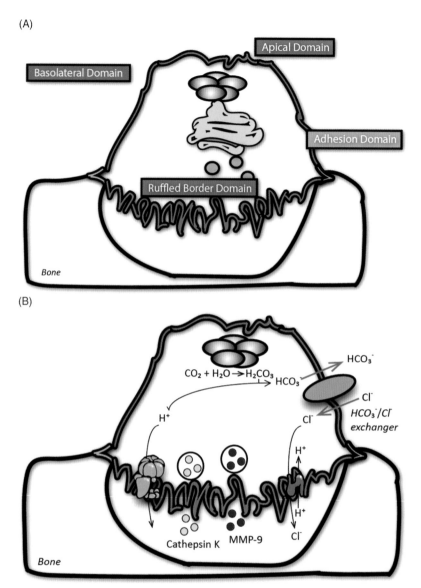

Figure 25.1 (A) Osteoclasts undergo polarization and use exocytosis to insert proton pumps into the plasma membrane facing the bone surface (the ruffled border). (B) Acid and proteases are delivered across the ruffled border into the resorption lacunae by exocytosis and direct transport.

Clinical Features of Malignant Infantile Osteopetrosis

MIOP commonly presents within the first year of life and is a severe disease that is fatal if left untreated. Patients typically present with symptoms of hematologic abnormality due to bone marrow failure associated with a reduced or absent medullary cavity and therefore extramedullary hematopoiesis resulting in hepatosplenomegaly. There is low serum calcium associated with secondary hyperparathyroidism and hypocalcemic seizure, and tetany may be the presenting feature as early as in the neonatal period.

Increased bone density results in macrocephaly despite a generalized growth retardation and failure to thrive. Other characteristic facial features include frontal bossing, exophthalmos, and micrognathia, so there are characteristic facies of the MIOP patient.

The increased bone density can be identified radiologically with classic features of bone in bone most commonly noted in the pelvis, vertebrae, and the ends of long bones (Figure 25.2). Bone overgrowth also results in defective formation or encroachment of cranial nerve foramina causing compression of the optic, auditory, and facial nerves. Calvarial thickening and abnormal cranial foramina lead to hydrocephalus,

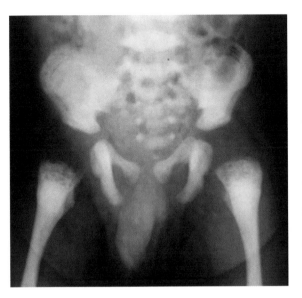
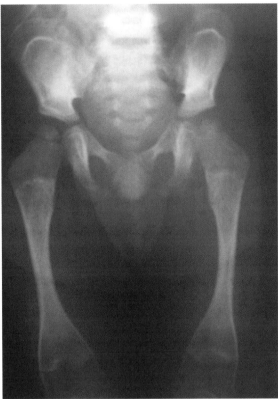

Figure 25.2 MIOP radiographs before and after HSCT.

and often patients with MIOP develop type 1 Chiari malformations, in which the cerebellar tonsils extend through the foramen magnum. Sclerotic changes also can lead to choanal stenosis resulting in respiratory and feeding difficulties. The MIOP child is typically snuffly.

Pathologic fractures after minor trauma occur mainly after the infantile period, and there is poor healing of the fractures. Tooth eruption can be delayed, and there may be severe dental caries. Osteomyelitis of the jaw is reported to be common after tooth extraction.

There are additional intrinsic symptoms present in specific types of MIOP. There are neuronopathic subtypes in which seizures, developmental delay, hypotonia, and primary retinal atrophy may be present. In patients with such neuronopathic MIOP, there may be changes on the electroencephalogram (EEG) detectable before either cerebral atrophy or white matter abnormalities are seen on magnetic resonance imaging (MRI) and before such neurodegeneration is apparent clinically. If it can be detected, neurodegeneration is a contraindication to HSCT.

Genetics of Osteoclast-Rich and Osteoclast-Poor Osteopetrosis

A bone marrow trephine or bone biopsy will distinguish osteoclast-rich from osteoclast-poor osteopetrosis, and the genetic defects responsible for autosomal recessive osteopetrosis can be classified into those which cause osteoclast-rich disease, in which there is a defect in the resorption function of the osteoclast, and those which lead to activated osteoclast-deficient osteopetrosis.

The mutations identified in osteoclast-rich disease are associated with the transporter proteins of the ruffled border, which result in the inability to resorb bone. The mutation identified in activated osteoclast-deficient disease is a mutation in the *TNFSF11* gene, which codes for the RANKL protein found on the osteoblast surface. Binding of the RANKL protein to RANK, a cell surface receptor found on the surfaces of osteoclasts, results in the activation of osteoclasts. Therefore, loss-of-function mutations in the *TNFSF11* gene result in activated osteoclast-deficient

173

disease, in which the increased bone density is caused by a lack of the ability to activate osteoclasts. For these patients, bone marrow transplantation of hematopoietic stem cells will not be curative because the osteoblast on the surface of which the RANKL protein is found derives and differentiates from mesenchymal stem cells, unlike osteoclasts, which differentiate from hematopoietic stem cells. Similarly, loss-of-function mutations in the *TNFSF11A* gene, which codes for the RANK receptor on the osteoclast surface, result in activated osteoclast-deficient osteopetrosis. However, these cases are curable by HSCT because the RANK receptor is found on the osteoclast surface.

Mutations have been identified in five genes associated with osteoclast-rich osteopetrosis. These genes code for proteins that are involved in acidification of the resorption lacunae; therefore, loss-of-function mutations within these genes result in defective osteoclast function. Mutation in the *TCIRG1* gene accounts for 50 to 60 percent of MIOP cases. The *TCIRG1* gene codes for the α_3 subunit of the V-type H^+-ATPase pump. The H^+-ATPase pump, which is inserted into the plasma membrane as part of formation of the ruffled border, pumps H^+ ions across the border to acidify the resorption lacunae (Figure 25.1). The second most common mutation, which accounts for 10 to 15 percent of MIOP cases, occurs in the *CLCN7* gene. The *CLCN7* gene codes for the protein transporter CLC-7, which is responsible for transporting Cl^- ions across the ruffled membrane to maintain the electroneutrality of the secretion into the resorption lacunae (Figure 25.1). The *OSTM1* gene codes a single-pass glycoprotein that influences the function of the previously mentioned CLC-7 transporter. Mutations in the gene coding for SNX10 also have been identified in MIOP cases. SNX10 belongs to a group of proteins involved in protein trafficking in endosomes. SNX10 is specifically thought to regulate the intracellular trafficking of the V-type H^+-ATPase protein. Loss-of-function mutations in the *SNX10* gene therefore interfere with osteoclast function by inhibiting the insertion of the H^+-ATPase pump into the ruffled border. The fifth gene in which mutations have been identified is the *PLEKHM1* gene, which codes for a protein involved in intracellular vesicular trafficking that could affect the incorporation of transporters into the ruffled border.

TG1RG1 mutation MIOP is not typically associated with neurodegenerative disease. Some, but not all, cases of *CLCN7* mutation MIOP and all cases of *OSTM1* mutation MIOP are associated with neurodegeneration. *SNZ10* and the osteoclast-poor MIOP associated with mutations in *RANK* or *RANKL* are not associated with neurologic disease.

Investigation and Management of the Newly Presenting Child with MIOP

1. The diagnosis should be made with

    a. X-ray of the long bones
    b. Blood film, which will show the features of extramedullary hematopoiesis, including nucleated red blood cells (RBCs), myelocytes, (leukoerythroblastosis) and teardrop poikilocytes
    c. A bone marrow trephine or bone biopsy performed by the pediatric orthopedic surgeon (It is critical to distinguish osteoclast-rich from osteoclast-poor osteopetrosis. Usually the marrow will be very difficult to aspirate.)

2. The genetics of the disease should be elucidated as quickly as possible. There should usually be a national reference laboratory for this disease. The genetic etiologies of osteoclast-rich osteopetrosis are distinct from those of osteoclast-poor osteopetrosis, and this can focus the search somewhat.

3. Associated neurodegenerative disorder should be excluded as far as possible by a pediatric neurologist or by retinal examination by a pediatric ophthalmologist, by MRI of the brain, and by an EEG.

4. The complications for the disorder should be assessed and managed. A CT scan may be used to examine the bony foramina of the skull. The pediatric opthalmology team should assess the residual vision of the child, including by visual evoked response (VER) analysis. Any electrolyte disturbance should be corrected and nutritional support given to infants who are often significantly failing to thrive.

5. The patient should be referred early to the specialist bone marrow transplant team, and a search for a stem cell transplant donor should be initiated immediately by tissue typing the patient and immediate family members. Where there is consanguinity, it is useful to look beyond siblings

and into the extended family, including grandparents, for potential matches. A concurrent unrelated donor including cord blood search should be initiated.

Specific Transplant Considerations in MIOP

Stem cell transplantation is difficult in MIOP but can restore bone mineral density (Figure 25.2), preserve organ function, and restore normal life expectancy. In the preceding sections, several contraindications to transplantation were noted. Transplantation should not be performed where there is evidence of neuro-degenerative disease, and such a child should be managed palliatively, and appropriate genetic advice should be given to the family. Transplantation also should not be performed in osteoclast-poor MIOP, where the defect is in RANKL because this protein is osteoblast derived and therefore of mesenchymal rather than hematopoietic stem cell origin.

In addition to these difficulties of case selection in young, sick children, HSCT is also difficult and challenging in MIOP for the following reasons:

1. Affected individuals are often not doing well, with failure to thrive, respiratory difficulties from their narrowed airway, small thoracic cage, and abdominal splinting from organomegaly.

2. Engraftment of donor stem cells is difficult to achieve because the marrow cavity is obliterated by excess bone.

3. There is an increased risk of veno-occlusive disease (VOD), and it has become customary in some institutions to give prophylactic defibrotide to reduce this risk. Cyclophosphamide is now usually replaced by fludarabine in conditioning regimens because this former agent will only add to the already considerable VOD risk.

4. With engraftment, there might be malignant hypercalcemia as the abundant disordered bone becomes rapidly remodeled. This can be managed with hydrations, steroids, furosemide, and bisphosphonates, but a monoclonal antibody directed at RANKL – denosumab – might have a role in particularly difficult disease.

5. For the child with impaired vision at the time of transplantation, the vision will not usually recover, and early referral to appropriate services for children with visual impairment should be made.

Hemophilia

1. Hemophilia is one of the most common inheritable bleeding disorders.

2. Prophylaxis with recombinant factor concentrates in severe hemophilia has significantly reduced the frequency of bleeding episodes and development of joint arthropathy and has improved quality of life.

3. Alloantibodies to factor VIII (FVIII) (i.e. inhibitor) and its treatment present the most serious challenges in the management of hemophilia.

4. Genetic counseling is an important component of care for families with hemophilia, and identification and counseling of women who are carriers are important, especially when they are in the adolescent age group and of childbearing age.

5. It is important to keep acquired hemophilia in the differential diagnosis of any patient who presents for the first time with musculoskeletal bleeding in the absence of a known bleeding disorder.

6. Long-acting recombinant products in different phases of clinical trials will revolutionize the treatment of severe hemophilia.

7. Gene therapy for hemophilia is likely to be a clinical reality in the next years.

Introduction

Hemophilia is an X-linked bleeding disorder in which there is a quantitative deficiency of factor VIII (hemophilia A) or factor IX (hemophilia B) coagulation factors. Of all patients with hemophilia, 80 to 85 percent have hemophilia A and 10 to 15 percent have hemophilia B. Both these disorders have common clinical

manifestations and diagnostic methods, but management slightly differs. Factor XI deficiency, which is referred to as *hemophilia C*, has a different clinical bleeding phenotype. The coagulation factor levels determine the severity of hemophilia: *severe* deficiency is defined as a level of less than 1 percent, *moderate* deficiency is a level of 1 to 5 percent, and *mild* deficiency is a level of 6 to 40 percent. The level of deficiency usually dictates the frequency of bleeding episodes. Those with severe deficiency have recurrent spontaneous bleeding or bleeding provoked by minimal trauma, whereas those with moderate or mild deficiency have bleeding in association with trauma or surgery. Hemophilia is seen in all racial and ethnic groups.

Hemophilia A

Hemophilia A is seen in 1 in 5,000 males. The factor VIII gene is located on the long arm of chromosome X at position Xp28, is 186 kb long, and has 26 exons. Factor VIII is produced in liver sinusoidal cells and vascular endothelial cells. The factor VIII protein has six domains – three A domains (A1, A2, and A3), a central B domain, and two C domains (C1 and C2). Factor VIII (FVIII) circulates in a noncovalent complex with von Willebrand factor (vWF). The FVIII in complex with vWF has a half-life of approximately 12 h. The role of FVIII in the coagulation cascade is discussed in more detail in Chapter 2. Briefly, FVIII is activated by thrombin, which causes release of activated FVIII (F VIIIa) from vWF. The cofactor FVIIIa binds to FIXa with Ca^{2+} to form the intrinsic Xase complex. In hemophilia, the intrinsic Xase complex cannot be formed, and the levels of FXa needed for thrombin generation are not produced, resulting in poor clot formation and a bleeding phenotype.

Hemophilia B

Hemophilia B occurs in 1 in every 30,000 males. The *FIX* gene, located on chromosome Xq27, is

33 kb in length and encodes a vitamin K–dependent single-chain glycoprotein consisting of 415 amino acids. The liver is the primary site of factor IX synthesis. Factor IX is proteolytically activated to FIXa by either activated factor VII (FVIIa) in the presence of tissue factor, calcium ions, and phospholipid or by factor XIa in the presence of calcium ions. Factor IXa then activates factor X in the presence of activated FVIII, phospholipid, and calcium ions. A deficiency of FIX, due to an inherited defect or to a liver disease, results in the reduction of a functioning intrinsic tenase complex leading to diminished thrombin generation and an inability to form and maintain a stable clot

Diagnosis of Hemophilia

A prolonged activated partial thromboplastin time (APTT) will often raise the suspicion of hemophilia, but isolated reduced levels of FVIII or FIX are diagnostic. The classification into severe, moderate, or mild disease is based on the factor levels. As with all coagulation tests, one should be cautious of labeling a patient based on one abnormal test, and repeat assays that demonstrate consistent results are usually required, especially for mild or moderate disease.

- FVIII circulates bound to vWF, and if vWF levels are low (as in type 3 von Willebrand disease [VWD]), then FVIII is also low, even though its production might be normal. In type 2N vWD, the association of FVIII with vWF is reduced in association with a specific mutation of vWF, and circulating FVIII levels are low.
- Mild hemophilia B may be missed in the newborn period because newborns may normally have low levels of FIX.
- Genetic testing in hemophilia confirms the diagnosis. This information can be used for carrier testing within families. In severe hemophilia A, inversion mutations are most common. Missense mutations cause mild or moderate hemophilia. Other mutations that occur in hemophilia are nonsense, frame shift, insertion/ deletion, and splicing mutations.

It is important to distinguish hemophilia from other bleeding disorders by their bleeding phenotype and FVIII levels:

- Musculoskeletal bleeding is the hallmark feature in hemophilia that distinguishes it from mucocutaneous bleeding seen in vWD and platelet disorders and similar to bleeding seen in severe deficiencies of other rare factors.
- Moderate to severely low FVIII levels can also be seen in other bleeding disorders such as severe vWD type III and type 2N.
- A rare combined FV and FVIII deficiency generally associated with consanguinity may be mistaken for hemophilia.

Clinical Presentation

The symptoms and signs are similar in both hemophilia A and B and are characterized by bleeding and excessive bruising. The site of bleeding varies with the age of the child and the severity of the hemophilia.

- Boys with severe deficiencies may present with bleeding in the newborn period (i.e. bleeding from venipuncture/heelsticks or during circumcision) or with intracranial hemorrhage (ICH). Not all babies with severe hemophilia will bleed with circumcision, so lack of this history should not exclude the diagnosis of hemophilia. The risk of ICH in babies with hemophilia is 3 to 4 percent. It is important to rule out hemophilia in any newborn male with ICH.
- In infancy and childhood, musculoskeletal bleeding is more common. The joints that frequently have bleeding are the elbows, knees, and ankles. The other joints are less commonly affected. Joint bleeds may be trauma related or spontaneous. The hallmark features of a joint bleed are pain, swelling, redness, and decreased range of movement. A joint with recurrent bleeds – approximately one bleed per month or four to six bleeds over 6 months – is referred to as a *target joint*. The other types of bleeds are soft tissue (i.e. hematomas) or muscle bleeds. A large muscle bleed can cause compartment syndrome and an iliopsoas bleed may lead to avascular necrosis of femoral head, and they require prompt evaluation and treatment.
- Those with mild to moderate hemophilia can present at any age with bleeding symptoms or frequent bruising at unusual locations such as the chest, back, abdomen, and face. They may present with excessive bleeding after trauma or surgery.

Management

The management of children with hemophilia is best carried out at hemophilia treatment center under the guidance of a multidisciplinary team. This approach is directed toward treatment and prevention of bleeds with factor replacement. Prophylactic factor replacement has considerably reduced the frequency of bleeds and thereby has improved the quality of life of children with hemophilia. The timing of initiation (i.e. primary versus secondary prophylaxis), the choice of product, and the frequency of administration of factor product are variable across countries.

Regular Review in Clinic

In a regular clinic setting, the following should be reviewed (at six month or annual intervals, depending on local resources and patient geographic factors):

- The bleeding history in order to ascertain whether prophylaxis is necessary or, if already given, is adequate
- To make a diagnosis of other medical conditions (e.g. ADHD, obesity, etc.)
- To investigate the impact of the bleeding disorder on school performance (specific nursing intervention and education in the school will be usual) (There will be many reasons that school performance will be affected in patients with hemophilia.)
- Joint examination by a physical therapist, especially if there is a target joint or recurrent bleeding into a joint (It is important to tailor prophylactic treatment to lifestyle/bleeding episodes, that is, every other day versus three times a week.)
- Counseling of family members who are pregnant and carrying out carrier testing for family members with a history of hemophilia (Age-based management is outlined later.)
- Dental review
- Regular blood draws for inhibitor exclusion
- Implementation of an age-based approach to management

Age-Based Approach to Management of Severe Hemophilia

1. *Newborn (NB) period*. There is no clear consensus that cesarean deliveries are preferable to vaginal births. It is recommended to avoid fetal scalp electrodes for clinical monitoring and avoid vacuum or forceps (instrumental) for vaginal deliveries. In the NB period, no arterial punctures should be performed, and circumcision should be performed under factor replacement. Routine vaccination should be carried out with small-caliber needles (e.g. 26 gauge). Consideration should be given to subcutaneous rather than intramuscular administration, application of ice and the inclusion of an observation period in the office to watch for hematoma development. Family support and counseling should occur with the help of a social worker.

2. *Infancy*. A protective environment for the child is necessary to prevent injuries and bleeding episodes (e.g., gates for stairs, protective covers for sharp corners, and a safe play area).

3. *Toddler*. Prophylaxis should be initiated for patients with recurrent joint bleeds. Good dental hygiene should be promoted to prevent caries and dental procedures that can present with bleeding complications.

4. *Childhood*. Logs of factor replacement and treatment of bleeding episodes should be maintained, and treatment should be tailored to the child's physical activity. Education should be supplied in an age-appropriate manner (e.g. identifying joint bleeds, seeking help early from school nurse, making safe sport choices, encouraging self-infusion of factor by ages 8 to 10 years). Target joints should be recognized, and early referral to orthopedics should occur. Joint health should be promoted by regular exercises and vitamin D therapy.

5. *Adolescence*. It is important to stress adherence to treatment. Initiate transition to adult service in early adolescence. Stress the importance of choosing jobs that are better suited to the bleeding disorder. Counsel regarding avoidance of high-risk behaviors (e.g. drinking and driving). Encourage patients to discuss their bleeding disorder with their friends.

Factor Replacement Strategies

The half-life of infused factor VIII is approximately 8 to 12 h. Younger children have faster clearance. Giving 1 unit/kg increases the factor level by 2 percent. The half-life of FIX is approximately 18 h. Giving 1 unit/kg

Table 26.1 Suggested Factor Replacement for Different Bleeds in Hemophilia A and B

Type of bleeding	Level of correction (%)	Dose in hemophilia A (units/kg)	Dose in hemophilia B (units/kg)
Oral mucosa/ epistaxis	40	20	40
Joint/muscle	80	40	80
Gastrointestinal	80	40	80
Intracranial	100	50	100

increases the factor level by 1 percent. The desired/suggested replacement strategies for different bleeds in hemophilia A and B are listed in the Table 26.1.

Adjunctive Therapies

Other adjunctive therapies used in the treatment of hemophilia include desmopressin (DDAVP), both intravenous and intranasal preparations. These act by release of vWF and FVIII from their endothelial sites. Its use is limited to mucocutaneous bleeding episodes such as epistaxis, oral mucous membrane bleeding, or menorrhagia. DDAVP tends to be of value only in mild disease, and tachyphylaxis is well described. Antifibrinolytics such as tranexamic acid and epsilon-aminocaproic acid (EACA) are also effective in controlling bleeding episodes, especially bloody noses or oral bleeding. However, they should not be used in urinary tract bleeding due to the risk of thrombosis formation in the bladder leading to urinary obstruction. Local hemostatic therapy such as fibrin glue is effective over surgical-site bleeding.

New Long-Acting Factor Concentrates

Both FVIII and FIX long-acting products are in different phases of clinical trials and have prolonged the duration of action and thus have resulted in less frequent dosing regimens. These include glycopegylation, FVIII-Fc fusion products, fusion to albumin, and tissue factor pathway inhibitors (TFPIs).

Surgery in Patients with Hemophilia

The most common procedures carried out in children with hemophilia are circumcision, placement of a Port-a-Cath, dental procedures, tonsillectomy, and adenoidectomy. There are no consensus recommendations for optimal therapy and monitoring for these procedures. The World Federation of Hemophilia (WFH) has released general guidelines for management during surgical procedures (WFH Treatment Guidelines Working Group, 2005), and there has been a published survey of European practices of invasive procedures in children with hemophilia (2009).

General Principles of Management in Hemophilia Patients Prior to Surgery

- Administer factor replacement preoperatively to obtain 100 percent correction.
- Maintain 80 to 100 percent correction for approximately 3 days postoperatively for minor surgeries, 7 to 10 days for major surgeries, and longer for intracranial surgeries.
- Given that the half-life of factor is shorter in younger children, they may need more frequent administration.
- Avoid surgeries in children with fewer than 20 exposure days to factor to avoid the occurrence of inhibitors.

Inhibitors in Hemophilia A and Immune Tolerance Therapy (ITI)

The overall incidence of inhibitors in hemophilia A is 10 to 15 percent, and in patients with severe and moderate hemophilia it is 20 to 30 percent. Inhibitors are seen when a child with hemophilia develops an immune response to treatment with the FVIII product, and the inhibitors are predominantly IgG4. Risk factors for the development of inhibitors include

- Severity of hemophilia
- Children with large deletions of the factor VIII gene
- Family history of inhibitors
- African and Latino ancestry
- Early intensive exposure to high doses of factor concentrates, particularly for the first 20 doses
- Major histocompatibility class (MHC) class polymorphisms of cytokine genes *TNF-A* (tumor necrosis factor α), *IL10* (interleukin 10), *CTLA4* (cytotoxic T-lymphocyte-associated protein 4)
- Bacterial/viral infections, vaccinations, surgery

To detect the presence of an inhibitor and to determine the strength (titer), the Bethesda assay is used. Inhibitors are classified as either low titer (i.e. <5 BU) or high titer (i.e. >5 BU). Those with low-titer inhibitors can be observed, whereas those with high-titer inhibitors need immune tolerance induction (ITI) for inhibitor eradication.

Management of Bleeding Events in Hemophilia Patients with Inhibitors

Management of bleeding in a patient with an inhibitor is a common clinical scenario and should form part of that patient's ongoing treatment plan. The options for any patient will depend on

- The patient's inhibitor titer
- The likelihood of an anamnestic response. The anamnestic response is the rapid rise in inhibitor level after renewed exposure to FVIII therapy. Such a response will render the child refractory to further FVIII therapy
- The site and severity of bleeding
- Whether ITI is going to be initiated

Options include

- *High-dose factor concentrates.* Administering factor concentrates at higher doses and/or more frequent intervals or continuously is the preferred treatment for acute bleeding in low responders.
- *Recombinant activated FVII or Novoseven (rFVIIa)*: Recommended dose: 90 micrograms/kg every 2–3 hrs. Repeat dose every 2–4 hrs for minimum of 3 doses and maximum of 5 doses. This is often used in those with a high inhibitor

level or those with a risk of an anamnestic response to administered FVIII.
- *Activated prothrombin complex concentrates (aPPCs).* Recommended dose: 50 to 100 units/kg every 6 to 12 hours, not to exceed 200 units/kg per day.

Consensus Guidelines for ITT

There has been significant advance over recent years in optimizing the protocols for ITI, which in reality only became possible with the widespread availability of recombinant factors. Patients are classified as good-risk patients (i.e. patients with a historical inhibitor titer < 200 BU, pre-ITI titer < 10 BU, and <5 years since inhibitors were diagnosed). For these patients, a number of ITI regimens are likely to be effective, and daily factor exposure likely will induce immune tolerance and enable effective use of factor concentrates in the future.

In contrast, poor-risk patients (i.e. those with peak historical titer > 200 BU, pre-ITI titer > 10 BU, and/or >5 yrs since inhibitor diagnosis) are likely to have more problems being induced, and current recommendations are for the use of a high-dose regimen (i.e. FVIII > 200 IU/kg per day).

In general, one should delay initiation of ITI until inhibitor titers are <10 BU, but 10 BU is not an absolute cutoff. One can consider initiating therapy if levels are >10 BU after 1 to 2 years of close monitoring or if life/limb-threatening bleeding occurs. Monitor FVIII recovery when titer falls to <10 BU.

Most patients are tolerized with the same product that was being used at the time of inhibitor development.

If effective prophylaxis is required during ITI, then additional treatment with either FEIBA (50 to 200 units/kg daily to twice weekly) or rFVIIa (90 to 270 μg/kg daily) for patients undergoing ITI who experience early joint bleeding or intracranial bleeding is recommended.

Measures of Successful ITI

- Undetectable inhibitor level (<0.6 BU)
- FVIII plasma recovery ±66 percent of predicted
- FVIII half-life ±6 h after a 72-h FVIII washout period
- Absence of anamnesis on further FVIII exposure

Inhibitors in Severe Factor IX Deficiency Patients

The frequency of inhibitor formation in hemophilia B patients is lower than in hemophilia A patients and is approximately 3 percent. Most are high-titer inhibitors, and development is frequently associated with the development of severe allergic/anaphylactic reactions to factor XI product. ITI is not routinely recommended, and if it is initiated, it needs to be performed with caution, and patients should undergo monitoring for nephrotic syndrome.

Acquired Hemophilia

This is a rare autoimmune condition characterized by acquired autoantibodies against factor VIII. There are differences in presentation, clinical features, and management from those in alloantibodies seen in congenital hemophilia, as listed in Table 26.2. The overall incidence is approximately 1 per 1 million population. It has a biphasic age distribution, with peaks occurring in the 20 to 40 age group (women of childbearing age) and >60 years. It rarely occurs in children. Most cases are idiopathic, and some are associated with malignancy, collagen-vascular disorders, postpartum, medications, or infections.

The antibodies are IgG antibodies directed against a single target on the factor VIII molecule. The antibodies follow second-order kinetics, in which there is rapid inactivation followed by slower inactivation of factor VIII activity. There is no correlation between inhibitor titer and residual factor VIII level. Severe spontaneous bleeding can occur even with factor VIII levels > 5 percent.

Patients without a prior bleeding history present with severe unexpected bleeding and bruising. Bleeding is usually subcutaneous, deep muscle, retroperitoneal, gastrointestinal, or intracranial. Hemarthroses almost never occur.

Acquired hemophilia is suspected when the APTT is prolonged. It is important to rule out the lupus anticoagulant by specific tests or heparin contamination. In the presence of autoantibodies to factor VIII, the APTT partially corrects with a mixing study (1:1 patient to normal plasma). After 1 or 2 h of incubation, the APTT is further

Table 26.2 Characteristics of Patients with Congenital and Acquired Hemophilia

Characteristic	Congenital hemophilia	Acquired hemophilia
Age of presentation	Infancy/ childhood	Older age; biphasic
Sex	Only in males	Males or females
Family history of hemophilia	Usually present	Absent
Bleeds	Hemarthroses common	Hemarthroses rare
Inhibitors	Alloantibodies	Autoantibodies

prolonged compared with the immediate mix. The diagnosis is confirmed by a low factor VIII activity level and detection of inhibitor by a Bethesda assay. It is important to remember that because this assay was developed to quantify alloantibodies to factor VIII, it may not accurately estimate the potency of the inhibitor.

Clinical management is directed toward management of the bleeding and eradication of the inhibitor. For acute management of bleeding, bypassing agents (i.e. recombinant activated factor VII [rFVIIa]) or activated prothrombin complex concentrates (aPCC) are used. There is no advantage of one agent over the other, and use depends on drug availability and physician preference. Side effects such as thrombosis, stroke, myocardial infarction, and disseminated intravascular coagulation have been reported, but these are rare and not specific to either agent. The benefits of using bypassing agents to control acute bleeding outweigh the risks. Several strategies have been used to eradicate the inhibitor with a success rate of approximately 70 to 80 percent. These include steroids alone or steroids with other immunosuppressants. There is no randomized trial with individual agents, but commonly used agents in conjunction with steroids include cyclophosphamide, cyclosporine, rituximab, and immunoadsorption. Intravenous immunoglobulin (IVIG) is not indicated in eradication of autoantibodies to factor VIII. Once antibodies are eradicated, the patient should be monitored for recurrence for 2 to 3 years.

Chapter 27

Congenital and Acquired von Willebrand Disease

1. Von Willebrand factor (vWF) plays a major role in initiating the hemostatic process.

2. Von Willebrand's disease (vWD) can present both as an absolute (type III, no protein) and a relative quantitative (type I) deficiency and qualitative function defect (various type 2 vWDs).

3. In vWD testing, an enzyme-linked immunosorbent assay (ELISA) is used to measure *quantitative* levels of the protein, and vW:RCo measures the *functional* activity of the protein in binding platelets. These tests and factor VIII determination are the essential laboratory tests for the diagnosis of vWD.

4. Type I vWD is the most common subtype and can present with variable bleeding manifestations and can be difficult to diagnose.

5. Several physiologic and pathologic conditions can influence vWF levels.

6. Recurrent iron deficiency anemia (IDA) and menorrhagia/dysmenorrhea merit screening for vWD in young women.

Introduction

Von Willebrand's disease is the most common inherited autosomal bleeding disorder. The protein is synthesized in endothelial cells and megakaryocytes and thereafter is stored in the Weibel-Palade bodies in the endothelial cell and the alpha granules of the platelet. vWF has an important role in primary hemostasis by binding platelet glycoprotein GPIb–IX receptor complex to initiate platelet adhesion, activation, and aggregation. It is also a carrier protein for the procoagulant factor VIII, stabilizing it and preventing its premature degradation.

The *VWF* gene is located on the short arm of chromosome 12, spans 178 kb, and comprises 52 exons. This results in an 8.5-kb message that directs synthesis of a 22-amino-acid signal peptide and a 2,791-amino-acid pro–von Willebrand factor monomer that is cleaved into a vWF propeptide (VWF pp) and a mature VWF monomer. Figure 27.1 shows the relationship between the 8.5-kb complementary DNA to structural and functional regions of the vWF protein and the mutation locations in the different subtypes of vWD.

Subtypes of vWD

Subtypes of vWD are defined by structural, functional, and molecular genetic techniques. Broadly, type 1 (partial) and type 3 (complete) are quantitative deficiencies of the protein, whereas the different type 2 vWDs (types 2A, 2B, 2M, and 2N) are qualitative deficiencies. Their frequency, inheritance, bleeding severity, and classification are described in Tables 27.1 and 27.2.

Clinical Features

Mucocutaneous bleeding is the predominant bleeding manifestation in vWD. This includes epistaxis, bruising, gum bleeding, and menorrhagia. In some children, excessive bleeding after surgical or dental procedures can occur. Other bleeding manifestations include bruising with routine immunizations and bleeding after loss of primary teeth.

In pediatric patients, epistaxis and bruising are common complaints and also can be seen in normal children. A good clinical and family history is very important to help distinguish between children who merit screening for a bleeding disorder and those whose presenting features are within the norm and who therefore do not require such screening. Moreover, children who have a bleeding disorder may not have had surgery or – if girls – may not have achieved

Table 27.1 Frequency, Inheritance, and Bleeding Severity in vWD

Type	Inheritance	Prevalence	Bleeding severity	Percent of vWD
Type 1	Autosomal dominant (AD)	1:100–1:1000	Mild–moderate	75
Type 2A	AD/autosomal recessive (AR)	Rare	Moderate	10–12
Type 2B	AD	Rare	Moderate	3–5
Type 2M	AD/AR	Rare	Moderate	1–2
Type 2N	AR	Rare	Moderate	1–2
Type 3	AR	1:1 million	Severe	1–3

Table 27.2 Classification of vWD

Type	Description
1	Partial quantitative deficiency of vWF
2	Qualitative deficiency of vWF
2A	Decreased vWF-dependent platelet adhesion and deficiency of high-molecular-weight multimers
2B	Increased affinity for platelet glycoprotein 1B, thrombocytopenia
2M	Decreased vWF-dependent platelet adhesion without deficiency of high-molecular-weight multimers
2N	Markedly decreased binding affinity for factor VIII
3	Severe quantitative deficiency of vWF

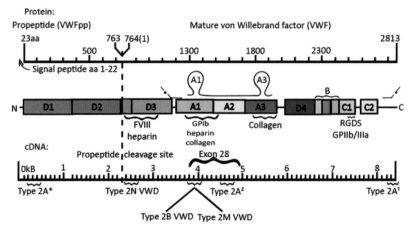

Figure 27.1 vWF protein structure and relationship to vWD subtype mutation location.

menarche yet, and therefore, their hemostatic system has not yet been fully challenged. To address these difficulties, 'bleeding assessment tools' have been developed and subsequently modified to optimize questionnaire administration to improve accuracy and to standardize evaluation of bleeding symptoms. The most recent International Society of Thrombosis and Hemostasis (ISTH) bleeding assessment tool (BAT) has refined previous bleeding tool assessments and published age- and gender-specific cutoffs for both adults and children for abnormal bleeding scores.

Clinical Scenarios That Merit an Evaluation for a Bleeding Disorder

A bleeding disorder workup should be considered if the following is reported in the history:

- Spontaneous nosebleeds lasting > 10 minutes, requiring medical attention or nasal cautery
- Bruising with trivial or without known trauma, especially on nonexposed parts of the body such as the chest or abdomen
- Prolonged bleeding from trivial wounds or recurring spontaneously several days after the injury
- Heavy, prolonged, recurrent bleeding with surgical or dental procedures, requiring medical attention or necessitating returning the patient to the operating room
- Bleeding causing anemia that requires a blood transfusion
- Heavy menses with clots > 1 inch in diameter, changing pads/tampons hourly, or resulting in iron deficiency/IDA
- Immediate family members with a blood disorder or needing medical attention for bleeding

Diagnostic Evaluation of vWD

The diagnosis of vWD is a combination of clinical symptoms, laboratory studies demonstrating a quantitative or qualitative vWF deficiency, and a family history of the disease. The diagnosis relies on standardized measurements of the vWF protein, vWF platelet-dependent functions, factor VIII level, and multimers. Tables 27.3 and 27.4 summarize the common terminology in vWD testing and the laboratory abnormalities in the different subtypes of vWD.

To summarize the laboratory tests:

- The quantitative level of protein is measured using ELISA
- The functional activity is measured using he vW: RCo assay
- In type 2B vWD, there is exaggerated increased binding of vWF to platelets with low levels of ristocetin. The clinical clue to type 2B vWD is the presence of vWD-type bleeding, vWD laboratory tests, and the concurrent presence of thrombocytopenia during bleeding.
- Multimers are useful in confirming and distinguishing types 1 and 2 vWD – in type 1, there is a normal multimer profile, and this is abnormal in type 2 disease.

Diagnostic testing is complicated by several physiologic factors influencing vWF levels:

- vWF is an acute-phase reactant, and thus, stress, anxiety, and mechanical difficulties in obtaining blood sample may falsely increase the level.
- The level increases with increasing age and may be especially difficult to interpret in individuals with a mildly reduced plasma level.
- The level is increased in pregnancy and use of hormonal contraception and is influenced by phases of the menstrual cycle.
- Individuals with blood group O have a 25 to 35 percent lower level of VW: Ag compared to other blood groups.

Therefore, testing for vWD may require repeated testing to ensure that true values are obtained. In

Table 27.3 Different Components of the vWF Assay and Functions

Test	Function/property	Assay
VWF	Multimeric protein promoting platelet adhesion and aggregation and carrier for FVIII	Assays described below
VW: Ag	VW protein level	ELISA
VW: RCo	Binding activity of vWF to platelets	Ristocetin cofactor activity
VW: CB	Ability of collagen to bind to collagen	Collagen-binding activity
vWF multimers	Size distribution of vWF multimers	Agarose gel electrophoresis
FVIII	Circulating level of coagulation protein bound to vWF	Plasma clotting test
Radio-immunoprecipitation assay (RIPA)	Binding to platelets with different concentrations of ristocetin	Platelet aggregation test

Table 27.4 Laboratory Abnormalities in the Different Subtypes of vWD

Test	Normal	Type 1	Type 2A	Type 2B	Type 2M	Type 2N	Type 3
VW: Ag	N	L, ↓ or ↓↓	↓ or L	↓ or L	↓ or L	N or ↓	Absent
VW: RCo	N	L, ↓ or ↓↓	↓↓ or ↓↓↓	↓↓	↓↓	N or ↓	Absent
FVIII	N	N or ↓	N or ↓	N or ↓	N or ↓	↓↓	↓↓
RIPA	N	Often N	↓	Often N	↓	N	Absent
LD-RIPA	Absent	Absent	Absent	↑↑↑	Absent	Absent	Absent
Platelet count	N	N	N	↓ or N	N	N	N
vWF multimers	N	N	Abnormal	Abnormal	N	N	Absent

some types of vWD, the only defect is in collagen binding, and this may be missed if testing is done with the platelet-binding function of vWF (i.e. vW: RCo). Hence, a collagen-binding assay may need to be performed in some patients. In addition to physiologic factors, several clinical disorders such as hypo/ hyperthyroidism, collagen-vascular disorders, *ventricular septal defect* (VSD), and disseminated intravascular coagulation (DIC) can alter vWF levels.

vWD Type 1 versus Low vWF

A level of <30 IU/dl of VW: Ag or VW: RCo is designated as a level for the definitive diagnosis of vWD. Thus, a diagnosis of vWD can be difficult for individuals with a VW: AG or VW: RCo level between 30 to 50 IU/dl, especially in type I vWD, where the diagnosis relies solely on VW: Ag/VW: RCo level. As noted earlier, vWF levels can vary and are a continuous variable. Thus, individuals with these levels may be at risk of bleeding but not necessarily have vWD. These individuals may benefit from therapy in clinically high-risk bleeding situations to raise the plasma level of vWF.

Role of Genetic Testing in vWD

The utility of genetic testing in subtypes of type 2 and type 3 is better defined. As illustrated in Figure 27.1, the mutations for types 2B, 2M, and 2N are located in discrete areas of the *VWF* gene, and genetic testing to confirm the diagnosis may be useful. Knowledge of the gene mutation for individuals with type 3 vWD is useful for prenatal diagnosis and care in the immediate newborn period. The role of genetic testing in type 1 vWD is less clear and not recommended because a fair proportion of individuals do not have *VWF* mutations

or the presence of polymorphisms makes it difficult to distinguish them from pathogenic mutations.

Management

Management includes local measures, pharmacologic agents, and adjunctive therapies.

Local Measures

Epistaxis can be a recurring symptom in some children with vWD and be disruptive in a school setting. Education of the family/individual and school nurse regarding correct maneuvers to stop a nosebleed and guidelines for how long to wait before seeking medical attention are useful. Local application of estrogen creams or salted pork has been used effectively in some children. Similarly, application of direct pressure and biting down on a piece of gauze to stop bleeding from a tooth are other effective strategies.

Pharmacologic Agents
Desmopressin (DDAVP)

This is used to treat muco-cutaneous bleeding and as prophylaxis to prevent bleeding before minor procedures or surgeries. DDAVP causes release of stored VWF from endothelial cell W-P bodies and stabilization of FVIII. It is not useful where sustained increase in VWF is required – once VWF is released from stores no further VWF is available. DDAVP can be given via intravenous or intranasal route. The reduced efficacy of DDAVP with repeated administration is known as tachyphylaxis.

- DDAVP is usually well tolerated with minor side effects of headache or flushing, but the main limitation of its use is tachyphylaxis, and the drug cannot be administered for more than two to three doses. Rarely, it can cause hyponatremia and seizures.

- DDAVP is most effective in type I vWD, where it increases the quantity of a protein that is functionally competent. Occasionally, in types 2A and 2M it might have a role. It is ineffective in type 3 and usually ineffective in types 2B and 2N.
- Individuals in whom DDAVP may be useful should undergo a test dose of the drug and post-DDAVP measurement of levels of VW: Ag, VW: RCo, and FVIII activity. Those who might benefit are therefore identified before its therapeutic use.
- The therapeutic dose is usually an intravenous dose of 0.03 µg/kg.

vWF Concentrates

Several factor concentrates are available with varying ratios of vWF and FVIII, and they provide effective hemostasis and have comparable safety profiles. The doses are based on the VW: RCo units, but the optimal dosing schedule for surgical procedures is not well established. The report from the NHLBI has suggested the strategies listed in Table 27.5 for minor and major procedures.

Use of these products for prophylaxis in individuals with type 3 has occurred but is not routinely recommended. The recent development of a new recombinant product may make prophylaxis possible and safe, but the dosing and frequency are not known.

Adjunctive Therapies

Adjunctive therapies include antifibrinolytic agents such as tranexamic acid and aminocaprioc acid (ACA). These are available in both oral and

Table 27.5 Suggested vWF Replacement in Minor and Major Surgeries

	Major surgery	Minor surgery
Loading dose	40–60	30–50
Maintenance dose	20–40 every 8 to 24 h	20–40
Monitoring	At least daily	At least once
Goal	Trough > 50	Trough > 50
Duration of replacement	7–14 days	1–5 days

intravenous preparations. Topical hemostatic agents such as fibrin glue to sites of bleeding are effective. Use of estrogen therapy to increase vWF and FVIII levels is helpful in young women experiencing menorrhagia.

Women and vWD

Women with VWD represent a significant health burden, and about 70 percent of them have menorrhagia, and half of them have dysmenorrhea. This can result in poor quality of life, school absenteeism, and sometimes depression. There is also a lack of a standardized way to assess menorrhagia, and pictorial blood assessment charts of the amount of menstrual blood loss have been used in the past. Clinically, the most feasible method of assessment is to ask about frequency of change of feminine care products, passage of clots, flooding, and past treatment of IDA.

Currently, there is no consensus on whether all women with menorrhagia should have vWD testing, but this should be considered in young women with recurrent IDA or a family history of abnormal bleeding or hysterectomy without an identifiable cause. Furthermore, diagnosis of vWD in women with menorrhagia is difficult because the phase of the menstrual cycle and possibly hormonal estrogen use can influence results. Diagnostic testing may need to be performed on more than one occasion if the degree of suspicion is high. Hormonal methods for regulation of the menstrual cycle and use of adjunctive treatments in the form of antifibrinolytics and intranasal desmopressin (Stimate) to decrease bleeding are effective.

Acquired vWD

Acquired vWD is an uncommon disorder but should be suspected when there is new onset of mild to moderate bleeding tendency or bleeding occurring after surgery that was previously tolerated. The pathophysiology is either antibody-mediated destruction, decreased production, adsorption to tumor, or shear stress in conditions such aortic stenosis that can cause proteolysis of the vWD multimers. Acquired vWD has been reported in several conditions, and the more commonly reported conditions are as follows:

- Hypothyroidism
- Wilm's tumor

- Systemic lupus erythematosus (SLE)
- Congenital heart defects

Acquired vWD can complicate management of the underlying disorders, and there is limited evidence for the management of bleeding symptoms in children with acquired vWD syndrome (AVWS). Children with an underlying diagnosis associated with AVWS should have vWF testing performed if they have bleeding symptoms or before surgical procedures. Correction of these abnormalities on treatment of the AVWS-associated disorder supports a diagnosis of AVWD.

Chapter 28

Rare Inherited Bleeding Disorders

1. The rare bleeding disorders are a heterogeneous group of conditions that combined comprise 3 to 5 percent of all congenital bleeding disorders.

2. The bleeding phenotype can be severe, but for some conditions, it does not correlate with the factor levels at all.

3. The diagnosis may be difficult but usually can be made by stepwise logical progression based on the pattern of abnormalities seen in the activated partial thromboplastin time (APTT)/prothrombin time (PT), fibrinogen, and thrombin clotting time (TCT) results.

4. Early intracerebral bleeding can complicate a number of these conditions, so rapid diagnosis and treatment are essential.

Introduction

Rare inherited bleeding disorders comprise deficiencies of fibrinogen, factor II, factor V, combined factors V and VIII, factor VII, factor X, and factor XIII and make up 3 to 5 percent of all inherited bleeding disorders. There is marked clinical heterogeneity even among those with the same factor deficiency, and together with the rarity of these disorders, the diagnosis and management can be challenging. Table 28.1 highlights important features of these disorders.

Fibrinogen

- Fibrinogen is produced in the liver and is composed of three polypeptide chains α, β, and γ. Fibrin is produced by proteolytic cleavage of fibrinogen by thrombin and the release of fibrinopeptides A and B and generation of insoluble fibrin monomer followed by polymerization.

- Besides its primary role in the formation of a blood clot, fibrinogen also plays an important role in primary hemostasis for normal platelet aggregation.

- Fibrinogen disorders are classified according to quantitative or qualitative defects. Afibrinogenemia is total absence of fibrinogen by an antigenic assay. Children with a fibrinogen level of <1 g/liter are classified as hypofibrinogenemia. Dysfibrinogenemia is characterized by structural abnormalities of the fibrinogen molecule resulting in altered function.

- The incidence of dysfibrinogenemia is unknown, but it is likely underdiagnosed and underreported.

Bleeding Manifestations

Afibrinogenemia has a variable bleeding tendency ranging from life-threatening or spontaneous bleeding events to long periods without any bleeding episodes. Bleeding from the umbilical cord is the most common presentation in the neonatal period. Mucosal bleeding, musculoskeletal bleeds, hemarthroses, and menorrhagia are some of the other bleeding manifestations seen in this condition. Spontaneous intracranial hemorrhage and intraabdominal bleeding have been reported. In hypofibrinogenemia, the bleeding pattern is similar but has a milder course. Afibrinogenemia and hypofibrinogenemia are associated with recurrent miscarriages, and in afibrinogenemia, impaired wound healing is reported. The clinical phenotype of dysfibrinogenemia is unpredictable. Paradoxically, certain phenotypes are in fact associated with a thrombotic tendency unrelated to replacement therapy, and unusual thrombosis at a young age may be the presenting feature.

Diagnosis

The screening tests – prothrombin time (PT), partial thromboplastin time (PTT), and thrombin time

Table 28.1 Characteristics of Rare Bleeding Disorders

Factor deficiency	Estimated prevalence	Inheritance	Half-life	Suggested hemostatic level	Licensed product/product of choice
Afbrinogenemia	1: 1 million	Autosomal recessive (AR) Autosomal dominant (AD)	3–5 days	0.5–1 g/liter	Plasma-derived fibrinogen concentrate
Dysfibrinogenemia	Unknown/ underreported				
II	1: 2 million	AR	3 days	20–30%	None, prothrombin complex concentrate (PCC)
V	1: 1 million	AR	12–36 h	15%	Fresh frozen plasma (FFP)
VII	1: 3 million	AR	3–6 h	10–15%	Recombinant FVIIa
X	1: 1 million	AR	40 h	10–20%	None, PCC
XI	1: 1 million 1:12	AR Ashekenazi Jews	50–80 h	15–20%	FXI concentrate
XIII	1: 1 million	AR	9–14 days	2–5%	Plasma-derived FXIIII concentrate/ recombinant FXIII concentrate in clinical trial

(TT) – are prolonged. Reptilase time can be used to distinguish between fibrinogen disorders and heparin contamination and is prolonged in patients with hypo- or dysfibrinogenemia. Fibrinogen levels are usually low. In afibrinogenemia, the fibrinogen level is undetectable by both the antigenic and functional assays. In hypofibrinogenemia, the antigen and functional level are reduced to the same degree. The TT is the most sensitive test for dysfibrinogenemia. Diagnosis depends on documenting a difference between functional and antigenic fibrinogen assays. A definitive diagnosis requires the demonstration of a molecular defect and these tests are commercially available. Family studies are helpful.

Management

The normal plasma concentration of fibrinogen is 1.5 to 3.5 g/liter.

1. *Fibrinogen concentrate.* Virally inactivated plasma-derived fibrinogen concentrate is the product of choice. The pediatric dose is 30 to 100 mg/kg administered intravenously depending on the severity and site of bleeding. The suggested amount of fibrinogen required is

$$\text{Dose(g)} = \text{desired increment in g/liter} \times \text{plasma volume}[0.07 \times (1 - \text{hematocrit}) \times \text{weight in kg}]$$

2. The aim in spontaneous bleeding is to increase the fibrinogen level above 1 g/liter until hemostasis is achieved and above 0.5 g/liter until wound healing is complete.
No recommendations for primary prophylaxis exist. Secondary prophylaxis is recommended after a life-threatening bleed. The frequency and dose of fibrinogen concentrate sufficient to maintain a trough level >0.5 g/liter may be used. Generally, weekly infusions are given in children with afibrinogenemia.

3. Anaphylactic reactions and neurologic complications (specifically strokes) have been reported as side effects of fibrinogen concentrate infusions in children with afibrinogenemia.

4. *Cryoprecipitate.* This is a good source of fibrinogen but is not first-line therapy because it is not virally inactivated. If fibrinogen concentrate is not available, 1 bag of

cryoprecipitate (containing 150 to 250 units of fibrinogen) is given per 5 to 10 kg of weight.

5. *Fresh frozen plasma (FFP).* The use of FFP in this condition is restricted to emergencies because large volumes are required.

6. *Antifibrinolytics/other supportive therapy.* These should be used with caution, especially in patients with additional risk factors for thrombosis. Combined oral contraceptive pills can be used in girls with menorrhagia, but it has been associated with precipitating thrombotic events in girls with dysfibrinogenemia.

7. Thrombosis associated with dysfibrinogenemia will require anticoagulation therapy and long term prophylaxis may be required.

Prothrombin

- Prothrombin is a vitamin K–dependent coagulation factor synthesized in the liver.
- Activated factor X (FXa) activates prothrombin on the surfaces of platelets, releasing an activation peptide fragment 1.2.
- Deficiency is either quantitative (hypoprothrombinemia) or qualitative (dysprothrombinemia). Hypoprothrombinemia is reported as an autosomal recessive disorder.
- Prothrombin deficiency is probably more commonly an acquired defect, occurring in some children with antiphospolipid antibodies, and it is associated with severe bleeding. Steroids are usually required to suppress the antibody to enable control of bleeding, and fortunately, the antibodies are usually transient.

Bleeding Manifestations

Severe deficiency is associated with levels of between 4 and 10 percent. The most common bleeding manifestations are hemarthroses and muscle hematomas. Bleeding from the umbilical cord, intracranial hemorrhage, menorrhagia, and oral bleeding after dental surgeries are also reported.

Diagnosis

Screening tests PT and PTT are prolonged, but the fibrinogen level is normal. Diagnosis is established by a prothrombin assay.

Management

No specific replacement products are licensed for use.

1. *Prothrombin complex concentrates (PCCs).* PCCs contain prothrombin. Thus, 1 unit of PCC/kg will likely raise the plasma prothrombin level by 1 IU/dL. Levels of 20 to 30 IU/dL are thought adequate for normal hemostasis, and doses of 20 to 30 IU/kg have been used. Higher doses may be required depending on the nature of the surgery and the bleeding event. The long half-life facilitates dosing every 2 to 3 days.

2. *Fresh frozen plasma (FFP).* In the absence of PCCs, FFP can be used. Prothrombin has a plasma half-life of approximately 3 days, and treatment can be effective without a significant volume overload. A dose of 15 to 20 ml/kg will raise the prothrombin level by 25 percent.

3. *Antifibrinolytics.* These can be used for mucosal bleeds, and combined with oral contraceptive pills may control menorrhagia. Antifibrinolytics should be used with caution when used in conjunction with PCCs because they can increase the risk of thrombosis.

Factor V

- Factor V (FV) circulates in the plasma as a single-chain polypetide.
- Platelet FV is partially proteolyzed and is stored in alpha-granules. Platelets contain 20 percent of total circulating FV.
- Factor V is activated by thrombin, and FVa acts as a cofactor for FXa in the conversion of prothrombin to thrombin. Factor V is inactivated by activated protein C.
- The gene for FV is located on 1q24.2.
- The North American Rare Bleeding Disorders Group classifies FV deficiency (based on FV levels) as mild (>20 percent), moderate (1 to 19 percent), and severe (<1 percent).
- Structural homology exists between FV and FVIII molecules.

Bleeding Manifestations

Homozygous FV deficiency is a moderately severe bleeding disorder, and patients present at an early age, generally before the age of 6 years. The usual presenting features of FV deficiency are bruising and mucous membrane bleeding. Bleeding after dental extractions and surgery has been reported. Hemarthroses and intracranial, umbilical stump, and muscle bleeding can occur in patients with severe bleeding. Menorrhagia is usually very problematic in the teenage years.

Diagnosis

PT and PTT are prolonged. Diagnosis is established by FV activity assay. Patients with low FV levels also should have their FVIII levels determined to exclude a combined FV and FVIII deficiency. Factor V genetic testing is not available for clinical use.

Management

1. *Fresh frozen plasma (FFP).* FFP is the only product available for replacement of actual factor V levels, but factor eight inhibitor bypass activity (FEIBA) and recombinant factor VIIa (rFVIIa) both have been used successfully in this condition. Recommended dose of FFP is 15 to 20 ml/kg. Close monitoring of the FV levels may be necessary to determine factor half-life in individual patients and guide further therapy. Daily infusions are required for patients with severe bleeding. Inhibitor development to FV is a potential complication of hereditary FV deficiency. This can occur after exposure to bovine thrombin or FFP. In this situation, FEIBA and rFVIIa are alternative treatments.

2. *Platelet transfusion.* If bleeding is not controlled with FFP, platelet transfusions can be considered because the transfused platelets will have FV within their alpha granules. Recent studies have suggested this might be a preferable treatment to FFP because Platelet associated FV is thought to be more hemostatic than plasma derived FV, as well as being resistant to inactivation by inhibitors.

3. *Antifibrinolytic agents.* Adjuvant therapies with antifibrinolytic agents (amicar and aminocarproic acid) can be used in children with mucocutaneous bleeding.

Additional Important Information

Combined deficiency of FV and FVIII is inherited as a rare autosomal recessive disorder. This is due to a single-gene defect encoding for the ERGIC-53 protein, which plays a role in the trafficking of FV and FVIII. The bleeding manifestations in these individuals are similar to individuals with deficiencies of either factor alone at similar levels. The treatment depends on the nature and severity of the bleeding and the FV and FVIII levels. Bleeding is treated with FVIII concentrates and FFP or both. For minor bleeding episodes, FVIII levels should be raised to at least 30 to 50 percent and for more severe bleeds, they should be raised to at least 50 to 70 percent.

Factor VII

- FVII is one of the vitamin K–dependent coagulation proteins.
- Inherited FVII deficiency is the most common of the rare coagulation disorders.
- The gene for FVII is located on chromosome 13q34. Nearly 120 different mutations have been described, of which missense mutations account for 70 to 80 percent of mutations.
- Factor VII levels are influenced by both environmental and genetic factors. Among the environmental factors, dietary fat intake and levels of fat triglycerides are positively correlated with FVII levels. Age, obesity, diabetes, and use of oral contraceptive pills also influence FVII levels.

Bleeding Manifestations

There is poor correlation between FVII levels and bleeding manifestations. Usually patients with plasma levels < 2 percent have severe bleeding and those with levels > 20 percent are asymptomatic. However, there are reported cases of patients with levels between 20 to 50 percent having severe bleeding and those with levels of <1 percent being asymptomatic. Epistaxis, gum bleeding, and menorrhagia are common. Joint bleeds have been reported. Intracranial hemorrhage can occur in the newborn period. Paradoxically, thrombotic episodes have been reported after surgery, but spontaneous thrombotic events also may occur.

Diagnosis

An isolated prolongation of PT points toward the diagnosis of FVII deficiency. Additionally, the diagnosis can be confirmed by estimating the FVII:C levels. Vitamin K deficiency or other acquired causes such as liver disease must be excluded before the diagnosis can be made. In cases of ambiguity, parental studies can be completed. Genetic testing for FVII deficiency is not readily available for clinical use.

Management

1. *Recombinant FVIIa (rFVIIa, Novoseven).* rVIIA is the treatment of choice for bleeding related to FVII deficiency. A smaller dose of 15 to 30 μg/kg is used for surgical procedures compared, with a higher dose used for FVIII deficiency with inhibitors. A FVII level of 10 to 15 percent is often sufficient to achieve hemostasis. For major surgery, the trough level should be maintained above 20 percent. However, given the previous discussion of the lack of correlation between plasma levels and clinical phenotype, the actual levels aimed for in any patient may need to be individually determined. Because of its short half-life, the dose needs to be repeated every 4 to 6 h. High-potency and long-acting FVII is in clinical trials.

2. *Fresh frozen plasma (FFP).* Due to the availability of rFVII product, FPP is not recommended for managing patients with FVII deficiency due to the risk of viral transmission and volume overload. In an emergency and where recombinant product is not available, the dose of FFP is 10 to 20 ml/kg.

3. *Supportive therapy.* Topical hemostatic agents and systemic antifibrinolytics are used either alone or in conjunction with factor replacement therapy.

Factor X

Factor X (FX) plays a key role in the coagulation pathway, being the first enzyme in the common pathway and the most important activator of prothrombin. Factor X is a vitamin K–dependent protein synthesized in the liver, and it circulates in the plasma as a two-chain protein. The gene for FX is located on chromosome 13q34.

Bleeding Manifestations

Classification of the severity of FX deficiency is based on FX: C activity measurements: <1 percent is severe, 1 to 5 percent is moderate, and 6 to 10 percent is mild. Levels above 20 percent are infrequently associated with bleeding.

The most frequent symptom is epistaxis, and it is seen with all severities of deficiency. Heterozygous individuals are usually clinically asymptomatic. However, some do have a bleeding tendency with easy bruising or menorrhagia. Moderately affected individuals may bleed only after hemostatic challenges such as trauma or surgery. Patients with severe deficiency tend to be more severely affected. Bleeding due to FX deficiency can present at any age; in the neonatal period, babies can present with umbilical stump bleeding. Hemarthrosis and intracranial hemorrhage have been reported, and recurrent joint bleeds may result in severe arthropathy.

Diagnosis

The diagnosis is suspected when both the PT and PTT are prolonged. Russell viper venom time (RVVT) is also prolonged. The diagnosis is confirmed by performing the FX activity assay. Exclusion of vitamin K deficiency, liver disease, and a consumptive process such as disseminated intravascular coagulation (DIC) is essential before the diagnosis of FX disease can be made. Family studies help in making the diagnosis in some cases.

Management

There is no FX concentrate available in the United States. Factor levels of 10 to 20 percent are generally sufficient for hemostasis. The half-life of FX is 40 to 45 h.

1. PCCs contain FX and are effective in controlling bleeding. Thus, 1 IU/kg raises the FX level by 1.5 percent, and a dose of 20 to 30 units/kg is adequate to control bleeding. In major bleeding, every-other-day dosing is sufficient. Children with repeated hemarthroses may benefit from prophylaxis once or twice a week.

2. *Fresh frozen plasma (FFP).* Because the half-life varies in individuals, postoperative dosing should be guided by measurement of FX levels. A loading dose of 10 to 20 ml/kg of FFP, followed by 3 to 6 ml/kg twice daily, will usually achieve trough levels above 10 to 20 percent.

3. *Supportive therapy* with antifibrinolytic agents – aminocaproic acid and tranexamic acid can be used to control mucocutaneous bleeding. Suppression of menstruation may be required in teenage girls.

Factor XI

- FXI is a serine protease whose function is to recruit the intrinsic pathway after the tissue factor pathway has generated thrombin.
- FXI deficiency occurs in all racial groups but is particularly common in Ashkenazi Jews, in whom the carrier frequency is 8 percent.
- The gene for FXI is located on chromosome 4q35.2. Three independent point mutations have been described. Mutations either disrupt normal mRNA splicing (type 1), cause premature polypeptide termination (type 2), or result in a specific amino acid substitution (type 3). Most individuals have a stop codon in exon 5 (type 2) or a missense mutation in exon 9 (type 3). Several other mutations have been reported in other racial groups.

Bleeding Manifestations

Children with FXI deficiency do not suffer from spontaneous bleeding events or hemarthroses. The bleeding with FXI deficiency is generally provoked by hemostatic challenges such as surgeries. The bleeding risk is also not as clearly influenced by the severity of deficiency. Additionally, bleeding tendency may depend on levels of other coagulation factors such as FVIII:C and von Willebrand factor (vWF). Heterozygous women may have menorrhagia and bleeding after childbirth. Severely deficient individuals may have a bleeding tendency after surgery, especially in areas with high fibrinolytic potential, such as the mouth and nose and the genitourinary tract. Paradoxically, some individuals do not have a bleeding tendency at all. This condition rarely presents in the neonatal period, and intracranial hemorrhage has not been reported, although infants may bleed after circumcision.

Diagnosis

The APTT is prolonged, and diagnosis is established by the FXI assay. Children with mild to moderate deficiency have FXI:C levels between 15 and 20 percent, and those with severe deficiency FXI:C have levels <10 to 15 percent. Genetic testing for known FXI mutations is available.

Management

The unpredictable bleeding nature of FXI deficiency makes management of this disorder challenging.

1. *FXI concentrates* (plasma derived) are available but have been reported to cause thrombosis, especially in older patients with other risk factors.
2. *Fresh frozen plasma* (FFP) 15 to 20 ml/kg that is type specific as an alternative is acceptable. A level of FXI of 30 percent is likely adequate for surgery, but for surgical patients with a bleeding tendency, a level of 70 percent is reasonable.
3. *Antifibrinolytic agents.* Dental extractions can be managed with antifibrinolytic agents such as tranexamic acid or epsilonaminocaprioc acid (EACA, Amicar). These have to be started the night before the surgery and continued for 7 days after the procedure.
4. *Recombinant FVIIa (rFVIIa, Novoseven)* has been used but is also known to cause thrombotic events and not recommended for use in these patients. No optimal dose is known.
5. *Desmopressin (DDAVP).* No clear role of DDAVP in the management of FXI deficiency has been established.

Factor XIII

- FXIII is a tetramer made of two catalytic A subunits and two carrier B subunits linked by noncovalent bonds. The A subunit has the thrombin cleaving site, and the B subunits are cleaved away when FXIII molecule is activated. The activated molecule stabilizes fibrin by cross-linking the strands.
- The gene for FXIII subunit A is present on chromosome 6p25.1, while the gene for FXIII subunit B is located on 1p13.3. Most mutations associated with FXIII deficiency have been described for the A subunit, and almost 50 percent of molecular defects responsible for a subunit deficiency are missense mutations.

Bleeding Manifestations

Heterozygous patients are asymptomatic, and homozygous individuals have a variable clinical severity. Homozygote neonates tend to bleed excessively from the umbilical stump and classically the bleeding is delayed to day 5-10. Affected infants are at high risk for intracranial hemorrhage. Bruising and bleeding are common, and affected patients have muscle and joint bleeding. Miscarriages can occur in affected women. FXIII deficiency also causes delayed wound healing. Patients with FXIII activity levels < 10 percent are at high risk of major spontaneous bleeding such as intracranial and gastrointestinal bleeding, suggesting that this is a target level for prophylaxis. Patients with levels > 40 percent remain largely asymptomatic, and those with levels between 10 and 40 percent only suffer minor spontaneous or triggered bleeding.

Diagnosis

The usual screening tests – PT, PTT, and TT – are normal. Hence, high levels of clinical suspicion are required in appropriate circumstances, and specific tests must be organized. Any infant with bleeding from the umbilical stump, especially if delayed to days 5 to 10, should be suspected of FXIII deficiency and tested. While there are other causes of umbilical stump bleeding, if not detected, the rate of intracranial hemorrhage in untreated FXIII deficiency is high. The clot solubility test is the most commonly available qualitative screening test. The principle of the test is that fibrin clots in the presence of FXIII and thrombin stay for at least 1 h in 2% acetic acid or 5 mol/liter urea solution; whereas clots in the absence of FXIII dissolve rapidly. The clot solubility test has poor sensitivity and only detects levels below 1 percent. However, because the level of activity required for adequate hemostasis is low, this is suitable for most cases. Confirmatory diagnosis is obtained by a direct assay of FXIII (enzyme-linked immunosorbent assay [ELISA]), and in many centers this is now the front-line test.

Management

Individuals with severe deficiency should be offered prophylaxis because of the risk of intracranial hemorrhage (ICH). The increase after infusion of 1 unit/kg of FXIII concentrate is by approximately 1.6 percent.

1. *Plasma-derived FXIII concentrate.* Virally inactivated and plasma-derived FXIII concentrate is the treatment of choice. A prophylactic dose of 20 to 30 units/kg is given every 4 to 6 weeks because of the long half-life of FXIII. Treatment of an acute bleeding episode requires administration of a dose of up to 35 units/kg. Further treatments at 24- to 48-h intervals should be given until bleeding has stopped. For ICH, FXIII levels should be maintained in the normal range for a minimum of 2 weeks.

2. *Cryoprecipitate.* Cryoprecipitate is used in the absence of FXIII concentrate availability. One bag of cryoprecipitate contains 75 units of FXIII and can be given for every 10 kg of patient weight.

3. *Fresh frozen plasma (FFP).* FFP is rarely used because of other safer alternatives and the large volumes required.

4. *Recombinant FXIII A2 subunit concentrates.* These are in phase III clinical trials (NCT00713648) and appear safe and effective for the prevention and treatment of bleeding. This product is available for compassionate use.

Chapter 29

Acquired Bleeding Disorders

1. Acquired bleeding disorders present unexpectedly in the absence of a previous history of bleeding.

2. Careful history, examination, and investigation help to distinguish between congenital and acquired bleeding disorders.

3. Acquired bleeding disorders can affect platelets, coagulation proteins, or both.

4. Laboratory tests of hemostasis test individual components of coagulation and have limited ability to predict overall bleeding risk when multiple components of the coagulation system are abnormal.

5. Thromboelastography (TEG) and rotational thromboelastometry (ROTEM) provide information on different phases of coagulation in whole blood simultaneously but there is little data to demonstrate their clinical utility outside of some specific circumstances in children.

Introduction

The physiology of coagulation is described in detail in chapter 2. However, to reiterate briefly, hemostasis is a complex process that stops bleeding after a cut/breach in the vessel wall. Hemostasis is traditionally divided into a primary hemostatic process that involves vessel vasoconstriction, exposure of endothelial prothrombotic materials, and platelet activation and adhesion resulting in the formation of a platelet plug. The secondary hemostatic process involves activation of the clotting cascade resulting in the formation of a fibrin clot. Tertiary hemostasis involves activation of the fibrinolytic pathway. Inhibitors of hemostasis include physiologic (protein C, protein S, and antithrombin), acquired, and iatrogenic (medications) causes. Multiple mechanisms can cause defects in the preceding pathways, resulting in acquired bleeding disorders. Specific acquired bleeding disorders (e.g. acquired von Willebrand disease (vWD) and acquired hemophilia) are covered in Chapters 26 and 27 respectively. This chapter will discuss other acquired bleeding disorders.

When to Consider an Acquired Bleeding Disorder

Acquired bleeding disorders usually present unexpectedly in children without a previous history of a bleeding disorder. Many specific acquired bleeding disorders, such as idiopathic thrombocytopenic purpura (ITP- described in Chapter 22), occur in previously well children without any particular clinical warning. However, other acquired bleeding disorders occur most commonly in children in whom there are substantial other medical or surgical problems. Thus, in a child with trauma, complex medical or surgical illness, organ failure, or on medications, the risk of bleeding from acquired hemostatic disorders should be considered. The history and physical examination provide important clues and should include

- Age at onset of bleeding. Generally, onset at an older age is suggestive of an acquired bleeding disorder. However, it is important to rule out milder congenital bleeding disorders (e.g. mild hemophilia A or B and vWD) because patients with these disorders may not yet have not had previous hemostatic challenges.
- What is the bleeding pattern? Spontaneous or secondary to surgical challenges, a single episode or recurrent bleeding, skin/mucous membrane bleeding (e.g. epistaxis, petechial), or muscle/joint bleeding/bleeding into an organ.

Table 29.1 Screening Coagulation Tests and Their Interpretation

Test result	Coagulation factors potentially responsible for clinical bleeding	Possible acquired causes
Prothrombin time (PT)/partial thromboplastin time (PTT) normal	Factor XIII deficiency vWD	Drugs (Na valproate) Acquired vWD (cardiopulmonary bypass [CPB] circuits)
PT prolongation	Factor VII deficiency, congenital, acquired, or with inhibitors	Vitamin K deficiency[a] Liver disease Warfarin therapy
PTT prolongation	Factors VIII, IX, XI, and XII deficiency, congenital, acquired, or with inhibitors	Heparin contamination Unfractionated heparin (UFH) therapy Lupus anticoagulant (LAC)/anti-phospholipid antibodies (APLAs)
Both PT and PTT prolongation	Factors V, X, and II, fibrinogen deficiency, congenital, acquired, or with inhibitors	Disseminated intravascular coagulation (DIC) Dilutional coagulopathy Vitamin K deficiency[a]
Mixing test 1:1 patient plasma and normal plasma	Complete correction in coagulation factor deficiencies	Partial correction with inhibitors; inhibitors may be specific factor inhibitors or LAC

Note: Further investigations, including fibrinogen, TT, D-dimers, and full blood evaluation (FBE), as well as clinical details, are helpful in differentiating between the alternatives.
[a] Vitamin K deficiency may initially prolong the PT alone, but as the disease progresses, both the activated partial thromboplastin time (APTT) and the prothrombin time (PT) are prolonged.

- Coexisting medical conditions, including liver disease and renal disease (which might be more occult).
- Medications that might cause bleeding.

Laboratory diagnostic testing will make the diagnosis, and the usual tests described in previous chapters will be employed in these disorders (Table 29.1).

Acquired Platelet Disorders

1. *Thrombocytopenia*. This is one of the most common causes of acquired bleeding. Neonatal thrombocytopenia and immune thrombocytopenia are discussed in detail in Chapters 7 and 22 respectively. Careful examination of the blood smear will help to distinguish spurious thrombocytopenia due to ethylenediaminetetraacetic acid (EDTA)–induced platelet clumping from true thrombocytopenia. Repeating the blood count in citrate will confirm EDTA-induced platelet clumping.

2. *Antiplatelet agents*. Aspirin use in pediatrics is restricted to selected medical conditions,

specifically stroke treatment and prevention and management of Kawasaki disease. However, other antiplatelet agents such as clopidogrel are used increasingly in pediatric cardiology patients. When used alone or in combination with nonsteroidal anti-inflammatory drugs (NSAIDs), antiplatelet agents can cause bleeding symptoms. The mechanism of action of different antiplatelet therapy is shown in Figure 29.1. Major bleeding is treated with transfusion of normal platelets and discontinuation of antiplatelet therapy. Aspirin inhibits platelets for their entire lifespan and needs cessation 10 days prior to elective procedures if its effect is to be fully reversed. Aspirin and NSAIDs are not as commonly associated with gastric irritation or ulceration as in adults, but especially in children on concurrent steroid therapy, consideration should be given to the potential for gastrointestinal blood loss.

3. *Uremia*. Bleeding in uremia is thought to be primarily due to a defect in primary hemostasis because both bleeding time and platelet adherence are altered in uremia. Other factors such as

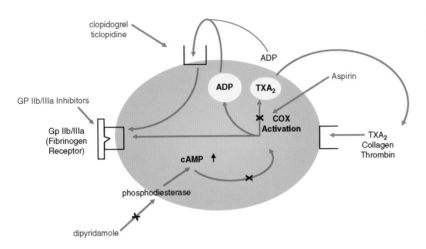

Figure 29.1 Mechanism of action of antiplatelet agents.

abnormal von Willebrand factor (vWF), abnormalities of platelet–platelet interaction, and parathyroid hormone abnormalities have been implicated but not substantially proven. Acute bleeding is treated symptomatically via red blood cell (RBC) transfusions, dialysis, or desmopressin (DDAVP) in a dose of 0.3 mg/kg. Conjugated estrogen has been used to treat subacute bleeding in a dose of 0.6 mg/kg intravenously for 5 days but is not helpful in the acute setting.

Acquired Coagulation Disorders

Just as congenital coagulation disorders can affect any component of the coagulation cascade, so can acquired disorders. Some affect individual factors, whereas many have broad effects on the plasma coagulation proteins, even if the bleeding manifestations are thought to be predominantly due to impact on specific factors (e.g. liver disease and vitamin K deficiency). A summary of acquired coagulation disorders is provided in Table 29.2.

Coagulation Factor Inhibitors

Acquired inhibitors can be seen with any coagulation factor, but the most common specific inhibitors are focused on FVIII, vWD, and FV. Acquired FVIII and vWD inhibitors are discussed in Chapters 26 and 27 respectively, and the others are listed in Table 29.1. Coagulation tests (PT/PTT) with a mixing study are performed to diagnose factor deficiency or the presence of an inhibitor. A mixing study is performed with a 1:1 mix of patient and normal plasma, which will correct in the presence of a factor deficiency but

will not in the presence of an inhibitor. On incubation for 1 h to 37°C, there will be further prolongation of PT/PTT in the presence of an inhibitor.

The most common cause of an acquired inhibitor is anti-phospholipid antibodies (APLAs) or a lupus anticoagulant (LAC), which are not specific to a particular coagulation factor but rather directed against a range of coagulation factor and phospholipid complexes. APLAs and LAC are rarely associated with clinical bleeding unless there is coexisting antiprothrombin antibody. Classically, APLAs and LAC are seen in children after minor viral infection, are transient (i.e. <3 months' duration), and are not associated with any bleeding or clotting tendencies. Less commonly in children, APLAs and LAC are autoimmune diseases that are longer lasting (i.e. >3 months) and may occur in isolation, in combination with ITP, or in combination with other autoimmune disease and in these cases are associated with a significant increased risk of thrombosis. Despite the prolonged APTT, there is no clinical bleeding. Following the positive mixing tests, confirmation of the LAC is achieved by a dilute Russell viper venom time (DRVVT) with a confirmatory phospholipid addition step. The principles of detecting a LAC are

1. Prolongation of a sensitive phospholipid-dependent coagulation test (different APTT reagents have different sensitivities to LAC)
2. Failure to correct on mixing with normal plasma
3. Correction with the addition of extra phospholipid

APLAs are detected by specific enzyme-linked immunosorbent assay (ELISA) against known epitopes and

Table 29.2 Acquired Coagulation Factor Deficiencies and Their Treatment

Acquired coagulation factor deficiency	Associated conditions	Laboratory tests	Bleeding	Treatment for bleeding
Reduced fibrinogen	Liver disorders Thrombolytic therapy DIC Dilutional coagulopathy	Prolonged PT and PTT	Usually with level < 1 g/l	Cryoprecipitate
Prothrombin (FII) inhibitor	APLAs Use of topical bovine thrombin	Prolonged PT and PTT Prolonged TT	–	Steroids for APLAs
FV inhibitor	Use of topical bovine thrombin	Prolonged PT and PTT	Variable	Fresh frozen plasma (FFP) and platelets
Reduced FVII	Vitamin K deficiency Liver disease	Prolonged PT	Variable	Recombinant factor VIIa (rFVIIa)
FXI inhibitor	Lupus	Prolonged PTT	Rare	FFP
Reduced FXIII	Drugs (e.g., valproate) Inflammatory bowel disease (IBD)	Normal PT and PTT, low FXIII level	Variable	FXIII concentrate

include β_2-glycoprotein and anti-cardiolipin and other antibodies.

Bleeding with Use of Anticoagulants

Bleeding can occur with the use of anticoagulants. Clinicians should remember that anticoagulants do not make a patient bleed. Patients bleed because they have a breach of their vascular endothelium. However, when on anticoagulation, breaches cannot be closed, and lesions that would otherwise be inconsequential can lead to life-threatening bleeding.

The two most commonly used agents in pediatrics are heparin (unfractionated and low-molecular-weight) and warfarin. Unfractionated heparin (UFH) has a narrow therapeutic window, and bleeding can also occur, even when in therapeutic range secondary to underlying comorbid conditions. Less common but potentially fatal bleeding can occur with inadvertent infusion of supratherapeutic doses of UFH or with errors in dilution and infusion rates. If bleeding with UFH is suspected, or if rapid reversal is needed, protamine is used as reversal agent along with

immediate discontinuation of the drip. See Chapter 33 for more details.

As with UFH, warfarin has a narrow therapeutic window and an unpredictable response to dose adjustments, making it difficult to maintain stable anticoagulation. Algorithms for reversal of the international normalized ratio (INR) in the presence or absence of bleeding are not specifically available for children and therefore are extrapolated from adult studies. See Chapter 33 for more details

Generally, patients presenting with major hemorrhage due to excessive warfarin anticoagulation require rapid reversal, usually achieved by either FFP (10 to 20 ml/kg) or Prothrombinex (30 units/kg). Vitamin K (30 µg/kg) should be administered to prevent rebound coagulopathy when the factor replacement wears off.

Asymptomatic patients (i.e. those with no bleeding symptoms with a high INR) are a challenge, and suggested guidelines are as follows:

INR > 8: Treat with an oral dose of vitamin K; usually 30 µg/kg is sufficient.

INR < 8: Discontinue warfarin; no other intervention but clinical and laboratory monitoring to follow decrease in INR is suggested.

Bleeding in Liver Disease

Bleeding is common in liver disease because it causes a disturbance in virtually all aspects of hemostasis.

- The liver is the major site of synthesis of procoagulants, anticoagulants, and components of the fibrinolytic system with the exception of vWF.
- It synthesizes thrombopoietin, which stimulates platelet production from megakaryocytes in the bone marrow.

There is a decrease in coagulation proteins that promote and inhibit coagulation, thrombocytopenia due to decreased production and from sequestration because of portal hypertension, and hypersplenism, as well as platelet function defects.

Fibrinogen, FVIII, and vWF levels are increased in inflammatory conditions, although whether their function remains normal is unclear. Although different causes of liver disease share the same general hemostatic pattern, there are differences between different types of liver disease. In both acute and chronic liver failure, there is a decrease in both procoagulants and anticoagulants, but the decrease is more pronounced in acute rather than chronic liver disease, and the abnormalities of INR are higher.

Laboratory tests of hemostasis assess individual components of the coagulation cascade and thus are severely limited in assessing the complex alterations that occur in liver disease (Table 29.3). Additionally, they do not measure the anticoagulants (protein S/protein C/antithrombin) or take into account the contribution of the endothelium. The INR is closely linked to liver synthetic dysfunction and has been used in algorithms that predict the severity of liver disease, but it is a poor predictor of bleeding risk. Whole-blood thromboelastography (TEG), rotational thromboelastometry (ROTEM), and thrombin generation are able to better assess hemostasis and especially to guide transfusion or predict the risk of postoperative thrombosis during liver transplantation. However, these tests are not available in all centers and require expertise to interpret. Whether they will have broader clinical value has yet to be tested.

Spontaneous bleeding can occur in liver disease, but more commonly there is variceal bleeding secondary to chronic liver disease/cirrhosis leading to portal hypertension and vascular alterations rather than coagulopathy. In acute liver disease, spontaneous bleeding is uncommon. Factors that may contribute to bleeding are the presence of infections and abnormal renal function. There are no consensus guidelines regarding blood product transfusion, transfusion parameters, or the goals to achieve in acute variceal bleeding episodes or prior to invasive procedures. Excess transfusion of packed RBCs may be deleterious because it can further increase portal venous pressure. Suggested ranges are hemoglobin > 8 g/liter, platelet counts > 50,000 to 60,000/liter, and fibrinogen level > 1 to 1.5 g/liter. Fresh frozen plasma should be used with caution because of the requirement of large volumes to correct suspected deficiencies.

Disseminated Intravascular Coagulation (DIC)

DIC is a syndrome of activation of the coagulation system causing consumption of clotting factors and platelets and increased thrombin generation. In reality, DIC is actually a disorder of the vascular endothelium that is most easily recognized by the resulting abnormalities in the coagulation system. There is widespread deposition of microthrombi, platelet activation, coagulation factor consumption, and secondary fibrinolysis. DIC may be associated with a hyperfibrinolytic state and bleeding or microvascular thromboses. In a specific patient, either bleeding or thrombotic tendency may predominate, but microvascular thrombosis causes progression to multiorgan failure.

Common causes of DIC in children include

- Sepsis
- Trauma
- Drowning
- Burns
- Acute promyelocytic leukemia.
- Neonatal asphyxia

DIC is diagnosed in the presence of an associated condition and coagulation laboratory abnormalities consisting of prolonged PT and PTT, decreased fibrinogen, and increased D-dimers and

Table 29.3 Common Tests of Hemostasis and Their Limitations in Liver Disease

Coagulation tests	Advantages	Disadvantages
PT	Readily available, quick, correlation with liver disease severity	Does not predict bleeding risk
PTT	Readily available, quick, inexpensive	Does not predict bleeding risk; does not correlate with liver dysfunction
Platelet function assay	Readily available, quick, inexpensive	Not studied in liver disease, can have false positives, not useful in the presence of thrombocytopenia
Fibrinogen level	Readily available, quick, inexpensive	Does not predict bleeding risk; low level can be seen in nonbleeding cirrhotic patients
Thromboelastography	Gives information on multiple components of hemostasis	Not readily available; requires expertise to interpret; not validated to predict bleeding or clotting risk
Thrombin generation	Gives information on both procoagulants and inhibitors	Not validated

thrombocytopenia. Scoring tools have been developed to assess severity, determine prognosis, and direct therapy. Early identification of DIC using scoring systems, as well as early and aggressive treatment of DIC and in particular the underlying disorder, can lead to improvements in patient outcome and reductions in mortality. The primary management of DIC is supportive and correction of the underlying clinical condition. Specific therapy should not be undertaken unless there is clinically significant bleeding or thrombosis. The role of blood component therapy is not to correct numbers but to address clinical bleeding or thrombosis.

Acquired Bleeding Disorders in the Intensive Care Setting

Acute Traumatic Coagulopathy (ATC)

This syndrome occurs as result of disruption of all components of hemostasis soon after trauma and is associated with a high mortality. Dysfibrinogenemia, impaired thrombin generation, hyperfibrinolysis, and platelet dysfunction are central to its pathogenesis and differ from DIC, which is primarily a consumptive process. Although prolonged coagulation tests, PT, and PTT poorly reflect the diagnosis of ATC, their presence nonetheless indicates a poor prognosis. Platelet counts may be normal because ATC primarily causes platelet dysfunction. TEG and ROTEM that evaluate global viscoelastic mechanical properties of whole blood are more commonly used assays and are

considered a more accurate measures of ATC in adults.

Resuscitation efforts using massive transfusion protocols have gained widespread acceptance in the management of ATC but are not well established in pediatrics. Management involves primarily paying close attention to the plasma-to-platelet-to-PRBC-transfusion ratio, and local institutional protocols should be followed.

Bleeding during Extracorporeal Membrane Oxygenation (ECMO)

Extracorporeal life support systems have evolved considerably during that last few decades, but bleeding complications can cause significant morbidity and mortality. The ECMO circuit causes activation of coagulation, including endothelial dysfunction, platelet activation, and thrombin generation and an acute inflammatory response. Bleeding complications in ECMO occur because of the following reasons:

1. *Systemic anticoagulation with unfractionated heparin.* The optimal test to monitor anticoagulation while on ECMO remains unknown. ACT, anti-Xa, APTT, and TEG have been used, but each test has limitations and variable applicability. Most centers use the activated clotting time (ACT) for monitoring, but values are influenced by factors other than UFH, including hemodilution, decreased clotting factors, thrombocytopenia, and platelet dysfunction. Because of the lack of an optimal

test for monitoring therapy, excess or not enough anticoagulation can result in bleeding complications.

2. *Thrombocytopenia and decreased platelet function.* There is platelet activation and aggregation due to shear forces and alterations in blood flow in the face of systemic anticoagulation. Microthrombi and continuous activation of coagulation lead to platelet consumption and thrombocytopenia and platelet dysfunction.

3. *Consumptive coagulopathy.* Interactions between blood and the circuit membrane cause activation of all components of hemostasis. Activation of the contact pathway occurs with adsorption of clotting proteins, mainly FXII, and ultimately the common pathway and thrombin generation. This, in turn, activates the fibrinolytic pathway. But both these pathways are not well regulated, causing thrombosis in the circuit and bleeding in the patient.

There may be generalized bleeding at multiple locations, including cannulation sites, chest tube insertion site, catheters, gastrointestinal, or localized to a particular organ. Management of the acute inflammatory response and dysregulation of hemostasis continues to be a challenge. Use of antifibrinolytic agents or prothrombin complex concentrates to control bleeding can cause thrombosis. Blood component therapy is frequently administered, and thresholds for transfusion in ECMO vary. Most centers target a hemoglobin > 100 g/l, platelet count > 100,000/liter, and fibrinogen concentration of > 1.5 to 2.0 g/liter.

Bleeding with Left Ventricular Assist Devices (LVADs)

Ventricular assist devices are increasingly used in children with end-stage cardiac failure refractory to medical therapy and as a bridge to heart transplantation. The choice of anticoagulation and monitoring depends on the type of LVAD implanted. High-intensity anticoagulant and antiplatelet therapy increases bleeding risk. Mechanisms of bleeding complications include aggressive anticoagulation/antiplatelet therapy, acquired vWD, gastrointestinal tract vascular malformations, and impaired platelet aggregation. Bleeding with LVADs is managed by deescalation of anticoagulant/antiplatelet therapy. Hemostatic agents are not commonly used because of the risk of increasing thrombotic complications.

1. Children appear to be protected from venous thrombosis compared with adults, in the sense that spontaneous thrombosis in children is rare, and the rates of thrombosis in children for similar stimuli are reduced compared with adults.

2. However, diagnosis of venous thrombosis is increasing in frequency, and it is predominantly a disease of tertiary pediatric care.

3. The most common precipitant of venous thrombosis in children is central venous access devices.

4. The role of primary prophylaxis to prevent venous thrombosis is often unclear and certainly is not similar to adult guidelines.

5. The most common use of primary prophylaxis is in children with congenital cardiac disease, although there remain many areas of controversy.

6. The natural history of venous thrombosis in many situations within pediatrics (especially neonates) remains unknown, so the risk-benefit ratio of treatment is difficult to judge. However, there is a clear morbidity and mortality associated with venous thrombosis.

7. Diagnostic algorithms used in adults cannot be directly extrapolated to children.

8. Pulmonary embolus is likely underdiagnosed in sick children.

9. There are almost no clinical outcome studies in children that confirm the optimal intensity or duration of anticoagulant therapy for venous thrombosis.

10. The significance of post-thrombotic syndrome in children remains unclear.

Introduction

The incidence of venous thromboembolism (VTE) in children at a population level is very low, reported to be 0.07 to 0.14 per 10,000 children. However, if one considers hospitalized children, the rate is 100 to 1,000 times increased to at least 58 per 10,000 admissions. Thus, despite some exceptions, VTE should be considered a disease of sick children. The most common age groups for VTE are neonates and teenagers, and this reflects the pattern of associated underlying diseases and interventions. The most common precipitating factor is the presence of central venous access devices (CVADs), which are related to almost 90 percent of VTE in neonates and more than 60 percent in older children. This association means that a large proportion of VTE in children occurs in the upper venous system (i.e. subclavian veins, internal jugular veins, brachiocephalic veins) in accordance with placement of CVADs as distinct from adults, in whom the overwhelming majority of VTE occurs in the ileofemoral system.

The natural history of VTE in children remains unclear in many circumstances. The reported VTE mortality from registry data is approximately 3 percent, in the context of approximately 16 percent of children dying from their underlying illness. The recurrence risk is variably reported up to 10 to 15 percent. Reports of post-thrombotic syndrome (PTS) vary from 10 to 60 percent depending on the tools used to assess for PTS, and there remains great controversy as to the clinical implications of PTS in many children.

Pulmonary embolus is likely underdiagnosed in sick children and, although rare, is often missed in well children who present with nonspecific, often transient symptoms. There are a number of organ-specific VTEs that are important to consider in children.

Clinical Presentations

For CVAD-associated VTE, the acute clinical symptoms, besides loss of CVAD patency, include swelling, pain, and discoloration of the related limb. If the CVAD is in the upper system, there may be swelling of the face and head with superior vena cava (SVC) syndrome. Venographic studies suggest that up to 20 to 30 percent of children with CVADs may develop VTE, and yet symptomatic VTEs occur in less than 5 to 6 percent of children. Respiratory compromise secondary to pulmonary embolism (PE) can occur, and stroke secondary to paradoxical emboli also can be the primary presentation in children with right-to-left shunts, such as children with congenital heart disease or neonates with patent foramen ovale. Right atrial thrombosis can present with signs of cardiac congestion. Children often do not present with any acute symptoms but rather long-term symptoms, including prominent collateral circulation in the skin over the related vessels, repeated loss of central venous line (CVL) patency, repeated requirement for CVL replacement, loss of venous access, CVL-related sepsis, chylothorax, chylopericardium, and PTS.

PE often presents in sick children with nonspecific cardiovascular compromise. In community-based children, the most common presentation is in teenage girls within the first 6 months of starting the oral contraceptive pill (OCP); the chest pain is often nonspecific, and shortness of breath or syncope may be transient. Persistent tachycardia may be a useful indicator, although more research is required to enhance clinical diagnosis.

Renal vein thrombosis classically presents acutely in neonates with a flank mass, hematuria, proteinuria, thrombocytopenia, and nonfunction of the involved kidney, or it may present later with renal dysfunction and hypertension

Portal vein thrombosis may present with acute abdominal pain but more often presents with portal hypertension, splenomegaly, and gastric and esophageal varices.

Diagnosis

Diagnostic algorithms and considerations of pretest probabilities have not been validated in children. VTE is a radiologic diagnosis, and ancillary tests (e.g. the presence or absence of thrombophilia and/or elevated D-dimers) should never be used as part of the diagnostic strategy. Objective radiologic studies must be used. There are numerous anecdotes of an apparent VTE actually being a mechanical obstruction or even an extravascular hematoma compressing the vessel. While sick children are often very difficult to image, every effort should be made to objectively prove a diagnosis of VTE before starting anticoagulant or other therapy.

Ultrasound (US) is the most common modality used in children, but its validity should be carefully considered. The low pulse pressure in premature newborns likely makes US more difficult to interpret. Similarly, the presence of CVADs makes compressibility difficult to assess, which greatly reduces the sensitivity of US. In the upper system, compressibility is not possible for veins below the clavicle, and the PAARKA study demonstrated US to have a sensitivity of 20 percent for intrathoracic thrombosis, yet it diagnosed jugular thrombi that were missed on venography. Linograms (contrast material injected through the CVAD) should never be used to diagnose VTE, most of which occur at the insertion site of the CVAD rather than at the CVAD tip.

In summary, for children with suspected upper system VTE, a combination of US (jugular veins) and bilateral upper limb venography (subclavian and central veins) is recommended. The temptation to extend US imaging below the clavicles should be resisted because of its reduced sensitivity in those veins. Magnetic resonance venography (MRV) may be a viable alternative to formal venography depending on local expertise. For children with suspected lower system thrombosis, US is a reasonable alternative for veins distal to the groin, based on adult experience. As in adults, serial US may be required to exclude VTE in specific circumstances. For more proximal veins, venography or MRV should be considered.

For renal vein thrombosis, US is the gold standard. For portal vein thrombosis, US is the most common modality used, although false-positive and false-negative results have been reported in comparison with contrast angiography.

A number of potential difficulties with interpreting ventilation-perfusion (V/Q) scans in children at risk of PE have been identified. In children following specific cardiac surgeries, such as Fontan surgery, total pulmonary blood flow is not assessed by isotope injected into an upper limb. Injection into both upper and lower venous systems is required, but even then the impact of intrapulmonary shunting may make interpretation difficult. In addition, there are concerns about the safety of perfusion scanning in children with significant right-to-left cardiac shunts because likely significant amounts of macroaggregated albumin will lodge in the cerebral circulation, and the impact of this is unknown. Reducing doses of isotope may be important in such children. Despite these concerns, V/Q scanning remains the recommended first-line investigation for PE in neonates and children. Pulmonary angiography remains the gold standard. Clinicians will frequently need to make a presumptive diagnosis based on clinical findings and the presence or absence of source thrombosis. Computed tomographic (CT) pulmonary angiography may be an alternative, but CT may miss small peripheral pulmonary emboli. Further, repeated CT angiograms may cause significant radiation exposure to breast tissue in young female patients. Adult-derived clinical probability scores and D-dimer measurements have not proven reliable in the only studies in children and should not be used.

Three studies have specifically compared transthoracic echocardiography (TTE) with transesophageal echocardiography (TEE) in the diagnosis of intracardiac thrombosis following Fontan surgery and found TTE to be significantly inferior to TEE. Despite this, right atrial thromboses, especially CVAD-related thromboses, are commonly diagnosed using TTE. Clinicians should consider the local expertise, availability of TEE, and the clinical situation before determining the diagnostic approach in any individual child. At present, there are no data to support the routine radiologic screening of asymptomatic children for VTE in any circumstance.

Treatment

The mainstay of treatment of VTE in children is anticoagulation therapy, and further details of this therapy are given in Chapter 33. Whether asymptomatic VTE requires treatment at all is unknown, and further studies are required. The current consensus is to treat all symptomatic VTEs, but in individual patients, especially neonates, where the bleeding risks of treatment may preclude safe therapy, observation and serial monitoring for extension may be optimal.

The three most common agents used in children to treat VTE are unfractionated heparin (UFH), low-molecular-weight (LMW) heparin (of which the most experience is with enoxaparin), and vitamin K antagonists (VKAs). A comparison of the pros and cons of these agents is provided in Table 30.1.

The duration of anticoagulation has been extrapolated from adult data, and for secondary VTE, 3 months of treatment is commonly used. In small infants with CVAD-related VTE, repeat imaging is often performed at 6 weeks, and anticoagulation is ceased at that time if there has been adequate resolution. There are currently no data to support this practice, although a multicenter trial is under way. Ongoing risk factors may require ongoing therapy at treatment or prophylactic levels. For spontaneous thrombosis, duration is often extended to 6 to 12 months.

Multiple new direct oral anticoagulants are currently being trialed in children, including direct factor Xa inhibitors such as rivaroxaban and apixiban, as well as direct thrombin inhibitors such as dabigatran. Until these studies are completed and safety and efficacy profiles are established, these agents should not be used outside of formal clinical trials.

Thrombolysis has at least a 10-fold increased bleeding risk over anticoagulation therapy and should not be used for VTE in children unless the VTE is life or limb threatening. While one study suggested reduced PTS with early thrombolysis, the risk-benefit ratio remains very questionable. If thrombolysis is considered, concurrent UFH and pretreatment with FFP have been suggested and seem reasonable. There seems little benefit of catheter-directed thrombolysis over systemic thrombolysis, and limiting the duration of infusion to less than 6 hours clearly reduces the bleeding rates.

Surgical thrombectomy is rarely indicated except in children with congenital heart disease who have obstructive VTE either within a venous shunt, circuit, or intracardiac. In some patients in whom anticoagulation may be contraindicated, surgical removal of thrombus may be indicated, although in general failure to anticoagulate as well leads to rapid recurrence.

The use of inferior vena cava filters in children remains controversial, and if required, removable filters should be used. These should be considered on an individual basis and in light of institutional experience, which clearly has an impact on success rates. In general, concurrent anticoagulation remains important.

Table 30.1 Common Anticoagulation Agents Used in Children

Agent	UFH	Enoxaparin	Vitamin K antagonists (VKAa)
Onset	Rapid onset/offset Ideal for critical children in whom surgical interventions may be required	Moderate onset/offset	Long onset/offset Requires heparinoid cover until levels are therapeutic
Mode of administration	Intravenous infusion only	Subcutaneous injection, usually twice daily	Oral daily
Excretion/ metabolism	Renal (beware renal impairment)	Renal (beware renal impairment)	Liver (beware liver impairment); critically dependent on vitamin K status of patient; beware changes from breast (vitamin K deficient) to formula (vitamin K replete) feeding
Reversibility	Easily reversible via stopping infusion or giving protamine; hence ideal for patients with very high bleeding risk	Not fully reversible even with protamine, so most useful in stable patients	Reversible with vitamin K (4–6 h) or more rapidly with fresh frozen plasma (FFP) or prothrombin concentrate
Monitoring	Bioavailability very variable; needs at least daily monitoring; venous blood required for APTT or anti-Xa	Relatively stable; can be monitored once or twice weekly once steady state; venous blood required for anti-Xa	Levels affected by multiple factors; requires regular monitoring (daily to 4 times weekly), which can be made easier by use of point-of-care capillary international normalization ratio (INR)
Duration	Suitable for short term only	Good safety data up to 3 months of treatment	Suitable for lifelong therapy, if required
Bleeding risk	Bleeding 1–24 percent depending on patient population; accidental overdose most common cause of fatal bleeding	Bleeding 1–20 percent depending on patient population; special precautions required around procedures, especially lumbar punctures	Bleeding 0.5–5 percent depending on service; formal anticoagulation clinics with high emphasis on patient/ parent education important
Other side effects	Osteoporosis reported with longer term use; heparin-induced thrombocytopenia (HIT) seems rare in children; allergic reactions; hair loss rare	Osteoporosis reported with longer term use; HIT rarely reported; allergic reactions uncommon; hair loss rare	Osteoporosis common in long-term patients, although cause-effect unproven; tracheal calcification and hair loss rare
Problems with current preparations	Wide range of concentrations used on same wards (50 up to 5,000 units/ml) and no standard packaging gives high probability of accidental overdose; calculation of infusion rates often difficult for inexperienced staff	Prefilled syringes in standard adult doses make weight-adjusted dosing difficult, especially for small infants	No oral suspension
Major current unknowns in children	Optimal therapeutic range; optimal monitoring test (APTT, anti-Xa, other)	Optimal therapeutic range and initial dosing strategies; safety and efficacy of once-daily enoxaparin	Optimal therapeutic range

Management of Post-Thrombotic Syndrome (PTS)

PTS is an important long-term complication of VTE, but it varies considerably in timing of onset and severity. Diagnosis can be difficult in the upper limb, where handedness often leads to subtle differences in limb size anyway. While many children have persistent collaterals and even some mild limb swelling, few seem to have functional impairment or pain. Currently, the Manco Johnson or modified Villata scales are recommended to assess the severity of PTS in children. While many children will have swelling and pain from the time of thrombosis onset, others will not develop symptoms until much later as the effects of gravity take over, for example, in toddlers who become upright in the months or year following their thrombosis. Other children first present with signs of PTS many years after the intervention that probably caused the VTE. All children with VTE probably require clinical follow-up for at least a number of years.

Early anticoagulation and limiting the size of the thrombus may be associated with reduced risk of PTS. The role of graduated compression stockings acutely is unknown, but they may be of benefit. In most centers, appropriate compression stockings are accessible for lower limb thrombosis, but for upper limb thrombosis they need to be specifically made for each child at considerable expense.

Once PTS is established, treatment is essentially supportive, including compression garments, elevating the limb when at rest or sleeping (for lower-limb PTS raising the foot of the bed by 3 to 4 centimeters is more effective than using padding under the specific affected leg), care to avoid injury (adequate footwear), and careful nail and foot hygiene to avoid infection. Encouraging activity to maintain fitness and optimal weight also may reduce symptoms. Monitoring for signs of venous eczema or ulceration and early aggressive treatment of any infection are important.

Prevention of VTE

In adults, there are numerous high-quality studies showing the benefits of primary thromboprophylaxis to prevent VTE in a number of clinical situations, including hospitalized patients, patients undergoing orthopedic and other surgery, and trauma patients. There are also many studies demonstrating the benefit of prophylactic anticoagulation to prevent intracardiac thrombosis and potential stroke in patients with conditions such as atrial fibrillation.

In neonates and children, the role of primary thromboprophylaxis is much less clear. The conditions for which thromboprophylaxis is commonly used in children include

1. Prosthetic cardiac valves
2. Pulmonary hypertension
3. Cardiomyopathy
4. Post-Fontan surgery and patients with artificial conduits
5. Children with long-term CVLs for infusion of home total parenteral nutrition (TPN)

There remains much controversy about the optimal strategy for a number of these groups.

Over recent years, there has been more interest in the broader concept of VTE prevention in hospitalized children, although the reported rates of VTE in hospitalized children makes widespread prophylaxis unlikely to be of benefit. Certainly there seems little rationale for thromboprophylaxis of any kind in pre-pubertal hospitalized children. For post-pubertal children, the illness-related factors that may need to be considered in risk stratification include the presence or absence of multitrauma and multiple fractures, hypotension or severe dehydration, and major surgery. The patient-related factors include morbid obesity, use of the OCP, positive family history, and potentially known thrombophilia. However, the optimal use of these risk factors to predict the need for prophylaxis and the risk-benefit ratio of mechanical prophyalxis (including early ambulation, compression stockings, and intermittent pneumatic compression) versus pharmacologic prophylaxis (usually LMW heparin) remains unknown. Further studies are required.

Conclusions

VTE in children is an important entity in tertiary hospital environments, but spontaneous VTE remains rare in children. There remains much to be learned about the optimal prevention strategies, diagnosis, and treatment of VTE in children. The clinical significance of asymptomatic VTE is particularly controversial. The mortality and morbidity from VTE justify significant efforts to improve our knowledge in these areas. The development of the direct oral anticoagulant drugs (DOACDs) and their successful introduction into adult clinical care will likely change the face of therapeutics in this field, but formal studies must be completed in children before these drugs can be used safely. In the meantime, UFH, LMW heparin, and VKAs remain the cornerstones of care. A better understanding of the natural history of VTE in neonates and children is arguably the most pressing research objective in the field.

Arterial Thrombosis in Children

1. Non-central nervous system (non-CNS) arterial thrombosis in children within tertiary pediatric hospitals occur with slightly less frequency than venous thrombosis.

2. Arterial thrombosis in children is predominantly iatrogenic - related to vascular access (arterial puncture or catheter placement).

3. Femoral artery thrombosis following cardiac catheter; peripheral artery thrombosis following arterial line placement, especially in neonates; and umbilical artery thrombosis, also in neonates, are the most common clinical situations encountered.

4. Thrombosis in arteries of transplanted solid organs is another significant clinical entity.

5. Spontaneous arterial thrombosis (including the aorta) can occur but is rare.

6. The degree of tissue ischemia depends on the degree of occlusion and the presence or absence of a collateral circulation.

7. Immediate removal of the catheter may restore blood flow and relieve distal ischemia, especially because any coexisting arterial spasm resolves over subsequent minutes to hours.

8. True rates of long-term consequences such as claudication or limb-length discrepancy (due to growth failure) remain unknown.

9. Peripheral artery disease as classically seen in vasculopathic adults is almost never seen in children.

10. Coronary artery thrombosis is almost always in the setting of giant aneurysms secondary to Kawasaki disease.

11. Initial anticoagulation with a heparinoid is often adequate therapy.

12. Thrombolysis or surgical intervention may be required if organ or limb infarction is imminent.

13. The optimal duration of anticoagulation therapy and the role of subsequent antiplatelet therapy remain unknown.

Introduction

The incidence of arterial thrombosis in children is reported to be less than that for venous thrombosis in tertiary pediatric populations, provided that one does not include CNS arterial events (see Chapter 32), which almost certainly are a separate entity. The factors causing arterial thrombosis in children are vastly different from those seen in adults, with iatrogenic arterial damage the overwhelming factor.

Arterial thrombosis is reported to occur in 1.2 percent of children in pediatric intensive care units secondary to arterial vascular access. Most data about incidence are specific to certain populations, with cardiac catheter–related femoral artery thrombosis being reported as a complication in 5 to 10 percent of procedures, with increased events in younger age groups. Clinically relevant peripheral artery thrombosis occurs in 1 to 3 percent of children requiring arterial access, but the actual rates of arterial occlusion may be much higher. The strong preference for only cannulating vessels that have dual supply (e.g. radial or ulnar arteries in the upper limb, posterior tibial or dorsalis pedis arteries in the lower limb) as distinct from end arteries such as the brachial artery means that many actual occlusions are asymptomatic and may never be diagnosed. Whether such asymptomatic occlusions have any long-term consequences for the patient remains unknown. In the neonates, aortic thrombosis secondary to umbilical arterial cannulation is well described. The natural history of iatrogenic vascular access is unclear, with initial (and ultimately self-resolving) vascular spasm a significant component in many cases. The true rate of long-term claudication or limb-length discrepancy remains uncertain, and this makes risk-benefit analysis for escalation of acute therapy very difficult.

The second most common iatrogenic situation in which arterial thrombosis occurs in children, after a complication of vascular access, is in the setting of solid-organ transplantation with thrombosis in the arteries of the transplanted organ (e.g. kidney or liver). Hepatic artery thrombosis is reported to occur as an acute complication of approximately 7 percent of pediatric liver transplants and has a significant impact on mortality and morbidity.

Of the non iatrogenic causes of arterial thrombosis, Kawasaki disease is by far and away the most important, with thrombosis in coronary artery giant aneurysms a significant concern. Spontaneous arterial thrombosis is reported, most commonly in neonates, and affecting either the aortic arch or distal aorta around the bifurcation, and whether this represents a developmental anomaly in these vessels remains unknown.

Symptomatic arterial vasculopathy related to hypertension, hyperlipidemia, and smoking is almost nonexistent in children. The pathogenesis of adult complications of these diseases clearly has its origins during childhood, with vessel changes detectable early in the teenage years. Attention to lifestyle during childhood and the need for population-based early interventions are obvious. However, with the exception of children with homozygous low-density lipoprotein (LDL) receptor deficiency, who, if untreated, often develop significant coronary artery lesions by their late teenage years, these long-term and important diseases of modern society do not have symptomatic presentations during childhood.

Femoral Artery Thrombosis

Cardiac catheterization, usually performed through the femoral artery, is the most common indication for gaining arterial access in children. In the absence of any prophylaxis, the rates of femoral artery thrombosis were said to be 40 percent, but since the seminal studies by Freed in the 1970s showing the benefits (thrombosis rates reduced to 8 percent) of unfractionated heparin(UFH) prophylaxis (and no benefit from aspirin prophylaxis), most children receive 100 units/kg bolus UFH at the start of the procedure. There have been studies suggesting that 50 units/kg is similarly effective, but most centers continue to use a 100 units/kg bolus, with further doses if the procedure continues beyond 60 to 90 minutes. In recent years, the rates of symptomatic femoral artery thrombosis have been reported to be 5 to 10 percent depending on patient size, patient hemodynamic status, operator technique, larger catheter size, total time of arterial cannulation, and procedural versus diagnostic catheters, which are all factors that affect the risk for arterial thrombosis. Long-term follow-up studies have suggested that up to 30 percent of children who have cardiac catheter will have evidence of occlusion of the relevant artery 5 to 14 years later or will have difficult access on subsequent procedures. Whether this long-term occlusion relates to thrombosis, stenosis or chronic scarring of the vessel from the traumatic puncture remains unknown.

Femoral artery thrombosis usually presents as a cold and pulseless limb following cardiac catheterization. Pulses may be absent or diminished. In severe cases, pain from limb ischemia may develop. Often the predominant symptoms are due to arterial spasm, and there is clinical resolution within hours of removal of the catheter. However, in this initial instance, distinguishing spasm from true thrombosis can be difficult, even with ultrasound imaging, and it is not unreasonable to start anticoagulation therapy immediately and observe carefully over the ensuing hours.

Long-term consequences of femoral artery thrombosis include leg-length discrepancies, muscle wasting, claudication, and loss of arterial access. Symptomatic ischemia may occur at times when the child experiences rapid growth, as occurs in the first year of life and during puberty.

Descriptions of treatment of femoral artery thrombosis in neonates or older children with thrombolytic therapy, anticoagulation, thrombectomy, or observation (no active therapy) consist exclusively of case series without comparison groups. The general practice in most children's hospitals is to initiate therapy with UFH, often just

209

starting an infusion without a bolus dose. Previous studies have reported that 70 percent of thromboses will resolve with UFH alone. Low-molecular-weight heparin (LMWH) may be a safe alternative in this situation, although the possible need for thrombolysis or surgery makes LMWH a less attractive option until after a couple of days of UFH therapy. In acute limb-threatening thrombosis, indirect evidence from adults supports the use of thrombolytic or surgical intervention.

The optimal duration of anticoagulation is unknown. Common practice is to treat for 7 to 14 days with heparinoid therapy and then cease, presuming that there are no ongoing major temperature or color differences between the limbs. Some centers subsequently transition to aspirin for 3 months. Recently, there has been some interest in monitoring the vessel with weekly ultrasound and continuing therapeutic LMWH until resolution of thrombus or for 3 months' duration, although there are no comparative studies, and the value of longer-duration therapy is unproven.

Peripheral Artery Thrombosis

Peripheral artery thrombosis usually presents with ischemic limb distal to the site of vascular interruption. A cold, pulseless distal limb, with or without impending gangrene and distal digit necrosis, is very common. This is most commonly seen in neonates but can be seen in any child in whom intraarterial access has been performed or attempted. Arterial access should at all times be restricted to dual-supply vessels unless there is no other way and the child's life cannot be saved without arterial access. When end vessels such as the brachial artery must be used, the most senior and skilled operator should be involved because there is no doubt that increased number of attempts to access the vessel dramatically increases the risk of acute thrombotic complications.

In terms of prophylaxis, most studies have examined interventions to prolong catheter patency as distinct from avoiding occlusive arterial thrombosis. Catheter patency was significantly prolonged for an UFH concentration of 5 units/ml compared with 1 unit/ml, UFH with normal saline versus dextrose flushes, and papaverine-supplemented compared with placebo-supplemented solutions. Thus, most guidelines recommend UFH 5 units/ml

as a continuous infusion through any indwelling peripheral artery cannula, but this purely relates to patency of the catheter and not to preventing arterial occlusion.

Once a symptomatic occlusion has occurred, immediate removal of the offending cannula often will lead to rapid improvement. The role of ultrasound or imaging in diagnosis and dictating therapy is unknown, and often decisions can be adequately made on clinical grounds. There is a suggested algorithm for ongoing assessment and management of these thromboses. In neonates especially, a surgical approach has fewer risks than thrombolysis, but this depends on the available local expertise. Local glyceryl trinitrate (GTN) patches are of no proven benefit (see Figure 31.1).

Aortic Thrombosis Secondary to Umbilical Artery Catheterization (UAC)

Aortic thrombosis secondary to UAC placement is said to occur in 1 to 3 percent of UACs placed. Duration of catheter insertion and the positioning of the UAC tip are important predictors of the rate of thrombosis. In general, it is recommended that the tip sit at the level of the T6 to T9 thoracic vertebral bodies. In this position, the catheter tip is placed above the celiac axis, superior mesenteric artery, and renal arteries and is therefore above the diaphragm on x-ray.

The clinical presentation of UAC-related thrombosis depends on the extent of the thrombosis but includes lower-limb ischemia, congestive cardiac failure, impaired renal function, and hypertension. Embolic events are also reported, and UAC thrombosis has been linked to the development of necrotizing enterocolitis (NEC). Longer-term outcomes include, persistent renovascular hypertension, and lower-limb growth abnormalities, and death.

Similar to the peripheral artery catheter situation, a number of studies have demonstrated that UFH infusion at 1 unit/ml enhances catheter patency, but there are no data on appropriate prophylaxis with respect to large-vessel thrombosis.

Treatment for UAC-induced aortic thrombosis includes acute anticoagulation with UFH followed by LMWH. The optimal duration of therapy remains unknown. If there is acute renovascular insufficiency or the lower limbs are threatened, thrombolysis or acute surgical thrombectomy may be appropriate

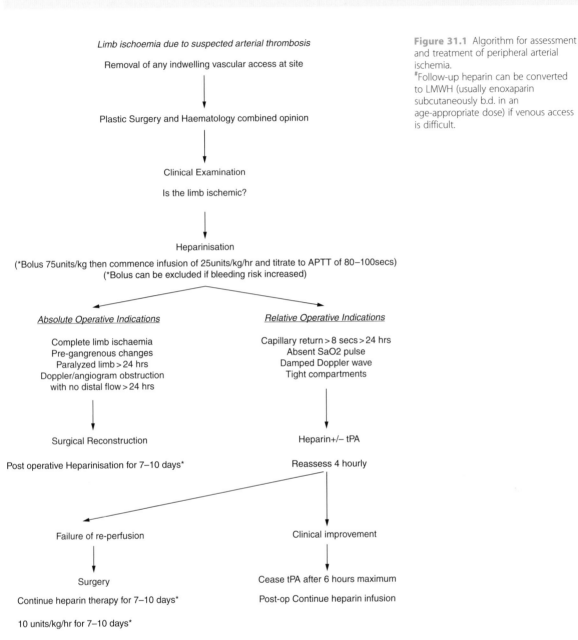

Limb ischoemia due to suspected arterial thrombosis

Removal of any indwelling vascular access at site

↓

Plastic Surgery and Haematology combined opinion

↓

Clinical Examination

Is the limb ischemic?

↓

Heparinisation

(*Bolus 75units/kg then commence infusion of 25units/kg/hr and titrate to APTT of 80–100secs)
(*Bolus can be excluded if bleeding risk increased)

Absolute Operative Indications

Complete limb ischaemia
Pre-gangrenous changes
Paralyzed limb > 24 hrs
Doppler/angiogram obstruction
with no distal flow > 24 hrs

↓

Surgical Reconstruction

Post operative Heparinisation for 7–10 days*

Failure of re-perfusion

↓

Surgery

Continue heparin therapy for 7–10 days*

10 units/kg/hr for 7–10 days*

Relative Operative Indications

Capillary return > 8 secs > 24 hrs
Absent SaO2 pulse
Damped Doppler wave
Tight compartments

↓

Heparin +/– tPA

Reassess 4 hourly

Clinical improvement

↓

Cease tPA after 6 hours maximum

Post-op Continue heparin infusion

Figure 31.1 Algorithm for assessment and treatment of peripheral arterial ischemia.
#Follow-up heparin can be converted to LMWH (usually enoxaparin subcutaneously b.d. in an age-appropriate dose) if venous access is difficult.

depending on local expertise. Whether there is a long-term role for subsequent antiplatelet therapy remains unknown.

Transplanted Vessel Thrombosis

Hepatic artery thrombosis after liver transplantation and renal artery thrombosis after kidney transplantation are acute and often devastating complications that immediately threaten graft viability. Factors involved include the grafting of adult-size vessels in smaller children and significant periods of hypotension in the postoperative period. These thromboses usually present with signs of acute graft failure or may be detected on routine imaging after the procedure. Acute renal artery thrombosis is often clinically indistinguishable from hyperacute rejection.

211

Often acute surgical intervention is required with thrombectomy and reanastomosis of the relevant vessels and subsequent anticoagulation to prevent recurrence. Thrombolysis is usually contraindicated due to the recent transplant surgery. Mortality rates can be high.

Kawasaki Disease

Kawasaki disease is the leading cause of acquired heart disease in children in Western populations, surpassing rheumatic heart disease, which remains more prevalent in developing countries. Classical Kawasaki disease has fever for more than 5 days, cervical lymphadenopathy, bilateral nonexudative conjunctivitis, rash, and peripheral desquamation. However, many children have atypical presentations that are nonspecific and involve fewer than all five classic features, making diagnosis difficult. During the acute phase, Kawasaki disease causes a medium- to large-vessel vasculitis that can result in coronary artery aneurysms in 20 to 25 percent of patients without initial treatment. Thrombosis of these aneurysms and subsequent coronary artery occlusion leading to myocardial infarction is common.

Initial therapy for Kawasaki disease includes intravenous gammaglobulin (single dose, 2 g/kg) and high-dose aspirin (100 mg/kg per day for 14 days), which dramatically reduce the risk of coronary artery aneurysm development to approximately 5 percent. However, once coronary artery dilation or giant aneurysms have formed, ongoing anticoagulation (UFH or LMWH followed by warfarin, target INR of 2.5 [range 2 to 3]) is often used in conjunction with long-term low-dose aspirin (3 to 5 mg/kg per day) until such time as resolution of the coronary artery abnormalities. Regular echocardiography is effective for monitoring the resolution of the coronary artery abnormalities.

Spontaneous Arterial Thrombosis

Arterial thrombosis not associated with vascular access or surgery for transplanted vessels is very rare in children. Anti-phospholipid antibody syndrome and nephrotic syndrome have rarely been described as presenting with spontaneous arterial thrombosis (e.g. mesenteric artery thrombosis). Spontaneous aortic thrombosis has been described in small numbers of neonates and usually mimics a coarctation of the aorta in clinical presentation. Thromboses of the aortic arch and the bifurcation have been described, and there are no known associations. Anticoagulation and thrombolytic therapy have been used depending on the degree of tissue ischemia, and the role of acute surgical or interventional radiologic procedures remains unknown. Initial aggressive anticoagulation with UFH seems a reasonable first step while more thorough assessment is being made, and the risk-benefit analysis of thrombolysis can be determined.

Chapter 32

Stroke in Children

1. Arterial ischemic stroke (AIS) is one of the top 10 killers of children in Western societies, occurring at approximately the same frequency as brain tumors.

2. AIS is associated with a high rate of long-term neurologic deficits, approximately 60 percent, which varies according to site and size of the lesion.

3. The etiology of AIS in children is totally different from that in adults, with approximately 50 percent being due to arteriopathy, 25 percent to cardioembolic events, and 10 to 15 percent to unknown etiology.

4. The diagnosis of AIS in children is often delayed because of the nonspecific presentations, and the lack of distinguishing features from stroke mimics, such as migraine, Bell's palsy, seizures, and in older children, conversion disorders and syncope.

5. Magnetic resonance imaging/angiography (MRI/MRA) is the most sensitive and specific diagnostic tool for AIS.

6. There is debate as to the role of acute anticoagulation versus antiplatelet therapy for AIS in children.

7. Acute arteriopathy may require immune modulation therapy as well as anticoagulation.

8. Progressive arteriopathies such as moyamoya syndrome are associated with very high rates of recurrent stroke and usually require neurosurgical intervention.

9. Perinatal AIS may be a separate entity, and recurrence rates are much lower than AIS in older children.

10. Cerebral sinovenous thrombosis (CSVT) often presents with headache or nonspecific symptoms, and the spectrum of clinical presentation is very large.

11. CSVT can be associated with local infections such as mastoiditis or systemic issues such as nephrotic syndrome or L-asparaginase therapy in children with acute lymphocytic leukemia (ALL).

12. The rate of long-term sequelae is less for CSVT than for AIS and depends on the degree of associated brain infarction or hemorrhage.

13. MRI/MRV is the most appropriate imaging for diagnosis of CSVT.

14. There is better consensus that even in the presence of some hemorrhage, anticoagulation therapy is warranted for CSVT.

15. Hemorrhagic stroke (HS) in children does occur and often presents with sudden-onset headache, vomiting, and coma.

16. HS usually requires neurosurgical management and consideration of vascular abnormalities as well as congenital bleeding disorders and nonaccidental injury.

Introduction

Over recent years, childhood stroke has been increasingly recognized as a significant cause of long-term childhood morbidity and mortality. Childhood arterial ischemic stroke (AIS) occurs with a frequency of approximately 3.3 per 100,000 children per year, whereas cerebral sinovenous thrombosis (CSVT) has an incidence of 0.67 per 100,000 children per year. Childhood stroke differs from adult stroke in many facets, including clinical presentation, etiology, and

213

treatment. In fact, perinatal/neonatal stroke differs from childhood stroke in clinical presentation, etiology, and treatment as well. Much of our knowledge about childhood stroke has come from the International Pediatric Stroke Study (IPSS) Group, which is a collaborative network of investigators throughout the world who have accumulated prospective data on over 4,000 children with AIS or CSVT over the last decade and continue to gather data on new cases, long-term follow-up, and potential etiologic factors. As a disease entity, it was not until high-quality MRI became available that AIS and CSVT were reliably diagnosed in neonates and children. Much literature to date varies in description, classification, and outcome measurement, so there remain many unanswered questions. The relative infrequency and the heterogeneity of the patient population have hampered effective study. Long-term outcome data are only recently emerging. Primary hemorrhagic stroke will not be discussed in this chapter.

Cerebral Vascular Anatomy

The impact of childhood stroke, either arterial or venous, is closely related to the area of the brain affected. Hence, a brief discussion of the vascular anatomy of the brain is helpful. Figure 32.1 identifies the major arterial supply of the brain. The internal carotid ('anterior circulation') and vertebra basilar ('posterior circulation') systems join to form the circle of Willis. Figure 32.2 identifies the venous drainage of the brain. The right internal jugular vein and transverse sinus (lateral and sigmoid components) are usually larger than the left and drain the superficial hemispheres via the superior sagittal sinus, whereas the left jugular vein and lateral sinus usually drain the deep structures via the straight sinus. Obstruction of the dominant (usually right) system can increase the risks of pressure-related complications due to an inability to drain cerebrospinal fluid (CSF) adequately. The torcular is the junction of the superior sagittal sinus, the straight, sinus and the two transverse sinuses.

Perinatal/Neonatal AIS

Perinatal/neonatal AIS occurs with an incidence of 1 per 2,800 to 1 per 5,000 live births, making it the most frequent form of cerebral infarction in children. About 40 percent of the children do not have specific symptoms in the neonatal period and are only

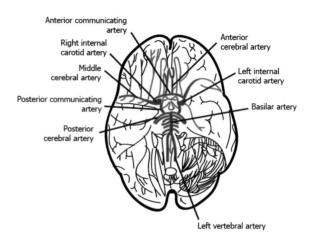

Figure 32.1 Physiologic arterial supply to the brain, which comes from two main circulations, the anterior and the posterior. The anterior circulation is comprised of paired carotid arteries, and the posterior is comprised of paired vertebral arteries that join to form the basilar artery (the vertebra-basilar system).

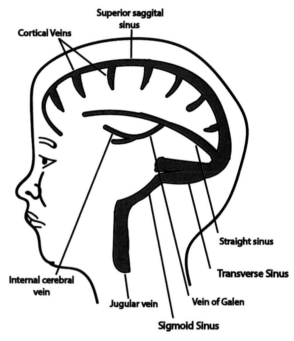

Figure 32.2 Physiologic venous drainage of the brain. The sagittal sinus usually drains to the right transverse and sigmoid sinus, which terminates in the right jugular bulb and internal jugular vein. The straight sinus usually drains into the left transverse and sigmoid sinus.

recognized later with the emergence of motor impairment, developmental delay, specific cognitive deficiency, or seizures. In the remaining 60 percent, children present with early symptoms, mostly seizures and nonfocal neurologic signs during the first 3 days of life. The seizures are often focal in nature. The diagnosis is initially made by cranial ultrasound but usually needs to be properly characterized and confirmed by MRI. Early MRI not only confirms the diagnosis but also might be useful in dating the injury and, most important, in providing important prognostic value to predict the motor outcome of the child. Of the infants who present symptomatically in the newborn period, over half will have evidence of persistent neurologic deficit at the time of discharge.

The mechanism of stroke in the different groups of newborns with stroke (term versus preterm, symptomatic neonates versus those with a delayed presentation, sick versus well) is likely to be different, and as yet, risk factors remain poorly defined.

Recurrence rates for most perinatal/neonatal AIS are extremely low, and hence there is no justification for anticoagulant or antiplatelet therapy once the diagnosis is made. In cases of cardioembolic stroke (with the proven embolic source remaining in the heart) or traumatic major vessel dissection, anticoagulation or antiplatelet therapy is usually warranted. Neonatal supportive care remains the mainstay for all infants, including managing seizures, glucose, and blood pressure and preventing infection.

There is no specific evidence that early rehabilitation therapy improves long-term outcome, but it is a very reasonable extrapolation given the role of early intervention in improving the neurologic outcome for many other infants who suffer neurologic insults in early life. Physical, occupational, and speech therapy may be required as well as specific learning assistance in later life. The recurrence risk for subsequent pregnancies appears to be low in most cases.

Childhood AIS

Stroke is the most common cause of brain attack (focal neurologic deficit) symptoms in adults, accounting for approximately three-quarters of cases in patients presenting to the emergency department. In contrast, there is a much lower a priori probability of stroke in children presenting with brain attack symptoms. Migraine is the most common cause of sudden-onset focal neurologic symptoms and signs, first febrile or afebrile seizures the second most common diagnosis, and then Bell's palsy before ischemic or hemorrhagic stroke and conversion disorders.

Thus, fewer than 10 percent of children who present to an emergency department with acute focal neurologic symptoms and signs will have stroke. More common presenting features of stroke include hemiparesis (22 to 100 percent), headache (16 to 45 percent), altered mental state (12 to 24 percent), speech disturbance (28 to 55 percent), altered consciousness (24 to 52 percent), and seizures (11 to 58 percent). Age at presentation influences the clinical presentation, with seizures, altered mental state, and nonfocal signs being more likely in infants. History should include any evidence of recent head/neck injury or chiropractic neck manipulation, varicella infection in the last 6 to 12 months, and history or family history of migraine and oral contraceptive pill (OCP) or illicit drug use in adolescents.

The nonspecific symptoms and alternative potential diagnosis often lead to delay in diagnosis of childhood stroke, with multiple studies reporting the average time from symptom onset to diagnosis to be in excess of 20 hours. This obviously has massive consequences in terms of the use of acute therapies such as thrombolysis or endovascular procedures.

Arteriopathies (vasculopathies) are the most common cause of AIS in children, accounting for about 50 percent of cases. Over 90 percent of unilateral anterior circulation strokes attributable to vasculopathy are caused by a transient cerebral arteriopathy (TCA) characterized by lenticulostriate infarction due to nonprogressive unilateral arterial disease affecting the supraclinoid internal carotid artery and its proximal branches. Approximately one-quarter of these children will have complete resolution of the vascular changes, with three-quarters having residual arterial abnormalities on follow-up. Of course, the neurologic deficit caused by the stroke is more often permanent, even if the vascular changes recover. About 40 percent of cases are preceded by chickenpox. Most infarcts are localized in the basal ganglia. In about 20 percent of TCA patients, transient worsening of the arterial lesion occurs before the arteriopathy stabilizes or improves. The recurrent stroke rate in these patients is about 20 percent. Many TCA patients have a good neurologic outcome. A smaller proportion of anterior circulation strokes is due to progressive arteriopathies, and while these can be initially unilateral in presentation, they often progress to bilateral disease. The classic progressive arteriopathy is moyamoya disease, and imaging often shows arterial occlusion, moyamoya vessels, and anterior cerebral artery (ACA) involvement. Cortical infarct localization was significantly associated with poor neurologic outcome, and there is a trend for occlusive arterial disease to predict poor outcome. Young children with bilateral cerebral arteriopathies have a malignant course, with frequent recurrent events, progressive disease, and poor outcomes. Current classifications are limited in characterizing disease in many cases. Symmetric involvement suggests that these arteriopathies may be developmentally determined, while systemic involvement suggests potential genetic etiology.

Cardioembolic strokes frequently occur in children with underlying congenital heart disease and most often around the time of major surgical procedures. These may be in the anterior or posterior cerebral circulations and are usually single events, although occasionally showers of embolic lesions can be seen on neuroimaging. Careful search for the source thrombosis needs to include not only the heart but also the venous system (especially around central venous access devices) because many children have right-to-left shunts. Distinguishing septic emboli from endocarditis from primary thromboembolism is important because the treatments are obviously different. The risk of recurrence usually relates to the flow abnormalities within the heart, the presence or absence of a further source clot, and the effectiveness of anticoagulation.

Dissection of major vessels including the extracranial carotid artery or the vertebra basilar system is not uncommon after minor trauma or twisting forces. Often formal angiography is required to exclude or confirm the diagnosis. Most protocols for initial imaging of pediatric stroke patients include extension of the vascular imaging to include the neck vessels to consider this potential diagnosis.

The role of thrombophilias in the etiology of pediatric stroke remains controversial. While many studies report associations between stroke and heterozygous thrombophilic states in children, the methodology of most studies is less than ideal, and the evidence that links the blood results to recurrence or outcome – and hence has an impact on potential therapy – is weak.

A significant proportion of childhood strokes are truly cryptogenic, occurring in otherwise well children without any precipitating factors. Multiple other associations have been suggested, including iron deficiency, but the reality is that many events remain unexplained. Fortunately, in these cases the recurrence risk appears to be lower, but it is difficult to be totally reassuring to patients and their families. Stroke is very common in children with underlying sickle cell disease, and this specific entity is covered in Chapter 17.

The diagnosis of stroke requires specific MRI/MRA of the head and neck vessels, and most tertiary centers have specific stroke protocols aimed at identifying not only the vascular lesion responsible but also at defining the areas of infarction and ischemia within the brain. Computed tomographic (CT) scanning is insensitive and will fail to detect 50 percent of AIS. Sometimes formal contrast angiography is required to accurately identify dissections. If anesthesia is required for appropriate imaging, this should be managed by an experienced pediatric anesthetist. Avoiding distress, dehydration, hypotension, and hypocapnia is particularly important in children with known arterial stenosis or moyamoya disease because perturbations of these parameters are known to precipitate further strokes. The risk-benefit ratio of each imaging episode in these children needs to be carefully considered.

Echocardiography including bubble studies with forced Valsalva to exclude patent foramen ovale and the possibility of paradoxical emboli is often required. Transesophageal echocardiography (TEE) may be required to look for intracardiac thrombus in children with congenital heart disease, especially with Fontan circuits. Blood work for thrombophilia may be appropriate, and in cases of arteriopathy/vasculitis, autoimmune workup also may be required.

The treatment of childhood stroke can be divided into five separate considerations:

- *Acute supportive care aimed at maximizing brain recovery and limiting any secondary brain damage.* This includes maintaining normovolemia and avoiding hypo- and hypertension. Maintaining normal blood glucose levels is particularly important. Airway management may be required and oxygen support to keep oxygen saturations above 96 percent. Any fever should be controlled with antipyretic agents, and if seizures occur, they should be managed aggressively with antiseizure medications to minimize further seizure activity. Feeding should occur only after adequate assessment of safe swallowing ability. Occasionally, raised intracranial pressure, especially with posterior circulation strokes, may require aggressive medical care or even neurosurgical intervention. Hemorrhagic conversion of AIS, which can occur in the first week after the AIS, may result in intraparenchymal bleeding that requires surgical drainage.

- *Anticoagulation or antiplatelet therapy.* This treatment is aimed at reducing the risk of recurrence and maximizing the recovery of the ischemic penumbra surrounding the infarcted area. The evidence supporting any specific approach is relatively low, and the risk of increasing secondary hemorrhage must always be considered. In general, arteriopathies are thought to require antiplatelet therapy, whereas cardioembolic and dissection-related strokes are thought to require formal anticoagulation. The question of whether, at presentation, anticoagulation therapy should be begun with conversion to antiplatelet therapy once cardioembolic causes or dissection has been excluded or, alternatively, whether antiplatelet therapy should be started with conversion to anticoagulation once cardioembolic causes or dissection has been proven remains unanswered. There are clear geographic differences in approach. In part, this relates to how comfortable some physicians are with anticoagulation therapy in small children and perceived bleeding risks, although most cohort data and case series suggest that anticoagulation can be administered safely in this patient population. The author prefers to start anticoagulation, usually with unfractionated heparin (UFH) due to its ease of reversibility should bleeding occur. UFH should be started as a continuous intravenous infusion, without an initial bolus, and then gently titrated to a therapeutic activated partial thromboplastin time (APTT) or anti-Xa. If ongoing anticoagulation is required (cardioembolic or dissection), then conversion to low-molecular weight heparin (LMWH) or warfarin can be done over the subsequent week of therapy. Once these causes have been excluded by appropriate imaging, conversion to aspirin at 3 to 5 mg/kg per day is reasonable. The optimal duration of these therapies is unclear, but anticoagulation is frequently used for 3 months, whereas antiplatelet therapy is often prescribed for 12 months after stroke. Aspirin is a relatively low-risk treatment,

and some children/families may choose to continue this therapy indefinitely. There are few data to support the use of thrombolysis in acute stroke in childhood. This relates primarily to the frequent delays in diagnosis and the subsequent inability to start thrombolysis within an acceptable 3- to 4-hour time frame from symptom onset. In cases of stroke in which this can be achieved, individual consideration of the risk-benefit ratio is required for each child, although one could argue that thrombolysis should only be given to children in the setting of an appropriate clinical trial.

- *Immunomodulation.* Specific arteriopathies, especially those showing signs of progression, may benefit from immunotherapy including prednisolone acutely or longer-term therapy with cyclosporine or other immunomodulatory drugs.

- *Surgical interventions.* Surgical interventions may be required for acute relief of raised intracranial pressure or for drainage of associated hemorrhage. In progressive arteriopathies such as moyamoya disease, revascularization procedures including multiple burr holes or direct revascularization surgeries are the mainstay of treatment.

- *Rehabilitation.* Obviously, optimizing recovery in terms of neurologic function is a key component of stroke treatment, and ongoing improvement may be made many months after the initial event. Tiredness is often a prominent feature during stroke recovery, and at times, this hampers the ability of the child to return to school or normal activities, as well as any specific physical or neuropsychological deficits. Physiotherapy, occupational therapy, speech therapy, and appropriate splinting of limbs may be required. Psychological support is also an important component of care. This is best coordinated by a specific pediatric rehabilitation unit.

The outcome of childhood AIS can be very variable but does relate to the size and site of the infarct. There is a small but definite mortality associated with AIS in children. In general, about 35 percent will be normal at long-term follow-up. Approximately 50 percent have mild to moderate deficits that will not stop them from becoming adults who can be independent in relationships, employment, and driving. However, 15 percent will have severe deficits that will affect their ability to be independent into adult life. The functional assessment at 1 year after the stroke is a strong predictor of longer-term outcomes. Recent studies have reported a significant proportion of children after AIS suffer from depression or anxiety, and early psychological/mental health support would seem to be appropriate. Overall recurrence rates are reported to be approximately 10 percent, but this is influenced significantly by the underlying etiology, with progressive arteriopathies having the highest recurrence rates.

Neonatal CSVT

Most neonatal CSVT presents during the first week of life, and seizures are the most common presenting symptom. Altered consciousness and focal motor deficits are other common symptoms. A significant group of infants may have relatively few specific neurologic signs but may have nonspecific symptoms such as apnea, irritability, poor feeding, hypotonia, and vomiting.

The etiology of CSVT remains unclear, and a number of risk factors have been suggested. These include a range of maternal pregnancy complications, including preeclampsia and maternal diabetes; fetal/neonatal complications including meconium aspiration, dehydration, and sepsis; and underlying fetal conditions such as congenital heart disease and thrombophilias. However, none of the associations is particularly strong, and it seems likely that CSVT is the result of a multihit pathogenesis.

Cranial ultrasound (CUS) is frequently used as a screening test for CSVT in the neonate, and CUS is often positive when the central sinuses are affected in this age group. However, CUS is insufficient to either confirm or refute the diagnosis, and if clinical suspicion is high, MRI/magnetic resonance venography (MRV) should be performed even in the setting of normal CUS. Similarly, if CUS is suggestive, confirmatory MRI/MRV is required. MRI is important to identify the venous occlusion but also to document any evidence of cerebral infarction and subsequent hemorrhagic conversion. While computed tomographic venography (CTV) has been used, the available data would suggest the MRI/MRV is the optimal imaging strategy.

There is significant geographic variation in treatment of neonatal CSVT most likely related to uncertainty about the true risk of bleeding when neonates with CSVT are given anticoagulation therapy. The American College of Chest Physicians (ACCP) guidelines suggest anticoagulation for all affected neonates unless there is substantial intracerebral hemorrhage. Alternatively, the American Heart Association (AHA) guidelines suggest monitoring with sequential imaging and anticoagulation only in the presence of thrombus progression. If anticoagulation is used, UFH without an initial bolus (the most easily reversible anticoagulation strategy) seems reasonable, with gradual titration to therapeutic doses in the absence of bleeding. Conversion to LMWH once the neonate has tolerated UFH without bleeding, to complete 3 months of therapy, seems a reasonable option. There is little evidence to support antiplatelet therapy for CSVT. There are no data to support thrombolysis.

The mortality from neonatal CSVT is probably less than 5 percent. In contrast, over 60 percent of infants are reported to be normal at long-term follow-up. The presence of cerebral infarction and/or hemorrhage is associated with long-term neurologic deficits, and these range in severity from mild to severe based on the size and site of the abnormalities.

Childhood CSVT

The presentations of childhood CSVT can be subtle and varied. Seizures, loss of consciousness or altered consciousness, focal neurologic deficits, headache, and symptoms of raised intracranial pressure all have been reported. Some children are in fact asymptomatic, and the CSVT is discovered on CNS imaging performed for other reasons.

The cause for many CSVTs in children remains unknown, but many are associated with local infections/inflammation. Otitis media and mastoiditis can be associated with sigmoid and transverse sinus thrombosis. Systemic causes such as severe dehydration are important to consider. Occasionally, CSVT occurs in children unwell from systemic illness (viral, bacterial, or inflammatory) without any apparent direct link to the cerebral circulation. CSVT is not an uncommon site for thrombotic complications in children with leukemia, especially when treated with L-asparaginase. Similarly, other conditions that can be associated with increased risk of thrombosis, such as nephrotic syndrome and anti-phospholipid antibody syndrome, will sometimes be associated with CSVT. The role of congenital thrombophilia remains controversial, and more data are required, but it would seem rarely to be the sole causative factor (but perhaps a minor factor in a multihit pathogenesis).

The diagnosis of CSVT in children is best achieved by either CTV or MRI/MRV. As stated previously, it is important not only to visualize the venous obstruction but also to detect evidence of venous infarction and associated secondary hemorrhage.

Supportive care – including hydration, blood pressure management, and management of raised intracranial pressure – is critical. In cases of mastoiditis, adequate drainage of the infection and hence removal of the thrombotic stimulus is important, followed by relevant antibiotic treatment. In L-asparaginase-induced cases, correction of the coagulopathy is also likely required. There may be a role for antithrombin replacement in some L-asparaginase-induced CSVT because antithrombin depletion is thought to be part of the coagulopathy.

In general, anticoagulation is an accepted component of therapy for all CSVT, but this must be managed around any early surgical interventions that are required. UFH is a reasonable first option, with no bolus, because this is the most reversible of the anticoagulant options, and if bleeding occurs or surgery is required, then it is the easiest therapy to manipulate around such things. While many authors suggest the use of anticoagulation in the presence of hemorrhage, unless it is severe, the amount of hemorrhage that should preclude anticoagulation is not well delineated, and it is probably better to err on the side of caution. Once the child is stable, conversion to LMWH or warfarin for a subsequent 3 to 6 months of anticoagulation is appropriate. There seems to be little role for antiplatelet therapy. There are few data to support thrombolysis.

The outcome of CSVT in children depends on the size and site of the thrombus and, in particular, the presence of venous infarction with or without hemorrhage. The underlying causes are important in the response to therapy and the likelihood of recurrence. In general, the mortality is approximately 3 percent. Long-term neurologic deficits including seizures are seen in 20 to 30 percent of children, but over 50 percent of children will be normal at follow-up. As with other kinds of CNS-related thromboses, appropriate rehabilitation services are an important component of care.

Chapter 33

Anticoagulation in Children

1. Anticoagulation in children is best managed by a dedicated pediatric anticoagulation service.

2. Basic assumptions about anticoagulants that are accepted in adult populations may not be true in children.

3. The enormous difference in weight across the pediatric population increases the potential for drug errors to be life-threatening, especially given the multitude of dose preparations of unfractionated heparin (UFH) maintained on many pediatric wards. Drug safety requires specific consideration.

4. While there remains great anxiety about the difficulty in using traditional anticoagulants in children, there is nothing to suggest that newer agents will be less problematic, and we have much less clinical experience with newer drugs in children. At this time, new oral anticoagulants should be used only in the setting of clinical trials to assess their safety and efficacy.

Introduction

Anticoagulation in children is used commonly now in tertiary pediatric hospitals for treatment and prevention of venous and arterial thromboses. The use of antithrombotic drugs in pediatric patients differs from that in adults for a multitude of reasons:

- The epidemiology of thromboembolism (TE) in pediatric patients differs from that seen in adults, altering the risk-benefit ratio of any drug.
- The coagulation system is a dynamic, evolving entity that likely affects the response to therapeutic agents.

- The distribution, binding, and clearance of antithrombotic drugs are age dependent.
- The frequency and types of intercurrent illnesses and concurrent medications vary with age.
- The need for general anesthesia to perform many diagnostic studies in pediatric patients has an impact on the ability to investigate and monitor TE and hence the confidence one can have in therapeutic decisions.

Limited vascular access reduces the ability to effectively deliver some antithrombotic therapies:

- Limited vascular access makes accurate monitoring of anticoagulant levels difficult.
- Specific pediatric formulations of current antithrombotic drugs are not available.
- Dietary differences make the use of oral vitamin K antagonists (VKAs) particularly difficult, which is especially true in neonates because breast milk and infant formulas have very different vitamin K levels.
- Compliance issues, for example, in small infants who cannot understand the need for therapy, adolescents who intellectually comprehend but emotionally are unable to cooperate, and children who experience the effects of inadequate parenting. The social, ethical, and legal implications of these issues frequently have an impact on anticoagulant therapy.

For all these reasons, anticoagulation therapy in children is best managed by a dedicated pediatric anticoagulant service, with nurse-led models of care being the most successful models reported to date. Despite all the differences, much has been extrapolated from adult use of anticoagulants to pediatric practice, and to date, the actual amount of specific pediatric data that support all current recommendations related to anticoagulant therapy remains very limited.

Currently, multiple new oral anticoagulants are being trialed in children, including dabigatran (direct thrombin inhibitor), rivaroxaban, apixaban, and edoxaban (direct factor Xa inhibitors). The results of pharmacokinetic and pharmacodynamic (PK/PD) studies as well as safety and efficacy data will become available over the next 5 years. Each agent will have specific pediatric preparations, which will be a new experience for pediatricians working in this field. Until such time as the appropriate studies are completed, off-label use of these drugs should be avoided. In the meantime, UFH, LMWH, and VKAs remain the mainstays of anticoagulant therapy in children.

Unfractionated Heparin

UFH remains a commonly used anticoagulant in pediatric patients. In tertiary pediatric hospitals, approximately 15 percent of inpatients are exposed to UFH each day. There are a number of specific factors that may alter the effect of UFH in children (see Table 33.1). The clinical implications of these changes on dosing, monitoring, and effectiveness – safety profile of UFH in children – remain uncertain.

There have been no reported clinical outcome studies to determine the therapeutic range for UFH in neonates or children, so the therapeutic range for all indications is extrapolated from those used in venous thromboembolism (VTE) therapy in adults. This equates to an APTT that reflects a heparin level by protamine titration of 0.2 to 0.4 units/ml or an anti-factor Xa level of 0.35 to 0.7 units/ml. There are multiple reasons why this extrapolation might be invalid, but the safety and efficacy of this approach, in experienced hands, seem reasonable.

Bolus doses of 75 to 100 units/kg result in therapeutic APTT values in 90 percent of children at 4 to 6 hours after the bolus. Maintenance UFH doses are age dependent, with infants (up to 2 months) having the highest requirements (average 28 units/kg/hr) and children over 1 year of age having lower requirements (average 20 units/kg per hour). The doses of UFH required for older children are similar to the weight-adjusted requirements in adults (18 units/kg per hour). However, boluses of 75 to 100 units/kg in children have recently been shown to result in excessive prolongation of APTT for over 100 minutes, implying that the recommendations may need to be reexamined. In many cases, especially where the bleeding risk is higher, therapy should be started with an infusion only and no boluses. Reduced doses are usually required in renal insufficiency.

Table 33.1 Factors in Children That Affect the Action of UFH

UFH factor	Age-related difference
UFH acts via antithrombin (AT)–mediated catabolism of thrombin and factor Xa	Reduced levels of AT and prothrombin Reduced capacity to generate thrombin Anti-Xa:anti-IIa activity of UFH
UFH is bound to plasma proteins, which limits free active UFH	Alterations in plasma binding
Endothelial release of tissue factor pathway inhibitor (TFPI)	Amount of TFPI released for same amount of UFH

Table 33.2 Nomogram for Managing Heparin Infusion According to Monitoring of APTT or Anti-Xa Levels

APTT (s)	Anti-Xa level (IU/ml)[a]	Bolus (units/kg)	Hold (min)	Rate change (percent)
<50	<0.1	50	–	↑ 20
50–59	0.1–0.34	–	–	↑ 10
60–85	0.35–0.70	–	–	No change
86–95	0.71–0.89	–	–	↓ 10
96–120	0.9–1.2	–	30	↓ 10
>120	>1.2	-	60	↓ 15

[a] This assumes that the APTT range of 60 to 85 s correlates to an anti-factor Xa level of 0.35 to 0.70 IU/ml. This will depend on the reagent and analyzer used in the laboratory.

Monitoring of UFH therapy is current standard practice, but there are difficulties with interpreting the monitoring assays related to a lack of correlation between the anti-Xa, APTT, and thrombin clotting time, as well as in making dosage adjustments. There are no published studies in children that establish the ideal frequency of UFH monitoring, and vascular access is a frequent limiting factor. Contamination of results when blood is taken from the same limb into which the infusion is being given is often a major issue. A typical nomogram for manipulating UFH doses in children is shown in Table 33.2. However, many experienced clinicians use small, incremental changes and no boluses to feel comfortable about

221

monitoring on a once-daily basis, which is often more practical. Given that there are no data to support the absolute advantage of a defined therapeutic range, and if one takes into account the rationale for treating and the clinical progress of the patient, this seems to be a reasonable approach.

Further studies are required to accurately determine the frequency of UFH-induced bleeding in optimally treated children, which is probably below 1 percent depending on patient selection and the experience of the managing team. Probably the most common cause of fatal bleeding secondary to UFH relates to accidental overdose, especially in neonates. While rarely reported in the medical literature, the number of deaths reported in the popular press appears to be increasing. This often occurs in children who are receiving low-dose UFH flushing of vascular access devices, intended, for example, to be 50 units/5 ml UFH. Errors in vial selection and failure of bedside checking procedures result in 5,000 units/5 ml UFH being injected, and in small infants this results in a massive and unexpected overdose of UFH. Figure 33.1 shows the range of heparin preparations found in a typical pediatric intensive care unit (PICU). It is not hard to see how such errors occur in busy units, which operate 24 hours per day. Units should actively manage the choices of UFH preparations available to their staff to minimize the risk of confusion. Staff should be educated in the dangers of UFH and encouraged to be vigilant at all times when administering a drug that consistently ranks in hospital lists of the drugs most commonly involved in medication errors. Rapid reversal of UFH can be achieved with protamine titration (Table 33.3), although in many instances simple cessation of UFH infusion is adequate.

Apart from bleeding, the other potential side effects of UFH include anaphylaxis and osteoporosis. Clinicians should be prudent to avoid long-term (weeks to months) use of UFH in children.

The true rate of heparin-induced thrombocytopenia (HIT) in children appears greatly reduced compared to adults. Many pediatric hematologists question its existence in children, although occasional cases are verified. Tests for HIT have high false positive rates which makes accurate diagnosis difficult. Presumed HIT is a frequent reason for children to receive less commonly used anticoagulant drugs, including danaparoid, hirudin, and argatroban, with poor clinical outcomes.

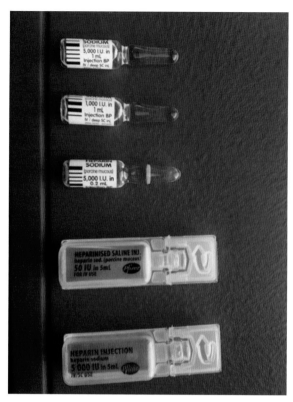

Figure 33.1 Heparin vials commonly used on the same wards in tertiary pediatric hospitals. The risk for confusion and dosing errors is high. Unexpected high APTT in patients who are meant to be receiving low-dose UFH flushing of vascular access should raise immediate suspicion of an error and may require removal of all UFH and remaking of infusions.

Table 33.3 Reversal of Heparin Therapy

Time since last heparin dose[a]	Protamine dose[b]
<30 min	1.0 mg/100 units heparin received
30–60 min	0.5–0.75 mg/100 units heparin received
60–120 min	0.375–0.5 mg/100 units heparin received
>120 min	0.25–0.375 mg/100 units heparin received

[a] Maximum dose of 50 mg. Infusion rate of a 10 mg/ml solution should not exceed 5 mg/min.
[b] Hypersensitivity reactions to protamine sulfate may occur in patients with known hypersensitivity reactions to fish or those previously exposed to protamine therapy or protamine-containing insulin.

Low-Molecular-Weight Heparin

LMWH has become the anticoagulant of choice in many pediatric patients for a variety of reasons. However, the predictability of the anticoagulant affect with weight-adjusted doses is less than in adults, presumably due to differences in binding to plasma proteins. Most clinical data of LMWH in pediatric patients used enoxaparin.

Therapeutic ranges for LMWH are extrapolated from results in adults and are based on anti-Xa levels, the guideline for subcutaneous administration twice daily being 0.50 to 1.0 anti-Xa units/ml at 2 to 6 h following injection. Most studies in children have used this therapeutic range, although one study used a lower maximal level (0.8 units/ml) with good efficacy and safety outcomes. Once-daily regimes are described much less commonly, and intravenous use has also been reported, but rarely. Reduced doses are required in renal insufficiency.

While initial doses that most likely attain the therapeutic range have been described (Table 33.4), considerable interpatient dose differences exist, suggesting that routine monitoring of anti-Xa levels in children and neonates remains necessary. Monitoring protocols have been suggested (Table 33.5). Whether clinical effectiveness will be altered by having multiple age-related initial and maintenance dose recommendations is unclear. Recent studies have suggested that even higher initial doses may be required for neonates to achieve therapeutic range, but given the absence of evidence that the therapeutic range extrapolated from adults is required in neonates, clinical outcome data would be more useful in driving changes to current therapy.

Major bleeding rates with LMWH in children appear to be low in stable patients, and although reports of bleeding rates vary from 0 to 19 percent. Patient selection is critical, and in many cases of bleeding, titratable and more readily reversible UFH would have been a better therapeutic option (e.g. immediately postoperative patients). LMWH is only partially reversed by protamine. There are no data on the frequency of osteoporosis (although case reports exist on extended use of LMWH, especially in premature infants), HIT, or other hypersensitivity reactions in children exposed to LMWH. Temporary hair loss is reported.

Vitamin K Antagonists

Warfarin is the most commonly used and studied VKA worldwide. Acenocoumarol is administered with high frequency in some European and South American countries, and phenprocoumon is the preferred VKA in some parts of Europe. The current therapeutic international normalization ratio (INR) ranges for children are extrapolated from recommendations for adult patients because there are no clinical trials that have assessed the optimal INR range for children. For most indications, the therapeutic target INR is 2.5 (range 2.0 to 3.0), although the therapeutic ranges for prosthetic valves vary according to the type and position of the prosthetic valve.

Table 33.4 Therapeutic and Prophylactic Dosing of Enoxaparin, Tinzaparin, and Dalteparin According to Age

Drug	Therapeutic dose	Prophylactic dose
Enoxaparin		
• ≤2 months of age	1.5 mg/kg SC b.d.	1.5 mg/kg SC o.d.
• >2 months of age	1 mg/kg SC b.d.	1 mg/kg SC o.d.
Tinzaparin		
• ≤2 months of age	275 units/kg SC o.d.	75 units/kg SC o.d.
• 2–12 months of age	250 units/kg SC o.d.	75 units/kg SC o.d.
• 1–5 years	240 units/kg SC o.d.	75 units/kg SC o.d.
• 5–10 years	200 units/kg SC o.d.	75 units /kg SC o.d.
• 10–16 years	175 units/kg SC o.d.	50 units /kg SC o.d.
Dalteparin		
• ≤ 2 months of age	150 units /kg SC b.d.	150 units/kg SC o.d.
• > 2 months of age	100 units /kg SC b.d.	100 units/kg SC o.d.

Table 33.5 Adjustment of LMWH According to Monitoring of Anti-Xa Levels

Anti-Xa level (IU/ml)	Withhold next dose?	Dose change?	Timing of next anti-Xa level
<0.35	No	Increase by 25 percent	After next dose
0.36–0.49	No	Increase by 15 percent	After next dose
0.5–1.0	No	No	After 1 week if hospitalized, 1 month if outpatient
1.01–1.25	No	Decrease by 15 percent	After next dose
1.26–1.5	No	Decrease by 25 percent	After next dose
1.51–2.0	Yes	Decrease by 30 percent	When next dose is due; if >1.5, continue to withhold dose and repeat after 12 h
>2.0	Yes	Decrease by 40 percent	When next dose is due; if >1.5, continue to withhold dose and repeat after 12 h

Warfarin is usually started at 0.1 to 0.2 mg/kg, capped at 5 mg maximal starting dose. Patients with liver impairment or after Fontan surgery require lower doses. A typical nomogram for guiding dosing is shown in Table 33.6.

Monitoring oral anticoagulant therapy in children is difficult and requires close supervision with frequent dose adjustments. Only 10 to 20 percent of children are safely monitored monthly. Studies in children comparing point-of-care (POC) monitors to venipuncture INR confirm their accuracy and reliability. The major advantages of POC devices include the reduced trauma of venipunctures, minimal interruption of school and work, ease of operation, and portability. However, all POC devices are operator dependent, and considerable family education is required to ensure accurate use. An ongoing quality-assurance program is recommended as well.

VKAs are often avoided in infants for several reasons:

- The plasma levels of the vitamin-K dependent coagulation factors are physiologically decreased in comparison with adult levels.
- Infant formula is supplemented with vitamin K to prevent hemorrhagic disease, which makes formula-fed infants resistant to VKAs.
- Breast milk has low concentrations of vitamin K, making breast-fed infants sensitive to VKAs, which can be compensated for by feeding 30 to 60 ml of formula each day.

- VKAs are available only in tablet form in most countries, thus being unsuitable for newborns even if suspended in water.
- VKA requirements change rapidly across infancy because of rapidly changing physiologic values of the vitamin K-dependent coagulation proteins and changes in diet.
- There is little efficacy or safety information specific to VKA use in neonates.

However, for prosthetic valves, homozygous protein C deficiency, and long-term therapy (beyond 3 to 6 months), VKA is probably superior to LMWH and can be managed in this age group by experienced teams and with adequate parental support.

Bleeding is the main complication of VKA therapy, but in experienced hands, the bleeding rates are reported to be less than 0.5 percent per patient-year. Approximately 30 percent of teenage girls on VKA will have menorrhagia and proactive management of menstrual bleeding, often involving gynecology services, and attention to iron status is critical. A high proportion of teenagers who start VKA during their teenage years will develop clinical depression or anxiety related to the psychosocial challenges involved in lifestyle restrictions. Proactive psychological support of these patients is important. Nonhemorrhagic complications of VKA, such as tracheal calcification and hair loss, have been described on rare occasions in young children. Reduced bone density in children on

Table 33.6 Adjustment of VKA Dose According to INR during Initiation and Maintenance Phases of Therapy

Initiation	**Day 1:** If the baseline INR is 1.0–1.3, give 0.1 to 0.2 mg/kg orally (maximum 5 mg)	
	Days 2–4:	
	INR	**Action**
	1.1–1.3	Repeat initial loading dose
	1.4–1.9	50 percent of initial loading dose
	2.0–3.0	50 percent of initial loading dose
	3.1–3.5	25 percent of initial loading dose
	>3.5	Hold until INR < 3.5; then restart at 50 percent of initial loading dose
Maintenance	**INR**	**Action**
	1.1–1.4	Increase dose by 20 percent
	1.5–1.9	Increase dose by 10 percent
	2.0–3.0	No change
	3.1–3.5	Decrease dose by 10 percent
	>3.5	Hold until INR < 3.5; then restart at 80 percent of dose

warfarin for greater than 1 year has been reported in a number of studies, and many programs routinely monitor bone density in all children on long-term VKAs.

Patient and family education protocols are major factors in reducing bleeding events in children on VKA therapy. Key age-related concepts of patient education that need to be addressed are listed in Table 33.7.

One of the important aspects of long-term VKA therapy is to manage interruptions of therapy required for procedures. One suggested approach (devised at RCH Melbourne by Dr. Sally Campbell and Prof. Fiona Newall) is shown in Table 33.8. The underlying principles are that management of anticoagulant therapy around invasive procedures such as surgery and lumbar puncture is determined individually according to each patient's risk for thrombosis and/or bleeding; Patients are stratified according to risk: low, medium, or high. Patients on anticoagulation for less than 3 months (i.e. being acutely treated for thrombosis) should have non urgent procedures delayed until cessation of therapy, if possible. Interruption of therapy requires planning in advance, especially in patients with complex surgical procedures.

Using this guide, if on the day of surgery the INR is <1.5, then surgery can proceed, and if INR is >1.5,

then surgery should be delayed or VKA reversed with vitamin K ± prothrombin complex concentrate (PCC), unless the surgeon believes that the bleeding risk is very low and surgery can proceed regardless of the INR. This usually requires a direct discussion between hematologist and surgeon.

In cases where emergency reversal of VKA is required due to bleeding or the need for urgent surgery, the required doses of PCC are shown in Table 33.9. If PCC is unavailable, then fresh frozen plasma (FFP) 10 to 20 ml/kg is usually adequate.

Thrombolysis

No study has compared the efficacy, safety, or cost of different thrombolytic agents in children. However, tissue plasminogen activator (tPA) has become the agent of choice in pediatric patients. There is minimal experience with other thrombolytic agents in children. There is little consensus in indications for thrombolysis, dose, mode of delivery, or duration of therapy, reflecting the lack of good-quality studies. At this time, there is no evidence to suggest that there is an advantage of local over systemic thrombolytic therapy in children with thrombotic complications.

Success rates for thrombolysis in pediatric patients vary. Thrombolysis is usually used when there is

Table 33.7 Age-Appropriate Warfarin Education

Education topic	<1 year	1–5 years	6–10 years	10–15 years	15+ years
Warfarin action and indication					
Warfarin acts against vitamin K	✓	✓	✓	✓	✓
Warfarin slows down body's ability to form clots (i.e. anticoagulant)	✓	✓	✓	✓	✓
This increases risk of bleeding/bruising	✓	✓	✓	✓	✓
Indication: prophylaxis or treatment of blood clot	✓	✓	✓	✓	✓

Warfarin tablet presentation:
  Different trade preparations
    available
  Tablet strengths and color
  Once-daily dosing (pm)
  Administer every dose same way
	✓	✓	✓	✓	✓

Monitoring of warfarin					
Warfarin must be monitored regularly by blood test	✓	✓	✓	✓	✓
Test is called INR	✓	✓	✓	✓	✓
Normal INR	✓	✓	✓	✓	✓
Target INR	✓	✓	✓	✓	✓
Venous versus capillary	✓	✓	✓	✓	✓
Procedure for INRs at anticoagulation clinic	✓	✓	✓	✓	✓
Procedure for INRs performed externally	✓	✓	✓	✓	✓
Home INR monitoring program	✓	✓	✓	✓	✓
Warfarin dose based on INR result	✓	✓	✓	✓	✓
Confounders to stable therapy					
Bottle versus breast-feeding	✓				
Consistent dietary intake (vitamin K)		✓	✓	✓	✓
Alcohol intake				✓	✓
Changes in prescription medications (including antibiotics and dose changes of current medications)	✓	✓	✓	✓	✓
Over-the-counter medicines and herbal remedies (specific information regarding NSAIDs, aspirin)	✓	✓	✓	✓	✓
Missing doses of warfarin	✓	✓	✓	✓	✓
Other drugs: cigarettes or other substances				✓	✓
Illness: coughs or colds, gastrointestinal, deterioration in primary health	✓	✓	✓	✓	✓
Growth and development (increasing height and weight)	✓	✓	✓	✓	✓
Hormonal changes				✓	✓
Activity changes (e.g. school holidays)		✓	✓	✓	✓

Table 33.7 (cont.)

Education topic	<1 year	1–5 years	6–10 years	10–15 years	15+ years
Side effects and first aid					
Increased bruising compared with usual but should not bruise without injury (~20 percent)	✓	✓	✓	✓	✓
Increased risk of minor bleeding (e.g. nose bleeds, cuts)	✓	✓	✓	✓	✓
Major bleeding risk 0.5–3 percent per year (depending on individual service data)	✓	✓	✓	✓	✓
Potential changes to menstrual bleeding				✓	✓
Osteoporosis (encourage calcium intake + exercise; routine screening after 12 months of therapy)	✓	✓	✓	✓	✓
Rare: tracheal calcification, hair loss, purple-toe syndrome	✓	✓	✓	✓	✓
Teratogenic effects (risks of pregnancy)				✓	✓
First aid management	✓	✓	✓	✓	✓
Anticoagulation clinic contacts (first point of contact; pager and e-mail contact details)	✓	✓	✓	✓	✓
After-hours contact details	✓	✓	✓	✓	✓
Annual review in hematology outpatient clinic	✓	✓	✓	✓	✓
Medic-Alert bracelet	✓	✓	✓	✓	✓
School letter		✓	✓	✓	✓

limb- or life-threatening thrombosis of arterial or venous origin. In this context, while there are a number of relative contraindications, there are no absolute indications to thrombolysis in children, and careful discussion of the risk-benefit ratio should be had with parents prior to therapy.

Infants have a relative plasminogen deficiency compared to adults, and common practice is to give FFP 10 ml/kg prior to tPA, in an effort to provide better plasminogen substrate for the tPA and to reduce bleeding through improved fibrinogen levels. Thrombolytics may not inhibit clot propagation; hence thrombin inhibition is required as adjunctive therapy. Concurrent low-dose UFH (10 units/kg per hour) followed by therapeutic UFH is usually recommended.

The optimal dose of tPA is uncertain, but most protocols use 0.5 mg/kg per hour for a maximum of 6 h. Some centers recommend doses as low as 0.05 mg/kg per hour. Reports of accelerated tPA, especially in the setting of cardiac infarction associated with Kawasaki disease, are described.

Thrombolytic therapy has significant bleeding complications in children, with major bleeding reported in 10 to 30 percent of patients depending on patient selection. The intracerebral bleeding rate is probably less than 5 percent but may be increased in neonates. Thus, the bleeding risk from thrombolysis in children is at least an order of magnitude higher than the bleeding risk of anticoagulation alone. This risk needs to be weighed against the potential benefits of therapy in any child considered for thrombolysis. The bleeding rate may be related to duration of thrombolysis infusion, and many centers recommend limiting the time of infusion to less than 6 hours. If further lysis is required, further doses can be given over the next 24 hours.

Inferior Vena Cava (IVC) Filters

The purpose of IVC interruption is to reduce the risk of pulmonary embolism in patients with proven thrombosis in whom anticoagulation is

Table 33.8 Interruption of Warfarin Therapy

	Low risk	Medium risk	High risk
Patient populations	1. Primary thromboprophylaxis: a. Fontan (no thrombosis) b. CVL[a] c. Pulmonary hypertension (HTN)[b]	1. Primary thromboprophylaxis: a. Cardiomyopathy 2. CVL – secondary prophylaxis[a] 3. Aortic prosthetic valve 4. Fontan with thrombosis > 3 months ago *or* poor flow in Fontan circuit 5. VTE/PE > 1 months after diagnosis	1. PHx prosthetic valve thrombosis 2. Mitral prosthetic valve 3. Fontan with thrombosis < 3 months ago 4. VTE/PE < 1 months after diagnosis 5. Recurrent VTE 6. Moyamoya disease[c]
Cessation of warfarin	5 days prior to procedure	5 days prior to procedure	5 days prior to procedure
Preprocedure bridging therapy	No	Commence LMH 1 mg/kg b.d. when INR below lower limit of therapeutic target range (TTR) Last dose on morning of day before procedure	Commence LMWH 1 mg/kg b.d. when INR below lower limit of TTR Last dose on morning of day before procedure Commence UFH IV infusion at 20 IU/kg/h at time of last dose of Clexane or on admission to hospital *Not* for UFH bolus at any stage Continue UFH until 4 h prior to procedure, then cease
Coagulation monitoring assays preprocedure	INR on day of or day prior to surgery N.B.: If INR >1.5, see box below.[d]	INR 3 days after cessation of warfarin Commence Clexane when INR below lower limit of TTR No monitoring of bridging therapy required	INR 3 days after cessation of warfarin Commence Clexane when INR below lower limit of TTR. If UFH duration is <24 h, no need to monitor APTT
Postprocedure bridging therapy	No	Restart Clexane 1 mg/kg b.d. on evening of procedure if there are no bleeding concerns If bleeding risk is present, delay restarting Clexane until morning of day following procedure	Restart UFH 4 h after procedure, provided there is no significant bleeding risk, and continue overnight Restart Clexane the morning after procedure, and cease UFH with first dose
Restart warfarin	Recommence warfarin on night of procedure with standard maintenance dose	Restart standard maintenance dose of warfarin on evening of the procedure, provided no contraindications are present Check INR 3 days after restarting warfarin	Restart standard maintenance dose of warfarin on evening of procedure, provided no contraindications are present Do not restart warfarin until patient has resumed dietary intake

Table 33.8 *(cont.)*

	Low risk	Medium risk	High risk
		Continue Clexane until INR is above the lower limit of TTR	Check INR 3 days after restarting warfarin
			Continue Clexane until INR is above the lower limit of TTR

[a] CVL prophylaxis is usually only required for long-term home total parenteral nutrition (TPN) patients and is tiered depending on history of previous thrombosis, lack of remaining access for the patient.
[b] Patients with primary pulmonary hypertension may not require bridging anticoagulation, but they do require very careful planning around procedures requiring sedation and/or anesthesia.
[c] Children with moyamoya disease having warfarin interruption periprocedurally may also require intravenous hydration during the fasting period. Please liaise with neurology regarding periprocedural planning.
[d] In setting of renal impairment, earlier cessation of heparinoid therapies may be required and monitoring tests may be required prior to procedure to ensure adequate drug clearance. This should be determined individually with hematology consultation.
[e] For patients on concurrent antiplatelet therapy, separate decisions need to made depending on perceived thrombotic risk of underlying indication and perceived bleeding risk of procedure as to whether or not antiplatelet therapy is stopped. For aspirin, clopidogrel, and dipyrimadole, cessation of therapy is required 7 to 10 days prior to the procedure to reduce any bleeding risk. Whether the use of a short-acting antiplatelet agent such as tirofiban is indicated should be determined individually.

Table 33.9 PCC Dose to Reverse Anticoagulant Effect of Warfarin

Target INR	Initial INR			
	1.5–2.5	2.6–3.5	3.6–10.0	>10.0
0.9–1.3	30 units/kg	35 units/kg	50 units/kg	50 units/kg

contraindicated or who have failed anticoagulation therapy. They were developed for adults who primarily have venous thrombosis in the lower limbs. However, given that most VTEs in children occur in the upper system related to CVLs, the role of IVC filters is significantly reduced. However, there are reports on the use of IVC filters in children as young as 6 years of age.

Blood Transfusion: Indications and Safe Use in Children

Key Messages

1. Patient and sample identification are critical to safe blood transfusion practice.

2. All hospitals/health services should have well-documented policies and procedures around transfusion medicine, and physicians should be familiar with these and act accordingly.

3. Blood storage and handling are critical to the safety of blood products.

4. A number of blood products are available, and manipulations of those products have specific indications and risks/benefits.

5. Minimizing blood donor exposure to children is optimal.

6. Iatrogenic blood loss is a common cause of transfusion requirement in hospitalized children, and every effort should be made to minimize blood testing.

7. Transfusion volumes in children should be calculated in milliliters. One commonly used formula is desired hemoglobin (Hb, g/liter) – actual Hb (g/liter) × weight (kg) × 0.4 = volume for transfusion.

8. In general, transfusion of red blood cells (RBCs) should be based on an individualized assessment of oxygen-delivery requirements and projected course of anemia based on knowledge of underlying disease processes rather than a preset Hb level. Understanding the principles tissue oxygen delivery is fundamental to this assessment.

9. Tissue oxygen delivery = cardiac output × Hb × O_2 saturation × 1.34.

10. In oncology, chronic transfusion-dependent patients, and premature infants, the time course of anemia is very predictable, and standard transfusion triggers related to convenience or based on hemoglobin (Hb) or hematocrit (Hct) are reasonable.

Introduction

Blood transfusion therapy was a major advance in medicine in the beginning of the twentieth century, and much of the improved survival of patients with trauma, undergoing major surgery, or undergoing cancer therapy would not be achievable without adequate blood product support. Similarly, patients with inherited hemoglobinopathies that were previously fatal in early childhood can now lead long and productive lives due to blood support and iron chelation therapy. In hospitalized children, especially premature neonates, a major cause of anemia requiring transfusion is iatrogenic blood loss. In the latter part of the twentieth century, the spread of HIV infection and other viruses transmissible through blood products increased the emphasis on minimizing blood donor exposure and the safety of blood products. While the risk of transfusion-associated HIV infection is now miniscule in Western societies, fear of the next virus is ever present, and most clinicians still strive to limit blood donor exposure when at all possible. The mechanisms to achieve this include reducing unnecessary blood tests, blood conservation strategies during surgery, lowering of transfusion thresholds, the use of hematinic/erythropoietin support, and the use of Pedi-Packs that enable multiple transfusions over time from a single donor. Directed donation might not reduce donor exposure but rather dictate who the donor is, and this will be discussed in Chapter 35. Viral transmission remains one of the less common adverse affects of blood transfusion, and while minimization of donor exposure is a good principle, equally, there are times when rapid and aggressive transfusion therapy is required. However, fear of viral transmission is not the only driver behind minimizing transfusion exposure. The fact remains that blood donations are a precious and finite resource, and we are all impelled to ensure it is used to best effect.

Transfusion medicine is usually at the forefront of documentation and quality system processes within healthcare systems. Despite this, a major concern remains about the frequency of administrative and avoidable errors that contribute to the morbidity and mortality associated with transfusion therapy. The general public demands a safe blood transfusion service and is probably unrealistic in their expectations that zero harm should come from transfusion therapy. However, the general public is correct in assuming that strict adherence to patient identification procedures, blood ordering and checking procedures, and blood storage and handling procedures would drastically reduce the frequency of transfusion-associated adverse events. Thus, all healthcare professionals should be accountable in this regard.

Given the frequency of its use, one could argue that the evidence that supports many transfusion-related decisions is appalling, and it is true that there has been little effective research, especially in pediatric transfusion medicine. There are few other interventions that have as much accepted dogma with such little evidence in support. This is an area that needs ongoing significant research into very pragmatic and practical issues, such as the relative merits of liberal versus restrictive transfusion thresholds, as well as into questions of the immunomodulatory effects of transfusion, that may have an impact on survival.

Blood Components

While there are a multitude of fractionated products made from blood for specific clinical indications, we usually consider blood products for transfusion as being either packed red blood cells (RBCs), platelets, fresh frozen plasma (FFP), or cryoprecipitate.

Packed Red Blood Cells

RBCs are separated from the plasma and platelets by centrifugation. In many countries, packed RBCs are now filtered at the central blood bank to remove white blood cells (WBCs) and are thus termed leukodepleted RBC. Leukodepletion greatly reduces the rate of febrile nonhemolytic transfusion reactions but does not resolve all risks related to the WBC (see later). Standard packed RBCs have a volume of 260 ± 19 (>220) ml and a hemoglobin of 50 ± 6 (≥ 40) g/unit. The hematocrit (Hct, liter/liter) is usually on the order of 0.59 ± 0.03 (0.50–0.70), and the leukocyte count (10^6/unit) is 0.27 ± 0.07 (<1.0). Packed RBCs must be stored at 2 to 6°C and, when stored appropriately, have a shelf life of between 35 and 42 days. When stored correctly and without infection, there should be minimal hemolysis by the expiration date (hemolysis 0.37 ± 0.25 [<0.8] percent).

Pediatric RBC packs or Pedi-Packs are created when an original pack is divided into four subunits of approximately 60 ml each. They have a shelf life of 35 days and can be used for small-volume transfusions to reduce wastage or as sequential donations within that time frame to the same patient to reduce donor exposure.

Platelets

Platelets can be obtained in a number of ways. A standard adult platelet pack can be derived from the buffy coat (separated by centrifugation) from four identical ABO donors and then resuspended in nutrient-additive solution to produce a pooled platelet component.

Alternatively, platelets may be collected via apheresis of the donor along with some plasma, with the other blood elements being returned to the donor. An apheresis platelet unit can be further divided into four packs of equal volume to produce pediatric apheresis platelet components. This is to reduce donor exposure for small pediatric transfusions and to minimize product wastage.

In most countries, both apheresis and pooled platelets are leukodepleted at the source, and they are also often irradiated prior to dispatch from the central blood service. This is different from RBCs because routine irradiation of RBCs dramatically reduces their shelf life and would make the blood supply not viable in most countries. Platelets can be stored for 5 days at 20 to 24°C with gentle agitation.

Pooled leukodepleted platelets usually have a volume of approximately 326 ± 14 (>160) ml and a platelet count of 284 ± 40 (>240) $\times 10^9$/pool. The leukocyte count is usually 0.33 ± 0.02 (<0.8) $\times 10^6$/pool. Apheresed platelets usually have a volume of 180 ± 11 (100–400) ml/pack with a platelet count of 280 ± 34 (>200 to ≤ 510) $\times 10^9$/unit and a leukocyte count 0.21 ± 0.15 (<1.0) × 10^6/unit. Pediatric apher-esed platelet packs usually have a volume of 51 ± 2 (40–60) ml and a platelet count of 76 ± 10 (>60) × 10^9/unit.

Fresh Frozen Plasma (FFP)

FFP can be derived from centrifuged whole blood, with each pack from a single donor, or via apheresis, with the yield of each apheresis split into two or three units of equal volume prior to freezing. Pediatric FFP is derived from a single unit of whole blood. The plasma is separated and then divided into four packs of equal volume. This reduces donor exposure for small pediatric transfusions and minimizes product wastage. All FFP must be frozen to a core temperature below –30°C within 1 hour of starting the freezing process and can be stored for 12 months at –25°C or below. A unit of FFP contains all coagulation factors including the labile plasma coagulation factors VIII and V.

Packs of FFP from whole blood usually have a volume of 280 ± 14 (250–310) ml, a platelet count of 5 ± 4 (<50) × 10^9/liter, a leukocyte count of 0.04 ± 0.03 (<0.1) × 10^9/liter. Apheresis FFP usually has a volume of 273 ± 11 (250–310) ml, a platelet count of 12 ± 10 (<50) × 10^9/liter, and a leukocyte count 0.02 ± 0.02 (<0.1) × 10^9/liter. Pediatric FFP packs usually have a volume of 70 ± 4 (60–80) ml.

Cryoprecipitate

Cryoprecipitate is derived from whole blood or col-lected via apheresis and is prepared by thawing FFP between 1 and 6°C and recovering the precipitate. The cold-insoluble precipitate is refrozen. Cryopreci-pitate contains most of the factor VIII, fibrinogen, factor XIII, von Willebrand factor, and fibronectin from FFP. Whole-blood cryoprecipitate has a volume of 36 ± 2 (30–40) ml and has 153 ± 35 (≥0.70) IU/pack of factor VIIIc; 423 ± 120 (≥ 140) mg/unit of Fibrinogen and 275 ± 63 (> 100) IU/pack of Von Willebrand factor. Apheresis packs are approximately double in volume and amount of these factors.

Blood Product Compatibilities

Blood groups are proteins/glycoproteins on the RBC surfaces. There are many blood groups, including ABO, Rh, Kidd, Kell, Duffy, MNS, and Lewis. The most important of these are ABO and Rhesus (RhD).

Red Blood Cells

The ABO blood group is the most important of all the blood group systems, and the discovery of these blood groups in 1901 earned Karl Landsteiner the Nobel Prize for medicine in 1930. There are four different ABO blood groups, determined by whether or not an individual's RBCs carry the A antigen, the B antigen, both A and B antigens, or neither (blood group O). From early childhood, normal people make RBC antibodies against A or B antigens that are not expressed on their own cells. These naturally occur-ring antibodies are mainly IgM immunoglobulins. Transfusion with ABO-incompatible blood can lead to severe and potentially fatal transfusion reactions, even in the absence of a transfusion history. Blood group O is known as the *universal donor* for RBCs because it can be given to anyone without fear of ABO incompatibility – there is no antibody to O. Blood group AB is known as the *universal recipient* because it can receive RBCs of any ABO group without fear of ABO incompatibility because AB recipients will not have antibodies to A or B since they have these anti-gens on their own cells (Table 34.1).

The Rhesus blood group system was first dis-covered in Rhesus monkeys during the 1930s, and again, Lansteiner was instrumental. There are more than 40 different kinds of Rh antigens. The most significant Rh antigen is RhD. When RhD is present on the RBC surface, the RBCs are called *RhD positive*. Approximately 80 percent of a particular Caucasian population is RhD positive. The remaining 20 percent of the population that lack the RhD antigen are called *RhD negative*. These ratios vary considerably with ethnicity.

Antibodies to RhD develop only after an individ-ual is exposed to RhD antigens via transfusion, preg-nancy, or organ transplantation. Unlike in ABO, there are no naturally occurring antibodies. RhD is highly

Table 34.1 Blood Group Compatibilities for RBC Transfusions

Recipient blood group	Naturally occurring antibodies	Can receive RBCs from groups
A	Anti-B	A or O
B	Anti-A	B or O
AB	Nil	A, B, AB, or O
O	Anti-A and anti-B	O

Table 34.2 RhD Compatibility for RBC Transfusions

Recipient RhD status	Can receive RBCs of
RhD negative	RhD negative
RhD positive	RhD positive or negative

Table 34.3 Blood Group Compatibilities for Platelet Transfusions

Recipient blood group	First-choice donor platelets	Second-choice donor platelets	Third-choice donor platelets
A	A	B	O
B	B	A	O
AB	AB	A or B	O
O	O	–	–

Table 34.4 Blood Group Compatibilities for Plasma Transfusion

Recipient blood group	Compatible FFP/ cryoprecipitate
A	A, AB
B	B, AB
AB	AB
O	O, A, B, AB
Rh positive	Rh positive or negative
Rh negative	Rh positive or negative

immunogenic and can lead to RBC hemolysis in certain settings. This is of particular importance in pregnancy, where anti-D antibodies can cross the placenta from mother to unborn child and lead to hemolytic disease of the newborn (see Chapter 5).

As a general rule, RhD-negative individuals should not be transfused with RhD-positive RBCs, especially RhD-negative girls and women of childbearing age. If transfusion of an RhD-positive product to an RhD-negative recipient is unavoidable, the administration of anti-D immunoglobulin should be considered (Table 34.2).

Platelets

In transfusion of platelets, the use of identical ABO and Rh blood groups between donor and recipient is preferred. This is so because depending on how the platelets are prepared, there may be small amounts of RBCs in the pack and small amounts of plasma, which potentially could cause incompatibility reactions. However, often this is not possible due to supply issues, and compromises have to be made. Platelets from RhD-positive donors should be avoided for RhD-negative recipients. The small number of RBCs present may be sufficient to cause Rhesus immunization. If transfusion of an RhD-positive product to an RhD-negative recipient is unavoidable, consider giving Rhesus immunoglobulin. Transfusing platelets from group O donors to group A, B, or AB recipients may result in hemolysis (from anti-A and anti-B in group O plasma). Children and infants are more at risk than adults due to their small blood volume. If ABO-incompatible transfusion is unavoidable, the use of pooled platelets that are suspended in an additive solution, as distinct from apheresis platelets that are suspended in plasma, may reduce the risk of hemolysis. All these risks are relative, and the merits or benefits of the platelet transfusion must be weighed against the potential risks in the context of the product available at the time.

Platelets express class I HLA antigens; RBCs do not; they are the only cell in the body that does not. Therefore, patients may develop HLA antibodies after platelet transfusion, and they may become refractory to further platelet transfusions that have the same HLA. This is a major problem in platelet transfusion (Table 34.3).

FFP and Cryoprecipitate

In transfusion of FFP or cryoprecipitate, the consideration is what antibodies may be in the donor plasma and how they might react with the recipient cells. In terms of plasma, group AB now becomes the universal donor (no ABO antibodies), and group O becomes the universal recipient (Table 34.4).

Specific Treatment of Blood Products

Leukodepletion

As described earlier, many central blood services leukodeplete blood products at the source. This leads to at least a 3 log reduction in the number of WBCs in the product and dramatically reduces the rate of adverse events known to be associated with WBCs within blood products. For services that do not receive products leukodepleted in this way, bedside leukodepletion (using a filter that is based on cell size) remains an option.

Phenotyping

For patients who will require frequent transfusion (e.g. transfusion-dependent hemoglobinopathies), the likelihood of developing alloantibodies at some stage to a RBC antigen is high, and phenotyping the patient early in the course (preferably in anticipation and prior to the first transfusion) and providing phenotype-matched products (in which the RBCs are matched to blood group antigens other than ABO and RhD) is highly recommended. Similarly, in patients who have already developed clinically significant antibodies (usually HLA antibodies), ongoing provision of HLA-matched (as close as possible to the patient's own HLA type) products may produce both a better platelet increment after transfusion and reduce the development of further antibodies that may eventually compromise the ability to transfuse at all.

Washing of RBCs

Washing of RBCs and resuspending them in additive solution removes any plasma from the product, but at a cost of loss of some of the RBCs. This is indicated for patients who have had severe allergic reactions to blood transfusions. Most commonly, this involves IgA-deficient recipients who react against donor IgA, but other patients may have allergic reactions against known or unknown allergens in blood products that may be reduced by washing RBCs. The process requires time and must be completed in a sterile manner usually within a central blood service, so it is difficult to provide as an urgent request.

CMV-Seronegative Products

Cytomegalovirus (CMV) is an intracellular virus that can cause disease in transfusion recipients. Leukodepletion dramatically decreases the risk of CMV transmission but does not eliminate it. Thus, specific high-risk populations may require CMV-seronegative products, if they are available. Most guidelines recommend specific CMV-seronegative products (RBCs and platelets; this is not an issue for acellular components such as FFP and cryoprecipitate) for recipients of allogeneic or autologous stem cell, bone marrow, or solid-organ transplants; recipients of highly immunosuppressive chemotherapy (e.g. leukemia or lymphoma); recipients of intrauterine RBC transfusions; premature (<1500 g) or immune-compromised

neonates; and pregnant women regardless of CMV status. If CMV-seronegative products are unavailable, the risk of transfusion must be considered against the perceived benefits, and monitoring for CMV activation may be required after the transfusion.

Irradiation

Irradiation is designed to kill any remaining lymphocytes within the product (RBC or platelets) to prevent the possibility of transfusion-associated graft-versus-host disease (TA-GvHD). Leukodepletion never removes all lymphocytes. Adequate irradiation involves exposing the product to at least 25 to 30 Gy, and this reduces the shelf life of RBCs to approximately 2 weeks. In addition, the damage to the RBCs from the irradiation increases the extracellular potassium load of the product, and this may be clinically significant depending on volume and rate of transfusion. Immune-competent recipients will usually destroy any donor lymphocytes quickly and easily, so TA-GvHD occurs most likely when the recipient is immune compromised.

Every institution must have a policy for irradiated product use. In an immune-competent person, the patient's lymphocytes will reject the lymphocytes in the transfusion, which are few in number. Only cellular products (packed RBCs and platelets) ever require irradiation. The commonly used indication for irradiated products is when the patient has a poor cellular immune system:

- Premature neonates and those requiring an intrauterine tranfusion
- Children with known immunodeficiency
- Children with acquired immune deficiency, including high-dose chemotherapy and transplant recipients
- Children with Hodgkin lymphoma and children who have received lymphocyte-depleting chemotherapy with nucleoside analogues (e.g., fludarabine)
- Irradiation is also essential for directed donations because the frequency of TA-GvHD is markedly increased when the donor and recipient have a higher likelihood of homologous or semihomologous HLA phenotypes. In this situation, the HLA similarity between donor and recipient means that the transfused donor cells are less able to be recognised and rejected by the cells of the recipient immune system'.

Blood Ordering Including Volume Calculation and Transfusion Indications

In ordering blood products, strict adherence to institutional protocols and procedures should be observed. All institutions require strict governance around transfusion practice. Adequate attention to identification of the patient and identification of the appropriate and specific blood product to be given is critical.

The need to give packed RBCs and the urgency of the transfusion are guided by two factors:

1. The projected course of the anemia. For example, uncontrolled blood loss or ongoing hemolysis makes urgent transfusion likely. In the surgical setting, blood loss often can be reliably predicted from previous experience.

2. An understanding of the tissue oxygen delivery equation and the ability of the patient to maintain the required cardiac compensation.

This equation was detailed in Chapter 1:

Tissue oxygen delivery (ml/min) =
cardiac output (liter/min) × Hb (g/liter) × oxygen saturation (%) × 1.34 ml/g (constant : amount of oxygen per gram of normal Hb)

Cardiac output is the product of heart rate and stroke volume, and given that stroke volume rarely changes acutely, the cardiac compensation for rapid loss of Hb is reflected in the heart rate.

Thus, for example, if the cause of the anemia is iron deficiency, which causes a very slow reduction in hemoglobin, but the patient's heart rate indicates that he or she cannot sustain the compensatory increase, then transfusion would be indicated. At all times, transfusion should be used to prevent the patient from getting to the point where cardiac decompensation – and hence the possibility of tissue (particularly brain) hypoxic damage – might occur.

Packed RBCs may be ordered in three ways:

1. *Urgent*: Un-cross-matched blood group O negative can be used for all potential recipients and is the product of choice when urgent restoration of oxygen-carrying capacity is required. In most major hospitals, this product should be available within minutes of a request to the blood bank, and most trauma service units would have well-defined protocols for urgent blood release, even in the situation of unidentified patients.

2. *Semiurgent*: If the patient is stable in the short term, but transfusion is required within 30 minutes to restore oxygen-carrying capacity, then group-specific but un-cross-matched blood can be used. This requires a sample from the patient to have the blood group checked and then provision of appropriate blood. The advantage of this is that is saves O-negative blood, which can often be in short supply. Previous blood group data should never be used as the sole criterion on which blood group–specific blood is provided. A fresh sample, adequately identified and tested, is mandatory. Transfusion of incompatible ABO blood has disastrous consequences, and if there is any doubt about sample identity or insufficient time for testing, then un-cross-matched O-negative packed RBCs are safer.

3. *Nonurgent*: If the patient is judged to be able to tolerate more than 45 minutes before requiring transfusion, then fully cross-matched blood should be provided. This is especially the case in patients who have been or will be multiply transfused because antibody screening and avoidance of immunization against other common red blood group antigens is important. Samples for cross-match should be collected fewer than 3 days prior to transfusion, and once that time has elapsed, a fresh sample is required to ensure that no new antibodies have developed.

The volume required for transfusion is reliably calculated by the following equation:

Desired Hb (g/liter) − actual Hb (g/liter) ×
weight (kg) × 0.4 = ml packed RBCs required

This is often rounded to the nearest available unit size so as not to waste product. In urgent circumstances where Hb is unknown, estimations based on body weight and blood loss or empirical volumes such as 10 ml/kg are often used. In general, the aim is to restore oxygen-carrying capacity to either a safe or desirable level while minimizing the donor exposure for the recipient.

FFP and cryoprecipitate are usually given in doses of 10 to 20 and 5 to 10 ml/kg respectively. This may vary based on the situation and degree of coagulopathy and, where possible, should be guided by coagulation results. Cryoprecipitate is used predominantly to replace fibrinogen, whereas FFP is used for replacement of broader coagulation factors. In many circumstances (e.g. reversal of warfarin therapy [prothrombin complex concentrate] and congenital bleeding disorders [specific factor concentrates]), there are specific products that are more suitable and have the advantage of having undergone viral inactivation processes. FFP and cryoprecipitate should never be used for volume replacement in the absence of coagulopathy.

Blood Product Administration

Once again, strict adherence to institutional guidelines for the administration of blood products, especially with consideration to patient and blood unit identification; consent and documentation of transfusions; duration of transfusion (all blood products should be transfused within 4 hours of release from blood bank); use of appropriate giving sets, monitoring for acute complications; and reporting and management of adverse transfusion reactions are critical to enable the safe and effective use of blood products.

Conclusions

Transfusion therapy is an important component of modern-day tertiary care medicine, and many groups of patients, including oncology patients, surgical patients, those suffering trauma, and extreme prematurity, would not survive without safe and effective blood transfusion support. However, if not managed safely and within strict parameters, transfusion therapy can have disastrous consequences. Thus, adherence to institutional protocols and procedures is essential. There remains much to be learned about optimal indications for transfusion and alternatives to blood products, and there is a real need for ongoing active research in this field. This chapter has detailed the basics of the products available and how to choose the right product for each patient. Chapter 35 will discuss the potential adverse consequences of transfusion as well as some special transfusion circumstances.

Adverse Reactions to Blood Products and Special Transfusion Circumstances

1. Monitoring for complications of blood transfusions is important.

2. Acute transfusion reactions can be life threatening, and immediate action is often required.

3. If there is any concern that a transfusion reaction is occurring, stop the transfusion immediately, and repeat the pretransfusion checking of patient and blood identification and matching.

4. Acute hemolytic transfusion reactions (wrong blood to patient) and bacterial sepsis (potential errors in storage and handling) are the most devastating acute transfusion reactions.

5. For any complication of blood transfusion, immediate consideration must be given that other units from the same donor may be ready for use (at the same or at a different health service location), so potential implications for other recipients must be considered. A decision about the need to recall products should be made as a matter of urgency. This is especially the case for suspected infectious complications.

6. Viral infection from blood transfusion is a rare occurrence but is often of significant concern to the general public.

7. Massive transfusions are best managed according to a specific massive transfusion protocol.

8. Exchange transfusions may be required for specific indications.

Introduction

The only way to absolutely avoid a complication from blood transfusion is to avoid the blood transfusion in the first place. The need for transfusion should be justified in each and every case. However, there are times when transfusion therapy is required, and most institutions have well-documented processes and procedures to ensure maximum safety of blood transfusion. Clinicians should be aware of institutional policies, procedures, and practices and adhere to them carefully. Nonetheless, some adverse transfusion-associated events cannot be avoided irrespective of adherence to best practice. Appropriate education of patients and families should be provided in all but severe emergent situations and appropriate consent for transfusion therapy documented.

Adverse events from transfusions may be acute or delayed. Acute reactions are usually pretty obvious, with the patient becoming unwell usually during the transfusion. Delayed reactions require a high index of suspicion and an adequate transfusion history to have been taken.

Transfusion reactions can occur to all blood products, although the pathogenesis of reactions may differ between different blood products, as does the frequency of different types of reactions. For example, bacterial sepsis may complicate both red blood cell (RBC) and platelet transfusions, although the source and type of bacteria involved in each are usually quite different.

Increasing the transfusion volume, especially in an urgent scenario, increases the likelihood of specific complications such as hypothermia, metabolic derangement, coagulopathy, and potentially fluid overload. Thus, most institutions have specific protocols for massive transfusions in the emergency setting and for exchange transfusions that tend to be more semielective and planned. Irrespective of

Acute Transfusion Reactions

the transfusion scenario, adherence to strict identification checking, storage, and handling conditions and monitoring processes is the key to maximizing transfusion safety.

Acute Transfusion Reactions

The most feared immediate adverse event from transfusion are acute hemolytic transfusion reactions (AHTRs), which are usually due to ABO incompatability. Invariably, these reactions are due to errors in identification or labeling of either the pretransfusion sample or the actual transfusion itself. High-risk times include transfusion of the unidentified patient, usually in emergency departments or in situations where multiple patients have the same or similar names and finally where multiple patients are being transfused simultaneously (e.g., busy oncology day units). Staff inexperience are unfamiliarity with systems are also causative factors. Clinicians need to be aware of such situations and stick to established procedures and practices at all times.

Occasionally, hemolysis occurs for nonimmune reasons related to storage or administration of RBCs, for example, the mixing of RBCs with nonisotonic fluids during simultaneous infusion through a single intravenous access point. Compromises are often driven in pediatrics by lack of intravenous access, but in general, RBCs should not be co-infused with any other substance.

The initial symptoms of AHTR are often nonspecific, with fever, tachycardia, and chest pain, but there is rapid progression to hypotension, circulatory collapse, hemoglobinuria, multiorgan failure, and disseminated intravascular coagulation (DIC). Patients often describe a sense of impending doom and anxiety.

Immediate cessation of transfusion is essential. The blood pack should be returned to blood bank along with fresh blood sample for repeat grouping and checking. Urine for hemoglobin assessment and blood to assess general organ status (arterial blood gases [ABG]; urea, electrolytes, and creatinine [UEC] tests; liver function tests [LFTs]) may be required. Aggressive supportive care is often required.

Immediate consideration needs to be given that if this patient has received the wrong blood, then it is highly likely another patient in the facility is about to receive the blood intended for this patient, so the catastrophe may be repeated. Aggressive and emergent investigation of the source of the error and the need to avoid a second wrong transfusion is required.

As mentioned earlier, bacterial contamination is the most likely differential diagnosis for AHTR, and the clinical presentations are often identical. There may be higher fever and more prominent nausea and diarrhea in bacterial contamination, and profound hypotension and circulatory collapse usually occurs quite early. Bacteria may be introduced into the pack at the time of blood collection from sources such as donor skin, donor bacteremia, or equipment used during blood collection or processing. Bacteria may multiply during storage, especially if the recommended storage conditions are not rigidly followed. Individual blood products should never be infused over longer than 4 hours because this enables small numbers of bacteria contained during cold storage (of a RBC component) to multiple quickly at room temperature and reach pathogenic numbers. Grampositive and gram-negative organisms have been implicated. Platelets are more frequently implicated than RBCs, presumably because they are stored at room temperature.

In addition to the treatments described for AHTR, blood cultures should be taken and broad-spectrum antimicrobial agents started. Inspection of the pack to look for abnormal color, clumping, and so on of the blood should occur, and the pack should be sent for culture. Blood cultures also should be collected from the patient.

Fever, in the absence of signs and symptoms of circulatory failure, is more common. Acute nonhemolytic febrile transfusion reactions (ANHFTRs) are thought to be caused by recipient antibodies reacting with white blood cell (WBC) antigens or WBC fragments in the blood product or due to cytokines that accumulate in the blood product during storage. These reactions are greatly reduced if blood products are WBC filtered at source but also can be reduced by bedside filtering. Rigors can accompany the fever, and these reactions are more common with platelet transfusions than with RBCs.

Initial management of transfusion-associated fever should always be to stop the transfusion. Consideration of the underlying disease and potential for fever is important. Close observation for circulatory signs and rechecking of all procedures are essential. If the patient settles or stabilizes, then restarting the transfusion with acetaminophen cover is often acceptable. However, as stated previously, *no individual blood pack should be used more than 4 hours after removal from the blood bank.* 'Thus, if there are delays while assessing the patient, the pack should be removed and the need for transfusion be reassessed using another pack'

If patients have repeated febrile reactions, human leukocyte antigen (HLA) antibodies may have developed, and pretreatment before each transfusion may be required.

Acute Allergic Reactions

Acute allergic reactions occur when the patient is allergic to a protein in the donor's blood or the donor is allergic to a protein in the recipient's blood. The classic anaphylactic reaction occurs in recipients with IgA deficiency and IgA antibodies who react to IgA in the donor blood. Once these patients are identified, they usually need future transfusion with washed RBCs or with blood products collected from specific IgA-deficient donors.

Less severe allergic reactions can occur, ranging from bronchospasm and edema to urticaria. If urticaria occurs in isolation (without fever and other signs), slow the rate or temporarily stop the transfusion. If symptoms are bothersome, consider administering an antihistamine before restarting the transfusion. If the initial symptoms are associated with other symptoms, cease the transfusion and proceed with investigation, which primarily involves assessing IgA levels and the presence of IgA antibodies. More severe reactions may require epinephrine, usually given as a 1:1000 solution, 0.01 mg/kg subcutaneously, intramuscularly, or as a slow intravenous infusion. In the absence of IgA deficiency, many patients will not react to products from a different donor, but some will, and premedication for all future transfusions may be required.

Respiratory Distress

Volume overload can occur, especially with large-volume transfusions and especially if large amounts of colloid solution have been infused prior to blood products. Alternatively, patients who have had slowly developing anemia and have adapted to maintain their circulatory volume by expanding plasma volume are at risk. Anticipation of such events and careful monitoring, using diuretics as appropriate, often avoids this complication. Volume overload usually presents during the transfusion.

Transfusion-related acute lung injury (TRALI) usually presents within 2 to 8 hours after a transfusion and is a clinical diagnosis of exclusion characterized by acute respiratory distress and bilaterally symmetrical pulmonary edema with hypoxemia. Chest x-ray shows interstitial or alveolar infiltrates when no cardiogenic or other cause of pulmonary edema exists. TRALI is due to cytokines in the transfused product or to interaction between patient WBC antigens and donor antibodies (or vice versa). Oxygen support, with or without ventilatory support, is required, and most cases settle over the next few days.

Acute Metabolic Reactions

Large-volume transfusions, especially in small infants, can lead to a number of metabolic disturbances such as hypothermia, citrate toxicity, or potassium toxicity. The use of blood warmers during massive or exchange transfusions is important for avoiding hypothermia. Citrate is the anticoagulant used in blood products, which is usually rapidly metabolized by the liver. Hence, patients with liver failure or dysfunction are at most risk. Citrate toxicity causes hypocalcemia and hypomagnesemia, which may, in turn, cause myocardial depression or coagulopathy. Temporarily stopping the transfusion allows citrate to be metabolized. Replacement therapy may be required for symptomatic hypocalcemia or hypomagnesemia. Finally, stored RBCs leak potassium proportionately throughout their storage life. Irradiation of RBCs increases the rate of potassium leakage. Clinically significant hyperkalemia can occur during rapid, large-volume transfusion of older RBC units in small infants and children. This is avoided by using the freshest blood possible and irradiating (if required) immediately prior to transfusion.

Delayed and Long-Term Complications of Blood Transfusions

Blood transfusions are usually matched for ABO and RhD blood groups. However, there are many other RBC antigens that can cause alloimmunization. A delayed hemolytic transfusion reaction (DHTR) occurs when a patient develops an antibody directed against an antigen on transfused RBCs. The antibody may cause shortened RBC survival, with clinical features of fever, jaundice, and lower than expected hemoglobin following transfusion, often occurring 3 to 14 days after transfusion. In reality, many delayed hemolytic reactions produce few symptoms and may go undetected.

After RhD, the next most common antigen that causes alloimmunization is the Kell (K) antigens. Avoiding alloimmunization is critical for females with child-bearing potential because these antibodies can cause severe hemolytic disease of the newborn during pregnancy. Some centers, rather than expanding their pretransfusion testing panel from ABO and RhD to include Kell, just transfuse all young females with Kell-negative products when possible. Kell is often not expressed in African ancestry patients, so in sickle cell patients who need blood, Kell-negative blood is usually selected. In children on a transfusion program, blood with extended phenotype matching may be selected in any case.

Patients who are chronically transfused are at greatest risk of alloantibody formation. Prior to starting transfusion, patients with these conditions should have extended RBC phenotyping performed. Patients who are chronically transfused are also at risk of iron overload, and adequate iron chelation is a critical part of any chronic transfusion program.

Transfusion-associated graft-versus-host disease (TA-GvHD) occurs when donor lymphocytes in cellular blood products engraft in a susceptible transfusion recipient. TA-GvHD usually develops 8 to 10 days after transfusion (although it can be longer in infants) and targets bone marrow, skin, liver, and gastrointestinal tract. The clinical presentation includes fever, skin rash, pancytopenia, abnormal liver function, and diarrhea and is fatal in almost all cases. Irradiation of cellular blood products can prevent TA-GvHD and is important for at-risk patients, including all intrauterine transfusions, patients with known immune deficiency, patients receiving high-dose chemotherapy, and transplant patients. Some pediatric centers routinely irradiate blood for all neonates, congenital heart disease patients, and oncology and transplant patients. In addition, irradiation is required for all recipients of blood from biologically related (directed) or HLA-identical donors irrespective of their immune competence (see Chapter 34).

While bacterial infection is the most common infectious complication of blood transfusions and occurs as an acute complication, many patients and families are most concerned about the risks of viral and other infectious agents being transmitted via blood transfusion. Definitive evidence of viral transmission by transfusion requires demonstration of seroconversion or new infection in the recipient and isolation of an agent with genomic identity from both the recipient and the implicated donor. Suspected transfusion-transmitted infection of any agent (bacteria, parasitic, or viral) should be reported urgently in order to recall other potentially infectious blood products from the same donation.

The actual risk of viral transmission from blood transfusion varies from country to country based on the background rates of infection in the community, on whether blood donations are voluntary or paid, and on the donor screening procedures that are in place. The donor questionnaire about at risk situations is more important than the laboratory testing in excluding potential infected donors primarily because all laboratory testing strategies have a window period that reflects the time the donor is infected (and can transmit disease) and yet will have negative laboratory testing. Travel history to areas where parasitic blood infections such as malaria are endemic is an essential part of the screen. Hence, volunteer donations that provide little or no incentive to the donor other than altruism tend to be safer. Approximate estimates for risks of viral transmission are given in Table 35.1.

Special Transfusion Circumstances

There are a number of situations where transfusions require specific and special considerations. For example:

- The transfusion of an unidentified patient presents a particular challenge, and all institutions that offer emergency services need to have procedures for dealing with this situation. The key elements include that however the patient is identified, it must remain constant through the transfusion episode so that at all times the identification on the blood product matches that on the patient. Further, the method of identification must be robust (with more than one identifier) and able to withstand multiple

Table 35.1 Approximate Risks of Viral Transmission from Blood Transfusion in Volunteer Donor Programs in Westernized Countries.

Virus	Testing strategy	Window period (days)	Approximate risk per unit transfused
HIV	Antibody only	22	1 in 2.5 million
	Antibody plus nucleic acid testing	9	1 in 7 million
Hepatitis C virus (HCV)	Antibody only	66	1 in 300,000
	Antibody plus nucleic acid testing	7	1 in 3.5 million
Hepatitis B virus (HBV)	–	45	1 in 1.3 million
Human T-lymphotropic virus (HTLV) 1 and 2	–	51	<1 in 1 million
Variant Creutzfeldt-Jakob disease (vCJD)	–	Unknown	Rare

unidentified patients at the same time (as often occurs in multivehicle accidents).

- Use of cell salvage procedures intraoperatively (beyond the scope of this book).
- Directed donations. In general, there are no specific advantages over random donor transfusion in countries with high-quality and safe centralized blood banking services. The use of related donors is thought to reduce the validity of donor questionnaires because there is incentive to give the 'right' answers. The use of related donors significantly increases the risk of TA-GvHD, and all such donations should be irradiated.
- Autologous donations are used infrequently in children for volume reasons but may be useful in some older children having planned elective surgery in whom expected blood loss is very predictable.
- Exchange transfusion is most commonly used in neonates for the management of hyperbilirubinemia and in sickle cell disease to reduce hemoglobin SS in the setting of stroke or chest crisis. In neonates, the exchange transfusion serves two purposes. While phototherapy is the first-line treatment for hyperbilirubinemia in neonates, if jaundice levels continue to increase despite maximal phototherapy, exchange transfusion may be indicated first to remove circulating bilirubin (reducing levels and avoiding kernicterus) and, second, to replace antibody-

coated RBCs with antigen-negative RBCs. The bilirubin level at which exchange transfusion should be considered depends on the gestational age and weight of the infant, as well as the postbirth age and the presence or absence of other risk factors, including asphyxia, significant lethargy, temperature instability, sepsis, and acidosis. Irrespective of the bilirubin level, signs of bilirubin encephalopathy would demand urgent exchange transfusion. Most commonly, a double-volume exchange transfusion is used, and the volume is calculated on 80 ml/kg for term infants and 100 ml/kg for preterm infants. That is, a double-volume exchange for a term infant is 160 ml/kg. This will replace 85 percent of the blood volume and should reduce the bilirubin to 50 percent of preexchange levels. Rebound to two-thirds of preexchange levels can be expected within the subsequent 4 hours. Most tertiary hospitals will have specific protocols for exchange transfusion, and blood used should have a hematocrit of 0.5 to 0.6, be of the appropriate blood group for infants, and be negative for any antibodies detected in maternal serum. Leukodepleted, irradiated, and cytomegalovirus (CMV)–seronegative blood is optimal, and it should be as fresh as possible to reduce the biochemical disturbances. Use of a blood warmer is beneficial. In general, slower exchange transfusions are associated with better reductions in bilirubin and fewer metabolic complications.

241

Careful monitoring of the infant throughout is required. Hemodynamic and metabolic (temperature, glucose, calcium, potassium, acid-base) disturbances, coagulopathy, feed intolerance, and necrotizing enterocolitis are all well-described complications. Fresh frozen plasma (FFP) is given at 10 ml/kg halfway through and at the end of the procedure in many centers. Exchange transfusions can be performed via an arterial and venous line (two operators) or via a single venous access point such as umbilical vein (one operator), and careful use of three-way taps should control the blood flow so that small aliquots are withdrawn and replaced in sequence, and careful count of total volume of exchange is maintained.

- Massive transfusions are now very well defined as situations – usually related to trauma or massive blood loss – in which there is expected to be an urgent need to replace a large volume of blood quickly. This will necessitate not only adequate RBC replacement but also use of FFP and cryoprecipitate and platelets to avoid coagulopathy of massive transfusion.

The recognition that early and aggressive use of these products can improve outcomes has led to the development of massive-transfusion protocols that mandate the use of all these products in set ratios from early in the transfusion episode and adjusted according to the results of regular full blood count (FBE), activate partial thromboplastin time (APTT), prothrombin time/international normalized ration (PT/INR), and fibrinogen measurements. The effective management of massive transfusions requires clear and verified communication strategies among all team members, including clinicians, couriers, and blood bank staff. In children, massive transfusions often can involve relatively small absolute volumes of blood due to the size of the child involved, but the principles remain the same. With good management, avoidance of secondary DIC and transfusion-related coagulopathy can be achieved even in critically ill children who require replacement of multiple blood volumes until their bleeding is controlled.

Chapter 36

Acute Lymphoblastic Leukemia

Key Messages

1. There are general considerations when considering the diagnosis of any form of acute leukemia. An exact diagnosis is required, and there are different ways to classify and make the leukemia diagnosis – clinical appearance, morphology, immunophenotyping, cytogenetics, and molecular genetics.

2. At the same time as the diagnosis of acute lymphoblastic leukemia (ALL), an assessment of disease risk must be made so that appropriate therapy can be given – children with adverse-risk disease receive more intensive treatment than children with good-risk disease. Risk is assessed in ALL on clinical criteria (age and presenting white cell count [WBC]) and reassessed following quantification of response to standard therapy (including molecular – minimal residual disease [MRD] – quantification of residual disease) and following study of the cytogenetic and molecular genetic alterations in the patient's leukemia clone.

3. Although much is understood of the epidemiology and causes of ALL, such considerations are rarely of importance to the management of the individual child in the clinic.

4. There are different phases of ALL treatment, including remission induction therapy, consolidation of remission, central nervous system (CNS)–directed therapy, maintenance, and delayed intensification (or reinduction/consolidation) phases.

5. Specific consideration is given to management of relapsed disease, of infant ALL, and of ALL in children with Down syndrome.

6. Although most children with ALL are cured, there are significant late effects that are more manifest in children treated with a more intensive treatment schedule.

7. The future changes of ALL therapy are those of further treatment refinement to reduce toxicity, to deliver these treatment successes to children in the so-called developing world, and the better management – with new agents and new approaches – of children with relapsed and resistant disease.

8. Lymphoblastic lymphoma might be of precursor B-cell lineage or of T-cell lineage. In general, the therapy is similar to that for lymphoblastic leukemia. Management of a child with a mediastinal mass due to T-cell lymphoblastic leukemia is a particular issue in our wards and is dealt with separately in a Clinical Scenario 3.

Acute Leukemia in Children: General Considerations

On arrival in the hematology/oncology center, it is helpful to the family and child for the clinicial to state three things. Families are given hope and a framework for their child's management in the first days on the ward.

1. *They are in the right place.* This is the regional center for children with such blood illnesses, and there is concentrated expertise.

2. *An exact diagnosis will be made with appropriate investigation.* Such investigations include blood tests, bone marrow examination, lumbar puncture, and radiologic imaging.

3. *With the exact diagnosis, the appropriate therapy will be given, and this therapy will be of curative intent.* There is no possibility at the end of investigation that a diagnosis will be made for which nothing can be done.

a. Making an *exact* diagnosis is of paramount importance to the newly presenting child with acute leukemia.

b. It is helpful to consider five different classifications of leukemia in order to achieve this exact diagnosis (Table 36.1).

c. Making this *exact* diagnosis allows appropriate risk-directed therapy to be given.

d. Such therapies are derived from clinical trials, and the success of therapy of pediatric leukemia is the paradigm of large, multi-institutional phase III clinical trials in children.

e. Children with higher-risk disease are given more intensive treatment than children with lower-risk disease. Children with good prognoses are therefore not overtreated because such treatment carries the risk of toxicity, whereas the risks of treatment failure are minimized in children with adverse-risk leukemia.

Table 36.1 The Levels of Classification of Acute Leukemia

Clinical	What are the presenting symptoms? In acute leukemia, there is a short history of bone marrow failure.
Morphology	How do the leukemia cells appear? Cytochemistry might aid a morphologic diagnosis of leukemia. Do the enzyme reactions of the leukemic cell imply lineage commitment?
Immunophenotype	What antigen expression does the leukemic cell have, and what evidence is there of myeloid or lymphoid lineage commitment?
Cytogenetics	Are there nonrandom chromosomal changes that are associated with a particular leukemia?
Molecular genetics	Are there cellular genetic aberrations that are diagnostic of a particular leukemia, or is there is genetic change (e.g., immunoglobulin gene rearrangement) that is suggestive of lineage commitment?

Irrespective of whether the diagnosis is acute lymphoblastic leukemia (ALL) or acute myeloid leukemia (AML), the framework of initial diagnosis and management is similar. The leukemia is diagnosed according to the preceding classification. Prognostic information is sought so that appropriate therapy of curative intent can be given. There are certain emergency situations that must be managed, and these are dealt with separately. Management is specific to the particular leukaemia, but there is also generic supportive care such as management of infection and nutrition. The prognosis of acute leukemia in children is excellent, and the late effects of our treatments are therefore especially relevant because most patients will survive. For the minority in whom cure is not achieved, the research efforts of the community will be directed at furthering the efficacy of our therapies.

Acute Lymphoblastic Leukemia

Acute lymphoblastic leukemia (ALL) is the most common leukemia of childhood. It accounts for 30 percent of new cases of childhood cancer in the United States and Western Europe and in absolute numbers about 2,000 cases per annum in the United States and about 400 cases per annum in the United Kingdom or France.

The story of ALL is the story of childhood cancer. It is the story of improving treatment success through clinical trial. It is the story of childhood cancer epidemiology and pathogenesis. With increasing treatment success in ALL, it is also the story of treatment refinement, so treatment intensity reflects disease risk. The numbers of patients with ALL have allowed focus on the costs of treatment success in terms of late effects to be set against the risk factors that can be identified for failure of treatment.

Our job as clinicians in the management of childhood cancer is this juggling of risk. Without treatment, childhood ALL is a fatal disease. Our treatment also carries risk – both short-term morbidity and mortality during treatment and long-term morbidities. As clinicians, we need not apologize for these risks but ensure that they are proportionate to the disease; we must neither inadequately treat the disease and risk treatment failure nor overtreat the disease and risk unnecessary toxicity. Understanding the disease through careful scientific study and well-designed clinical trials over 40 years has allowed us to make these risk-based decisions and explain them, during treatment consent, to patients and their families.

Epidemiology of ALL

Incidence

ALL is the most common malignancy of childhood and accounts for 85 percent of childhood leukemias. In the United Kingdom, the incidence is 30 per 1 million children per year. The peak incidence is between the ages of 2 and 5 years, and ALL is more common in white than in black children. The incidence is greater in developed than developing countries. There are conflicting data as to whether ALL is becoming more common with time, but it is not thought that in developed countries there is much significant change.

Etiology

For any individual child, the cause of leukemia is seldom apparent and is little more than an interesting question to family and clinician. For that child and his or her family, this leukemia will represent a desperately unlucky chance and will not represent something that they as a family have done wrong or that is more likely to affect other of their children.

However, the etiology of ALL is a research field in its own right, and on a population level, it is possible to make some statements about the origins of this leukemia:

- Many cases of leukemia will have their clonal origin during fetal life. This is especially true of the ALL of early life, including the peak-incidence leukemias of early childhood. This can be shown by
    - The increased concordance rate of leukemia in monozygotic as compared with dizygotic twins. It can be shown that this increased concordance rate is a consequence of twin-to-twin leukemia metastasis through a shared circulation.
    - Backtracking leukemia-specific genotypic change to a blood sample (usually the Guthrie card) taken in early life. Using polymerase chain reaction (PCR), the leukemia-specific DNA (e.g. a leukemia-specific translocation such as TEL-AML) can be found in this neonatal sample and long before the clinical presentation.

The clinical relevance of this is that twins and especially monozygotic siblings of an index case diagnosed early in life should be regarded at high-risk of leukemia and screened as such after discussion and consent.

- Various possible causes of leukemia have been described:
    - *Infection.* In certain animal leukemias, it is clear that there is a direct relationship between virus infection, usually with retrovirus, and leukemogenesis. There is no such direct viral cause of leukemia in children. Epstein-Barr virus (EBV) is strongly associated with endemic Burkitt lymphoma/leukemia, but the molecular biology of this disease – *c-myc* translocation to the immunoglobulin gene – is the same as sporadic forms, demonstrating that the virus has a facilitating effect rather than a causative effect.

        However, the peak incidence of ALL strongly suggests an infectious etiology. This is not directly causal. Several other lines of evidence (e.g. international comparison, geographic clusters, inverse correlation with breast-feeding, decreasing incidence with birth order) suggest that ALL is a rare response to a common infection, and delayed exposure to the agent is critical to this aberrant response. Population mixing may bring this agent into a susceptible community, and some individuals are more prone genetically to such a response – as shown by an association with HLA type.

    - *Genetic causes.* Few cases of ALL have an association with a genetic syndrome. Down syndrome (DS), Bloom syndrome, ataxia telangiectasia (ATM), and neurofibromatosis (NF1) all have an increased incidence of ALL compared with the general population. In DS and NF1, the increased leukemia incidence is reduced for ALL compared with acute myeloid leukemia (AML). A search for AT with genetics and measurement of serum alpha-fetoprotein should be undertaken in any individual with cerebellar ataxia and ALL, however mild the former might be. As discussed earlier, there may be inherited differences that influence response to infection and that thus influence leukemia risk.

    - *Physical causes.* Undoubtedly exposure to ionizing radiation is a cause of ALL. This will include prenatal exposure during maternal x-rays, and there was an increase in the incidence of ALL following the nuclear bombs in World War II. However, there has been no detectable increase in ALL following the nuclear accidents and fallout at Chernobyl and Three Mile Island. Similarly, there has been no increase in ALL close to nuclear plants that cannot be explained by other factors such as population mixing. It is unlikely that low-energy electromagnetic fields produced by electricity supply pylons will cause ALL because it does not damage DNA in the laboratory, although it has been a matter of considerable public debate.

- *Exposure to certain chemicals and pesticides* has been associated with leukemia, but not usually ALL. The suggestion that parenteral vitamin K administration to neonates leads to an increased incidence of ALL has been disproved with further study.

Pathology of ALL

These are neoplasms of lymphoblasts committed to either B- or T-cell lineage. Our understanding of leukemia is that it is a clonal disease that originates by mutation in a single cell and that the remainder of leukemia cells within the clone are derived from this one cell.

About 80 to 85 percent of ALL in childhood is of B-cell lineage. ALL can be classified according to the features listed in Table 36.1 – clinical features, blast cell morphology, cytochemistry, immunophenotype, cytogenetics, and molecular genetics.

In employing any classification system in ALL, there are two questions to be answered:

- Am I certain that this is ALL, and can treatment be instituted?
- Does this classification of ALL tell me anything about the risk that this leukemia poses to the patient? This is the era of risk-based therapy (Table 36.2).

Table 36.2 Modalities of Classification of ALL and Their Influence

Classification mode	Question	Aid definitive diagnosis?	Risk stratification?
Clinical	What are the presenting features of this leukemia?	No	Yes (WBC)
Blast cell morphology	Do the blast cells appear as typical lymphoblasts using standard hematologic stains (FAB classification)?	Yes	No
Cytochemistry	Do the blast cells lack cytochemical evidence of myeloid lineage commitment (MPO) and/or show the typical cytochemical properties of lymphoblasts (B- or T-cell lineage) with PAS or AP stains?	Yes	No
Immunophenotype	Does the leukemia cell possess the membrane antigens that are present in normal precursor B and T cells?	Yes	No (There is no difference in the outcomes of precursor B and precursor T lymphoblastic leukemia.)
Cytogenetics	What are the chromosomal changes associated with the clone, and are these recognized findings in ALL?	Yes	Yes (Certain chromosomal changes are associated with adverse risk.)
Molecular genetics	Is there clonal immunoglobulin gene rearrangement (B-cell lineage ALL), or is there clonal T-cell receptor rearrangement (T-cell ALL)? Are there fusion genes that are described in ALL?	Yes	Yes (Useful in molecular monitoring of residual disease.)

Morphology

For all our sophisticated immunophenotype tools and cellular and molecular genetics, ALL is still diagnosed first by light microscopy of a blood and bone marrow smear taken from a child with a suggestive history and/or abnormal peripheral blood cell counts. Diagnostic immunophenotyping should only be performed on a morphologically abnormal blood or marrow sample, or mistakes will be made.

The FAB classification is a morphologic subclassification of ALL. It describes three types of ALL – L1, L2, and L3:

- In L1 disease, the blast cells are small and uniform with a high nuclear-cytoplasmic (N/C) ratio, inconspicuous nucleoli, and variable cytoplasmic vacuolation.
- In L2 disease, there is pleomorphism with larger and more variable blasts with variable cytoplasmic volume and vacuolation. Nucleoli may be multiple and prominent.
- In L3 disease, the blasts are large and uniform. There is intensely basophilic cytoplasm with prominent vacuolation, and there are multiple prominent nucleoli.

Only recognition of L3 leukemia has any modern relevance to diagnosis or therapy. L3 disease is mature B-cell leukaemia and the leukemic counterpart of Burkitt or large B-cell lymphoma. Translocation of the *c-myc* oncogene to the transcriptionally active heavy- or light-chain regions of the immunoglobulin gene defines the disease with typical clinical, morphologic (L3 morphology), immunophenotypic (mature B-cell markers including surface immunoglobulin), cytogenetic [t(2;8), t(8;14), or t(8;22)], and molecular genetic features (translocation of the *c-myc* oncogene). This disease will responds poorly to standard leukemia therapy but does responds very well to specific, abbreviated, and intensified therapy.

Otherwise, morphology alone does not distinguish T- and B-cell lineage ALL, nor does it necessarily distinguish lymphoblastic leukemia from certain myeloid leukemias, in which there is little maturation of the abnormal clone (FAB AML M0 and M1).

Cytochemistry

The principle of cytochemistry is that an apparently primitive and microscopically bland blast cell will show lineage commitment in its enzymes. The principal importance in ALL is that ALL blasts do not have myeloperoxidase and are therefore Sudan black negative and distinguishable from most cases of AML. ALL blasts of T- and B-cell lineage may be positive for periodic acid–Schiff (PAS) stain, often in a characteristic block pattern, and T-cell lineage leukemia may be positive in a characteristic polar pattern for acid phosphatase (AP).

Immunophenotyping

Immunophenotyping is the cornerstone of modern leukemia diagnosis. Just as cytochemistry assigns lineage commitment to an undifferentiated cell by its enzymatic capability, so immunophenotyping classifies leukemia by the membrane and cytoplasmic antigens it shares with cells of a certain lineage. In B-cell lineage leukemia, there are therefore B-cell lineage antigens, and in T-cell lineage leukemia, there are T-cell lineage antigens. These antigens are specific to the lineage and not to the leukemia.

During normal B- or T-cell ontogeny or development, there is serial and characteristic gain and loss of specified antigens. Thus, the developmental stage of a B-lineage cell from uncommitted stem cell to antibody-producing plasma cell can be defined by its pattern of antigen expression. Leukemia may arise as a clonal disease from cells of different developmental stages, and the antigen expression of the subsequent malignant clone reflects the antigen expression of the developmental stage at which the malignancy arose.

Usually immunophenotypic analysis in clinical laboratories consists of two stages:

- In the first stage, a broad panel of antibodies is employed. Such a panel includes antibodies directed at common T-lineage, B-lineage, and myeloid – including monocytic and erythroid – antigens. This will enable a broad immunophenotypic classification of leukemia to be made – in conjunction with morphology and cytochemistry.
- A second panel of more lineage-specific antibodies will enable a more exact diagnosis and subclassification of leukemia to be made.
  In the case of precursor B- and precursor T-lymphoblastic leukemias, this second panel of antibodies will allow classification according to the normal cell ontogeny.

It should be noted that several different classifications of B-lineage ALL can be attempted. In the modern

Table 36.3 An Immunophenotypic Classification of ALL

Leukemia	Immunophenotype, common antigens	Antigens used to discriminate this stage of precursor B-cell ALL	Leukemia frequency
Early pre-B, CD10$^-$	CD19, CD22, CD79a	TdT$^+$, CD10$^-$	8
Early pre-B, CD10$^+$	CD19, CD22, CD79a	TdT$^+$, CD10$^+$,surface and cytoplasmic Ig$^-$	70
Late pre-B	CD19, CD22, CD79a	Cytoplasmic Ig + I$^+$, SIg$^-$, CD10$^+$/CD10$^-$	18
Mature B (L3)	CD19, CD22, CD79a	TdT$^-$, CD10$^+$/CD10$^-$, SIg$^+$	4

treatment era, the importance of immunophenotyping is to make a certain diagnosis of precursor B-cell lineage leukemia and to make a certain diagnosis of B-cell leukemia because this has important treatment implications. The subclassification of precursor B disease has little impact on prognosis compared to other criteria of risk stratification, and little sleep should be lost by the practicing clinician in making such an exact diagnosis. Indeed, the World Health Organization (WHO) classification of acute B-cell neoplasms into precursor B-cell leukemia/lymphoma and Burkitt leukemia/lymphoma and further subgrouping are based on cytogenetic abnormalities (Table 36.3).

A similar subclassification of T-cell ALL can be attempted in which the leukemia immunophenotype reflects the stage of T-cell ontogeny where malignant change has arisen. As in subclassifications of B-cell lineage ALL, there is limited relevance to the treating clinician, and the WHO classification does not attempt any classification beyond this, even with cytogenetics. The frequency of T-cell ALL is about 12 percent of all ALL (Table 36.4)

Aberrant antigen expression is not uncommon in ALL and refers to the expression of antigens that are not associated with that leukemia's lineage. Aberrant antigens do not influence the diagnosis where there are immunologic, cytogenetic, and molecular features of a strong commitment to ALL. Over half of ALL cases will express some aberrant myeloid marker – usually CD13, CD33, or CD15. In these cases, blasts are myeloperoxidase (MPO) negative and have the other typical immunophenotypic features of B-cell ALL (CD19, CD22, and CD79a positive) or T-cell ALL (CD7 and cyCD3). Such aberrant antigen expression does not appear to independently influence

Table 36.4 An Immunophenotypic Subclassification of T-Cell ALL

Leukemia	Immunophenotype, common antigens	Antigens used to discriminate this stage of precursor T-cell ALL
Pro-T	cyCD3, CD7	TdT$^+$
Pre-T	cyCD3, CD7	TdT$^+$, CD5$^+$/ CD5$^-$
Cortical T	cyCD3, CD7	TdT$^+$, CD1a$^+$, CD5$^+$, CD4/8$^+$/ CD4/8$^-$
Mature T	cyCD3, CD7	TdT$^-$, sCD3$^+$, CD5$^+$, CD4 or CD8$^+$

outcome after treatment. Myeloid antigen aberrant expression is common in infant ALL with the t(4;11) translocation, which is associated with a poor prognosis.

Where there is coexpression of MPO and these typical ALL markers, this is a true biphenotypic leukemia. Mixed T-cell and B-cell ALL leukemias are also described. Gene rearrangement and expression may help to accurately classify these leukemias, which otherwise pose a therapeutic difficulty for the clinician. Rarely, there are two clear populations of blast cells expressing different antigens – this is termed *bilineage leukemia*.

Cytogenetics

Cytogenetics is the study of cellular chromosomal rearrangements associated with leukemia and may find typical rearrangements that both confirm the diagnosis and aid prognosis and therefore therapy. There are two techniques:

- *Conventional cytogenetics.* This remains the standard screening for karyotypic abnormalities in newly diagnosed leukemia. It will pick up abnormalities only in dividing cells (metaphase).
- *Molecular cytogenetics.* In *fluorescence in situ hybridisation* (FISH), a probe that is specific for normal (e.g. for a specific chromosome) or abnormal (e.g. for a particular translocation) part of the genome is applied to a cell that need not necessarily be dividing. This methodology cannot be readily used as a screen because it can only determine whether a particular probe binds or not, but it is useful for monitoring known abnormalities during therapy.

Two patterns of cytogenetic alteration are described – alterations of chromosome number and structural abnormalities. Both can confer prognostic information.

1. *Alterations of chromosome number.* ALL can be classified into five types according to the number of chromosomes:

   a. *Hyperdiploidy (>50 chromosomes).* This is a common finding, and as many as 30 percent of ALL cases have a chromosome number between 51 and 68. Such hyperdiploidy, especially where the number is 51 to 55 chromosomes, is associated with other good risk features and an improved cure rate. Rarely, there may be a near-tetraploid or, more rarely still, near-triploid karyotype. These do not appear in more recent analyses to have adverse outcomes. The pattern of chromosome gain in hyperdiploidy is not random, and the most common chromosome gained is chromosomes 21, and chromosomes 6, X, and 14 are also commonly gained. Hyperdiploidy also can be detected by flow cytometry – expressed as a DNA index – and this sometimes may be more sensitive than conventional cytogenetics.

   b. *Low hyperdiploidy (47–50 chromosomes).* This does not confer such a good prognosis as higher hyperdiploidy, but the prognosis is not adverse. Where only chromosome 21 is gained, then the prognosis is good, and where chromosome 8 is gained, it is usually

associated with T-cell disease, and the prognostic significance is uncertain.

   c. *Pseudodiploidy.* In this group, although there are 46 chromosomes, there are structural or numerical abnormalities. This is a heterogeneous group whose outcome with therapy will reflect the specific abnormality within the apparently normal chromosome number.

   d. *Diploidy.* In this group, there is apparently normal chromosome number and structure. About 10 to 15 percent of ALL is in this group. It may be more common in T-cell ALL. This group will contain children with cryptic translocations [e.g. t(12;21) in B-ALL and t(5;14) in T-ALL] that will themselves confer prognostic significance.

   e. *Hypodiploidy and near haploidy.* In this group, there are a reduced number of chromosomes. Where there is a near-haploid karyotype, there is a poor prognosis, even where there are relatively good presenting National Cancer Institute (NCI) features.

2. *Structural chromosome changes.* These are the more common structural abnormalities in ALL; their lineage specificity and prognostic significance are given in Table 36.5.

Molecular Genetics

Molecular genetics is the application of molecular biological techniques to determine the genes involved in ALL. Such techniques include analysis of the clonal origin of T- and B-cell leukemias and the acquired genetic origin of these illnesses.

- B and T cells generate the antibody and T-cell receptor diversity necessary for an adaptive immune system by rearranging the germ-line variable (V), diversity (D), and junctional (J) regions of the *IG/TCR* gene complexes. Each developing lymphocyte therefore obtains a specific VDJ combination, and diversity is further generated by nucleotide insertion and deletion during VDJ coupling. Because ALL is a clonal disorder arising from a developing lymphoid cell, this unique DNA – specific to that developing cell – will act as a DNA fingerprint' for all its progeny. There are two implications in terms of leukemia diagnosis and risk stratification:

Table 36.5 More Common Structural Chromosome Abnormalities in ALL

Structural chromosome change	Lineage specificity	Genes	Frequency (%)	Prognostic significance
t(1;19)	B	E2A-PBX1	5	Adverse[a]
t(17;19)	B	E2A-HLF	1	Adverse
t(4;11)	B	MLL-AF4	5 (higher in infants)	Adverse
11q23 trans, inv, deletion	Usually B	Variable	–	Adverse, except deletion or inversion; these are neutral
t(9;22)	B	BCR-ABL	<5	Adverse
t(12;21)	B	TEL-AML	25	Good
Tan dup (21)	B	AML1 amplification	2	Adverse
Del (6q)	Nonspecific	Unknown	10	Neutral
10q24, various partners	T	HOX11	0.5	Good
19p13, various partners	T	LYL1	1.5	Adverse
1p32	T	TAL1	6	Adverse
8q24	True B cell	c-myc overexpression	2	Good (with appropriate abbreviated and intensified therapy)[b]

[a] This adverse treatment outcome can be overcome with intensive therapy.
[b] Prognosis is good with short-term intensive chemotherapy.

- The presence of clonal TCR or IG gene rearrangement may aid diagnosis in difficult cases of leukemia such as bipheonotypic or bilineage leukemia.
- The unique DNA may be used as a target for monitoring the disappearance of the leukemia clone during therapy. Thus, primers for junctional regions are matched to either side of the junctions, generally within a distance of less than 500 bp. Usually consensus primers will be used that recognize virtually all V or J gene segments – germ-line DNA will not be amplified because of the long distance between these regions in unrecombined DNA. The PCR product – specific to the leukemia clone – can then be sequenced, and patient-specific (or allele-specific) primers can be designed for further monitoring of that leukemia clone during therapy. This is the basis of minimal residual disease (MRD) monitoring during ALL therapy and is strongly predictive of treatment outcome.

- The structural chromosomal alterations usually disrupt genes that encode transcription factors. Leukemia-specific translocations can activate transcription factors either by generating new fusion genes with oncogenic properties or by translocating those transcription factors to transcriptionally active portions of the genome – those coding for IG or the TCR. The importance to the clinician is twofold:

  - The chimeric gene is unique DNA and specific, within that patient, to the leukemic clone and can be monitored either by PCR or by FISH analysis of MRD in the same way as the IG/TCR gene rearrangement.
  - The action of the fusion oncoprotein or the translocated transcription factor will enable the clinician to better understand the molecular etiology of the leukemia and may in the future allow the leukemia to be targeted more specifically. In an analogous fashion, the BCR-ABL fusion oncogene is specifically

targeted in chronic myelogenous leukemia (CML) and ALL by tyrosine kinase inhibitors such as imatinib.

Clinical Presentation of ALL

Typical Presentation and Plan of Investigation

In most cases, the diagnosis of ALL is not difficult to make once there is sufficient clinical suspicion to merit investigation with blood tests. Leukemic blast infiltrate leads to marrow failure and the typical symptoms and signs of anemia, thrombocytopenia, and leukopenia. There is frequently bone pain and fever. On physical examination, there is frequently generalized lymphadenopathy and hepatosplenomegaly. The illness usually arises in a previously well child; there are few predisposing conditions (see earlier).

In this typical case, all institutions will have a standard series of investigations so that all information about the leukemia that might conceivably be useful can be gathered. Once therapy is initiated, the leukemia will soon be gone to sight, and this opportunity will be lost. Most institutions will do these and any subsequent invasive bone marrows and lumbar punctures under general anesthetic or deep sedation. A comprehensive clinical assessment of the fitness for such procedures should form part of the initial assessment of the child. Several points should be noted:

- In certain circumstances (e.g. large mediastinal mass; see below) causing respiratory compromise or superior vena cava (SVC) obstruction, it may not be possible to safely give anesthetic or sedation. In such circumstances, as much as possible must be done without anesthetic. Where there are circulating blast cells, diagnosis may be made and samples taken for MRD and cytogenetic tests using the peripheral blood alone. Treatment then may be initiated and invasive procedures requiring anesthesia or sedation deferred until anesthetic or sedation is safe. The safety of the patient must not be compromised for the sake of completeness of the diagnosis. This is sometimes a more critical issue in T-cell non-Hodgkin lymphoma (NHL), where there is no circulating disease but a large mediastinal mass. Steroid therapy may be given in these circumstances to shrink the presenting tumor, which is making

anesthetic unsafe. Often this mass will shrink over a matter of days, and the anesthetic will be perfectly safe. The child will require daily assessments by an experienced pediatric anesthetist to identify the window in which both anesthesia is safe and the tumor mass is not completely resolved.

- Tumor storage will require consent, in addition to the consent for anesthesia and investigations.
- It is clearly appropriate to do as many investigations under the same anesthetic as possible. It is usual practice to give intrathecal chemotherapy at the time of first investigation where there are unequivocally circulating peripheral blood blasts. This saves the child returning for a second procedure (therapeutic lumbar puncture) once a diagnosis is made on a first marrow and means that intrathecal chemotherapy is always given with lumbar puncture and there is a reduced risk of contamination of the cerebrospinal fluid (CSF) leading to later central nervous system (CNS) relapse via traumatic puncture (see CNS disease, below).

Other Presentations of ALL

Other organs might be involved. The most common site of involvement is clearly the lymph nodes, liver, and spleen. Involvement of these organs occur in a patient with typical features as earlier or be the site of presenting symptoms and signs.

CNS leukemia

Involvement of the CNS is more common in ALL than in other types of leukemia. It is more commonly a site of relapsed disease than presenting disease. It is more common in T-cell disease, true B-cell leukemia, and where the circulating WBC count is high. Its presentation may be on routine lumbar puncture, or there may be symptoms and signs of disease including headache, vomiting, papilledema, or cranial nerve palsies and abnormal eye movements (cranial nerves III, IV, or VI) or facial asymmetry (VII).

Diagnosis of CNS disease is on microscopic examination of a CSF cytospin in which the total WBC concentration has been counted. Three patterns of CSF are recognized:

1. *CNS-1*. No blast cells in the cytospin. Other cells may be present – often in considerable numbers either with infection or as a reaction to continuing intrathecal therapy. The frequent presence of

251

other cells underlines the importance of experience in making this diagnosis of CNS involvement. Immunophenotyping of CSF can be helpful in difficult cases – where there is limited material, the range of markers employed may be limited and will be guided by the immunophenotype of the patient's leukemia. Terminal deoxynucleotidyl transferase (TdT) is useful in this circumstance in precursor B- and T-lymphoblastic leukemias.

2. *CNS-2*. There are unequivocally blasts in the CSF, but their number is less than 5×10^6/liter.
3. *CNS-3*. There are unequivocally blasts in the CSF, but their number is greater than 5×10^6/liter.

Occasionally, the pattern of disease is predominantly parenchymal. The presenting features are related to mass effect, neurologic deficit, or seizures. Such a pattern of involvement is usually seen more at relapse, and parenchymal involvement is thought to be a later event in CNS invasion than meningeal involvement (which leads to CSF positivity). Epidural deposit of leukemia with spinal cord compression with a leukemic deposit is a rare presentation of ALL requiring urgent institution of appropriate therapy, including steroid therapy. The management of CNS leukemias is discussed separately (later).

Hypoplastic Presentation of ALL

Rarely, the diagnosis of ALL is preceded by an aplastic phase. This occurs in about 1 to 2 percent of these leukemias, and the pathophysiology of this process is unclear. Characteristically, there is fever with pancytopenia followed by restoration of normal counts and good health before, within 6 months, a diagnosis of overt leukemia. Uncommonly, there is no recovery of the peripheral blood counts, but usually in these cases there might be marrow fibrosis and foci of blasts expressing TdT and (usually) CD10.

Testicular Disease

Testicular disease is rarely overtly present at diagnosis in boys, although it is commonly present at a subclinical level – as was demonstrated by studies of testicular biopsy at diagnosis of leukemia of boys without clinically apparent disease – and is not associated with an adverse outlook. Overt testicular disease was formerly a not uncommon site of relapse, but the frequency of such relapse has diminished as protocol intensity has increased.

Lymphoma Including a Mediastinal Mass

In lymphoblastic lymphoma, the same cells as in ALL occur as a mass rather than occurring in the marrow or the blood. This mass may be nodal or extranodal. T-cell lymphoblastic lymphoma is more common than precursor B-cell disease and is commonly seen as a mediastinal mass, although it is described to occur in precursor B-cell disease rarely. It may be asymptomatic and simply noted on a posteroanterior (PA) chest x-ray that is done routinely on all children presenting with leukemia at the time of initial investigations. It may present, however, as respiratory compromise or a SVC obstruction. In these circumstances, management of the presenting emergency is the physician's priority, and investigations may be deferred while this is brought rapidly under control.

The treatment of lymphoma is similar to that of the leukemia. However, more intensive therapy is usually given as though the leukemia were presenting with a high WBC count or in an older child.

Bone and Joint Disease

Bone pain is common. In some children – usually with precursor B-cell lymphoblastic disease and often with a relatively normal blood count – the bone pain may be the dominant finding leading to presentation to orthopedic or rheumatology teams and diagnostic difficulty and delay. In addition to this feature, there may be characteristic x-ray changes including transverse metaphyseal radiolucent lines, osteolytic lesions, diffuse osteoporosis, and fracture. No specific orthopedic intervention is necessary in these circumstances – simply diagnosis and management of the underlying leukemia.

Ocular Disease

The incidence of eye involvement will depend on the intensity of the search. Overt involvement is only commonly seen at relapse and then more commonly in association with CNS disease. Like testicular disease, contemporary treatment protocols have reduced the incidence of relapse at this site.

Treatment of ALL

Historical Aspects

Treatment of ALL has proceeded from palliation to curative over the last 60 years. Most patients presenting with ALL can now expect to be cured of their disease. The obstacles to successful treatment that have been progressively overcome have included

- A lack of belief that anything other than transient responses and palliation of leukemia could be achieved with drug and radiation therapy.
- The lack of effective drugs capable of inducing response and the development of drugs that individually had some action in inducing response of the leukemia. The earliest drugs that had action were aminopterin (an early methotexate-like folate antagonist), corticosteroids, and the purine antagonists 6-mercaptopurine (6MP) and thioguanine.
- Primary and acquired resistance to applied antileukemia drug therapy. The use of multiagent drug schedules that form the backbone of ALL therapy today was first employed to overcome such acquired resistance in which children responded and achieved remission but later relapsed. Separate multiagent schedules are employed in remission induction, consolidation, and continuing therapy.
- CNS relapse leading to treatment failure even where there had been a medullary response. The development of strategies to prevent CNS relapse – initially this was achieved with prophylactic irradiation and subsequently with intrathecal administration of chemotherapy.
- The lack of a framework in which to test newer drugs and schedules. The concept of the randomized clinical trial in which new drugs or different scheduling of the same drug (e.g. methotrexate) or different combinations of drugs has allowed leukemia therapy to improve progressively and incrementally. These recent incremental steps of the large cooperative oncology groups studying ALL therapy are discussed in more detail later.

Principles of Treatment

- Treat of ALL is toxic, and an important component of therapy is supportive care. Improvements in outcome are partly due to improvements in supportive care. Supportive care components are discussed separately in this book, but any such care will require

  - Knowledge of the likely adverse effects of any applied therapy so that primary preventative therapy (prophylaxis) can be given.

  - Early detection of problems so that therapy can be given early in the course of any complication.
  - Effective drugs for the complications of the disease.

- Treatment of ALL is risk directed. The risk of treatment failure in ALL is influenced by clinical factors, and the NCI has developed a uniform classification based on age at presentation and presenting WBC count. Biologic features of the leukemia including cytogenetics and molecular genetics will further inform this risk assessment, and a treatment schedule will be selected. However, this risk assessment will be inaccurate, and some children with apparently good-risk disease by NCI criteria and disease biology will relapse during or after appropriate therapy, and conversely, some children with apparently poor-risk disease by these criteria will apparently be cured with such treatment. One reason for the incomplete relation between applied therapy outcome and pretreatment risk assessment is the individual response to drug treatment, so risk assessment can be improved by assessing the disease response to therapy, which will be influenced by pharmacodynamic and pharmacogenetic factors; this response may be assessed crudely by morphologic assessment of blast disappearance or using more sophisticated and quantitative measures of disease disappearance – flow cytometric or PCR molecular measures. This mode of disease assessment is summarized in Figure 36.1.

Results of Cooperative Studies in ALL Treatment

There are several large collaborative consortia that have performed randomized trials in the therapy of childhood ALL. These trials have sometimes asked not dissimilar questions. Progress has been incremental, with each successive national trial testing the proposed improved treatment strategy against previous best (standard) therapy.

Components of ALL Therapy

There is probably more randomized clinical trial information concerning the treatment of ALL in children than for any other human malignancy.

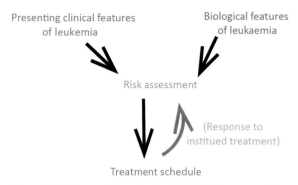

Figure 36.1 Determination of risk in ALL. Risk of treatment failure can be determined by (1) clinical features of the patient and the leukemia, such as age at presentation and the circulating blast count at presentation, (2) biologic features of the leukemia such as cytogenetics, and (3) the response of the disease to instituted therapy.

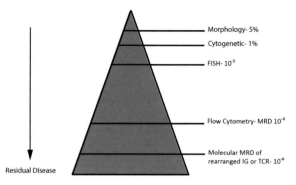

Figure 36.2 The iceberg concept of ALL – there is much more below than above the water. For children in remission by marrow microscopic examination (nothing to see above the water), there may be lots of disease left that can be detected by more sensitive methods of leukemia cell identification.

Treatment of ALL continues along the lines established in the early days of therapy:

- Remission-induction therapy
- Intensification/consolidation/reinduction therapy
- CNS-directed therapy
- Continuing/maintenance therapy

This section will review these treatment phases and summarize the objectives of each phase, the consensus treatment, and the evidence for that treatment.

Remission-Induction Therapy

Definition and Aim

This is the therapy that is given to a patient after a diagnosis is reached and once the patient's condition has been stabilized. Its aim is remission. Remission is defined as absence of detectable disease. The method of disease assessment needs to be defined in describing remission because different tools will have different sensitivities (Figure 36.2).

For any tool used, remission is defined as absence of detectable disease, and residual disease is disease that remains present but undetectable by that method. This is a difficult concept for families.

The level of remission is not an academic issue. About 99 percent of children will be in remission at the end of remission-induction therapy. Treatment failures will reflect a roughly equal mix of death due to toxicity and refractory disease. Patients with refractory disease have a dismal outcome with intensified therapy and transplantation. Patients with high-level MRD (above 1 percent) have similarly dismal outcomes despite morphologic remission.

MRD is currently estimated usually after induction (week 5) and after consolidation therapy (week 11). In current trials, high-risk disease by MRD is defined as disease levels greater than 0.01 percent (10^{-4}) at week 5 and low-risk disease as undetectable disease at week 11, having not been greater than 0.01 percent at week 5. Some disease is indeterminant by MRD (e.g. detectable disease but less than 0.01 percent at both time points). In the current UK trial, the risk of subsequent relapse is about 5 percent in the high-risk group and less than 0.5 percent in the low-risk group. MRD is therefore a highly useful tool, and it is hoped that treatment interventions based on MRD will improve overall survival – these interventions usually will be intensification of therapy in children with high-risk disease and reduction of therapy in those with good-risk disease as defined by MRD.

Drugs Used

Remission-induction therapy is a multiple-drug regimen following the earliest observation that multiple-drug use has higher rates of remission induction that were translated into improved rates of overall survival. The leukemic clone is rapidly diminished, so drug-resistant disease cannot emerge. Remission-induction schedules in all current regimens will include both vincristine and steroids and one or both of an anthracycline and L-asparaginase. In most studies, a three-drug remission induction will be employed in standard-risk disease, and four drugs will be reserved for those judged high risk by NCI criteria and those with adverse genotype or failing to respond appropriately to an instituted three-drug regimen.

- *Vincristine.* This is administered on a weekly schedule. The usual dose is 1.5 mg/m². Its toxicity is principally neuropathic. Excessive neurotoxicity is seen in hereditary sensorimotor neuropathies such as Charcot-Marie-Tooth disease, which may be expected based on family history and diagnosed genetically.
- *Steroids.* These are given by mouth. Several collaborative studies – Children's Cancer Group (CCG) and Medical Research Council (MRC) – have addressed the question of which steroid. There is evidence from these studies that use of dexamethasone has improved overall survival and reduced CNS relapse. It is unclear whether the dose of the steroids is equipotent or the improved results seen with dexamethasone reflect simply higher glucocorticoid effect with selected dose (in the UK trial, 6 mg/m²/day for 28 days). There is increased toxicity with this dose of dexamethasone. This toxicity is bony with increased osteopenia, behavioral disturbance, myopathy, and weight gain (both adding to the neuropathy of vincristine in reducing mobility of children during induction).
- *Asparaginase.* Asparaginase cleaves asparagines into aspartic acid and ammonia. It interrupts protein synthesis because asparagine is rate-limiting. Asparaginase is an important drug in the treatment of ALL, and children who are underdosed for asparaginase have an inferior outcome to those who receive a more intensive treatment schedule. There are different preparations – with several products of different potency derived from *Escherichia coli* and a single commercial product of reduced potency derived from *Erwinia.* If the different half-lives (and there is a pegylated version of the Medac *E. coli* asparaginase) and potencies of the different properties are taken into account in scheduling, comparable results will be achieved. While its importance in ALL treatment is undoubted, its timing in leukemia therapy is uncertain. It has considerable toxicity with thrombotic, infectious, and hepatic complications, and these are especially evident in leukemia induction therapy. The Dana-Farber Cancer Institute ALL Consortium has moved asparaginase into the postinduction period and demonstrated the importance of prolonged exposure while maintaining high remission-induction rates. The most appropriate timing,

therefore, of the drug will remain the subject of further study.
- *Anthracycline.* The most extensively used anthracycline in ALL treatment has been daunorubicin. It is myelotoxic and significantly increases infection risk during induction therapy. It has a cumulative cardiac toxicity when doses above 400 mg/m² are used. It may not be necessary to use an intensive four-drug remission-induction regimen in standard-risk patients in whom there is postremission intensification therapy.

Intensification Therapy

Definition and Aim

In the early days of leukemia treatment, remission was maintained by prolonged continuing antimetabolite (maintenance) therapy. Consolidation, intensification, and reinduction therapy is the therapy that follows achievement of morphologic remission and that interrupts continuing therapy. The addition of such intensification blocks improves the outcome of all types of ALL, even those of lowest risk. The intensity should be sustained over weeks rather than short blocks of chemotherapy with a prolonged interruption thereafter as a consequence of bone marrow aplasia.

Drugs Used

Different groups have evolved different schedules:
- Intensification therapy is delivered following achievement of remission and is used principally in high-risk leukemia. Usually cyclophosphamide, cytarabine, and mercaptopurine are given, which may be further intensified in those achieving remission more slowly by the addition of further agents, including vincristine and asparaginase. This approach of augmented intensification has been shown in CCG trials to be beneficial in improving outcome in these high-risk leukemias.
- In reinduction therapy, the induction drugs are repeated 3 months after achieving remission, and this was pioneered by the BFM Group. This can be done doubly,' with drugs repeated again at 32 weeks – which has been shown to improve outcome in higher-risk disease.
- Various other drugs are used after induction and have been shown to be of benefit. The replacement of induction asparaginase with postinduction

asparaginase was shown by the Dana Farber group to be beneficial, and asparaginase is an important component of the augmented delayed BFM consolidation therapy of CCG trials. Methotrexate after induction has been beneficial, especially in T-cell disease, where the blasts accumulate its active metabolites.

CNS Prophylaxis

Definition and Aim

This is therapy delivered specifically to the sanctuary site of the CNS. It is the story of leukemia therapy in that:

- CNS relapse was a huge problem in the early days, even when systemic leukemia control had been achieved – with as many as 50 percent of children suffering such relapse.
- There was identification of a therapy that reduced such relapse: craniospinal irradiation.
- There was identification of risk factors associated with CNS relapse (Table 36.6).
- There was a realization that radiation had long-term adverse sequelae on growth, neurocognitive function, and endocrine function.
- Craniospinal irradiation was gradually replaced with cranial irradiation and intrathecal therapy, reducing radiation dose. Then radiation was abolished, with only intrathecal therapy and improved systemic therapy.

Drugs Used

Effective prophylaxis of CNS relapse requires both effective systemic therapy and locally applied therapy. Local therapy is increasingly intrathecal therapy, and there is equivalence of each treatment in meta-analyses of different trials. Both St. Jude's and MRC treatment protocols no longer give any CNS radiation therapy. Intrathecal therapy is with either single-agent methotrexate or triple-agent therapy

with methotrexate, hydrocortisone, and cytarabine. There is no proven benefit to triple therapy.

Systemic therapy is better with dexamethasone, although this may reflect the fact that the trials that have shown a beneficial dexamethasone effect did not select equivalent glucocorticoid efficacy in the prednisolone arm. Where a higher dose of prednisolone was used, no advantage of dexamethasone was demonstrated. High-dose methotrexate reduces the systemic relapse rate but has little impact on CNS relapse – but perhaps the effect is only at higher doses of methotrexate (5 g/m^2).

Continuing (Maintenance) Therapy

Definition and Aim

ALL is unique in malignancies in its requirement for a prolonged period of low-dose but sustained and continuously delivered chemotherapy. Universally, it includes 6MP given daily and low-dose methotrexate given weekly. This phase of treatment proceeds from achievement of completion of remission to completion of therapy but is interrupted for intensification or reinduction therapy. Children are relatively well during this phase of treatment, and life can return to normal; however, children are significantly immune suppressed during this therapy, and viral infection can be significant, even overwhelming. Particular problems are seen with parvovirus and prolonged RBC aplasia, and transfusion need is seen.

Drugs Used and Duration

6MP and methotrexate are the synergistic backbone of maintenance therapy. Methotrexate inhibits *de novo* purine synthesis and thereby enhances the conversion of mercaptopurine to its active metabolite thioguanine. In maintenance therapy:

- There is considerable variation in the individual patient's response to the administered drugs.
  In everyday practice, the dose of drugs is adjusted so as to achieve myelosuppression – so that tolerant patients receive more drug. The effect on normal hematopoiesis is used as a surrogate for a presumed effect on malignant hematopoiesis. There is some evidence for such a strategy, with children interrupting therapy for neutropenia faring better.
- Some children are deficient in the enzyme thiopurine-S-methyltransferase, and these children show extreme sensitivity to 6MP.

Table 36.6 Risk Factors for CNS Relapse in ALL

High WBC count

T-cell immunophenotype

Traumatic lumbar puncture (LP) or CNS-2 LP at diagnosis

Adverse genotype – t(4;11) or t(9;22)

Heterozygotes may show some sensitivity to the drug.

- The 6MP is usually better given on an empty stomach and away from milk products. Methotrexate is as effective orally as parenterally.
- There is conflicting evidence about the benefit that the addition of pulses of vincristine and steroid beyond reinduction therapy brings, and it is probably not very significant. Such therapy brings continuing steroid toxicity.
- There is clear evidence that continuing therapy is necessary, and despite the increased intensity of earlier therapy and the evidence that such intensity is effective in improving cure rates, it has not been possible to reduce the duration of continuing therapy to less than 2 years. Some trials continue to offer increased therapy for boys – 3 years as opposed to 2 years for girls – but there is little evidence for such a strategy and evidence that prolonging maintenance therapy beyond 3 years is not helpful.

Treatment Failure: Predicting Treatment Failure

The factors associated with an increased risk of treatment failure are well described – clinical factors encapsulated by the NCI consensus criteria and disease-related factors, principally cytogenetic and molecular genetic factors. There is considerable overlap between these assessment systems – thus genotypically favorable leukemias typically have good clinical risk features. It is hoped that using gene expression profiles from an individual's leukemia might improve the sensitivity of risk determination by giving a molecular profile of the actual leukemia cells.

Some children with apparently good-risk disease relapse, and some children with apparently adverse-risk leukemia are cured with standard chemotherapy. Assessment of leukemia disappearance using morphology or MRD is an attempt to take account of this variation in expected response. Some of this variation in response is due to interindividual differences in drug metabolism. These pharmacogenomic differences mean that the drug dose delivered to leukemia cells is vastly different in some children than in others and will explain why those drugs delivered in a formulaic fashion are sometimes more effective than

expected and sometimes less so. Knowing these resistant mechanisms may mean that drug treatment can be more guided.

Special Situations

Infant ALL

Features

- The cell from which ALL in infancy arise is a primitive cell in the early stage of commitment to the B lineage. As such:
  - There is a high incidence of coexpressed myeloid antigens.
  - It is frequently of a null phenotype with $CD19^+$ and $CD10^-$.
- Eighty percent of cases have *MLL* gene rearrangement, with the most common translocation being t(4;11).
- Usually there are adverse clinical and genotypic risk factors, and there is frequently a poor response to steroid induction chemotherapy.
- Very young children do even worse.

Treatment

- Because of the primitive nature of the leukemia, because of the coexpression of myeloid antigens, and because of the *in vitro* sensitivity to cytarabine, a recently reported protocol, Interfant-99, attempted to improve treatment outcome by including myeloid as well as lymphoid treatment elements, such as cytarabine and high-dose cytarabine
- This protocol reports an event-free survival (EFS) at 4 years of about 50 percent, which is an improvement on previous reports.
- *MLL* gene, high WBC count, younger than 6 months of age, and poor steroid response were all independently associated with a poor outcome.
- CNS disease in infant leukemia is managed with intrathecal and systemic therapy only; radiotherapy is not employed in this age group.

ALL in Down Syndrome

The diagnosis and treatment of Down syndrome ALL is discussed in Chapter 6.

257

Relapsed ALL

The salient features of relapsed ALL include:

- It might affect about 15 percent of children in current leukemia protocols.
- It may involve the bone marrow or be extramedullary, or it may be combined.
- The CNS is the most common site of extramedullary relapse.
- The prognosis of relapsed leukemia depends on
  - The timing of relapse in relation to initial therapy, so relapse occurring earlier in relation to the initial leukemia treatment or even during such treatment does worse.
  - Site of relapse: isolated CNS relapse off therapy will have a prognosis as high as 70 percent.
  - Immunophenotype: T-cell disease will do worse.
- Even apparently isolated extramedullary disease should be regarded as a manifestation of inadequately controlled systemic disease and will require therapy with systemic treatment as well as locally directed treatment.
- The disease may show immunophenotypic, cytogenetic, or molecular clonal evolution compared to the original treated disease.

Many relapses will be predictable from adverse clinical or biologic factors at diagnosis or from an observed slow response to treatment. Relapse occurs most commonly in the first year after completing therapy and is uncommon, but not unheard of, 4 years after completing therapy. Relapse is managed as a systemic disease; even isolated extramedullary disease is regarded as a failure of systemic therapy and a harbinger of systemic relapse.

Isolated late CNS relapse has the best prognosis of relapse. As many as 70 percent of children will be cured with systemic therapy (including reinduction, consolidation, and maintenance therapy for 24 months) and local radiotherapy.

For higher-risk relapse – early, T cell, and poor response to relapse therapy (as assessed molecularly) – allogeneic stem cell transplantation will often form part of the relapse therapy. This is the major role for transplantation in ALL, although it may be offered to high-risk patients in first remission. Usually transplantation is applied in relapsed disease after remission reinduction therapy and consolidation therapy

and as continuing therapy otherwise would be starting. A chemotherapy approach alone may be adopted in lower-risk patients – usually in non-T-cell disease, where there has been a prolonged first remission.

Strategies for Follow-Up and Important Late Effects

Follow-up of treated ALL patients has two purposes:

- To monitor disease response and detect relapse
- To determine complications of applied treatment

During therapy, patients are usually seen at least weekly during intensive phases and fortnightly during maintenance. Most children who will go on to relapse will do so in the first year off treatment, and the remainder of relapses occur usually by the end of the fourth year off treatment. During this period, marrow relapse can be detected by marrow examination after abnormalities of the peripheral blood count. There is no need for serial bone marrow examinations, and these may even be confusing because lymphoblasts – even $CD10^+$ ones – may be seen in the marrow of normal children. CNS relapse will be diagnosed by examination of the CSF after suggestive symptoms are raised by the patient. Other extramedullary relapses will be diagnosed on biopsy of the affected organ after suggestive history or findings on clinical examination.

With time from completion of therapy, the focus of follow-up will gradually change from detection of relapse to monitoring for adverse and long-term complications of therapy. A spectrum of complications will be seen in the long-term follow-up clinic – with the least in those treated on low-intensity protocols and the most in those who have received intensive therapy including allogeneic stem cell transplantation and cranial or craniospinal radiation therapy (Table 36.7).

Summary and Future Directions

The treatment of pediatric ALL is a success story and a story that the wider field of oncology is trying to replicate. It is not yet a finished story. Some children relapse. Children still die of ALL. Some children are cured but affected by the long-term consequences of their treatment. Over the next 20 years of ALL therapy, we would all wish to see fewer relapses and fewer

Table 36.7 Late Effects of Therapy of ALL

Bone	1. Reduced bone mineral density in survivors of childhood ALL – especially in those who have received cranial radiotherapy. It can occur, but much less so in children treated with chemotherapy alone. 2. Avascular necrosis (AVN) can occur during therapy for ALL – and is more common in older children, girls, and those treated with dexamethasone. Avascular necrosis may present after completion of therapy and will cause ongoing problems in many cases for the affected child.
CNS	Complicated field. Imaging abnormalities can be seen. Global (e.g., IQ) and specific change in performance can be seen. Therapy might have impact on educational performance. This is probably more common in children receiving radiation and therapy at an early age. Changes are certainly seen with children receiving systemic therapy and intrathecal therapy only. Recognition, assessment, and support – including school support – are important
Cardiac	1. The principal risk in chemotherapy protocols is related to anthracycline. The cumulative dose in nonrelapsed patients is 200 to 260 mg/m^2 and is below the threshold for risk of cardiac damage. However, some reduction in cardiac function is seen (especially in patients with a young age at treatment, girls more than boys). 2. If there is reduction in cardiac function, then this might be increased during pregnancy and with isometric exercise and cocaine/alcohol misuse. 3. Relapse treatment will give more anthracycline. Total-body irradiation (TBI) and cyclophosphamide will contribute to cardiac dysfunction after treatment.
Growth and pubertal development	1. Cranial radiation is associated with a significant effect on final height due to growth hormone deficiency, abnormal growth, including early puberty, and hypothyroidism). 2. Bone marrow transplant with TBI causes significant effect on growth with irradiation of epiphyses of vertebral column and lower limbs and growth hormone deficiency. 3. There is probably little effect from chemotherapy only ALL schedules.
Pubertal development	1. Cranial radiation for ALL causes early puberty. This is more marked in treated girls than boys. 2. Allogeneic transplant may cause ovarian failure – and will be more marked with chemotherapy-only conditioning (e.g. busulfan and cyclophosphamide). Girls who enter puberty after cytarabine-TBI may subsequently experience premature menopause. Boys after TBI will retain hormonal function of testis. 3. Chemotherapy-only schedules should not affect puberty.
Fertility	Will be markedly reduced or absent after stem cell transplantation – regardless of conditioning regimen. In children treated with chemotherapy, fertility is preserved, and there does not appear to be an effect on subsequent pregnancy or offspring.
Second malignancy	Second malignancy is *not* common – perhaps 5 percent at 10 years. CNS tumors, particularly meningiomas, are the most common, and cranial irradiation is the usual cause. Possible relation with genetic defects in thiopurine metabolism. Risk of AML is low unless etoposide is used at regular scheduling and high dose.

long-term adverse consequences of therapy in cured children.

We contend that there are five areas where progress can be expected to take place in order to achieve these goals:

1. We need to be able prospectively determine children who are going to do well (better biologic definitions of good risk with gene expression profiles, etc.) or who are doing well with therapy (MRD that has been shown to be reliable in allowing treatment reduction) so that good-risk children receive even less treatment. No more children who are cured of their disease should die in delayed intensification blocks.

2. We need to be able to identify those who are going to do badly (better biologic definitions of poor risk with gene expression profiles, etc.) or who are doing badly with therapy (MRD that has been shown to be reliable in predicting subsequent treatment failure) so that appropriate therapy can be offered in first response to children who will later fail that therapy.

3. The benefits of leukemia cell therapy that have been developed in the so-called developed world should be available to children with similar disease in the so-called less developed world.

4. We need to find better therapies for high-risk disease, including defining better the role and strategies of allogeneic stem cell transplantation. Specifically engineered T-cell therapy (e.g. directed at B-cell antigens) of resistant disease has excited much interest in recent years but has yet to become generally available.

5. Basic scientific research into the mechanisms of leukemia needs to be translated into better and more specific drugs in the way that imatinib has transformed the therapy of CML.

Acute Myeloid Leukemia

Key Messages

1. The general considerations discussed in Chapter 36 apply to the newly presenting child with acute myeloid leukemia (AML). Exact diagnosis must be made. Several classifications of AML are used, particularly those of the French-American-British (FAB) and the World Health Organization (WHO).

2. AML arises either *de novo* or is associated with other disorders such as a constitutional bone marrow failure syndrome or previous therapy for another malignancy. *De novo* disease is much more common, but recognition of the latter is important because the prognosis is adverse, and hematopoietic stem cell transplantation (HSCT) will usually be required.

3. The prognosis of AML depends on the cytogenetics, molecular genetics, and response to therapy. There are recurrent cytogenetic and molecular changes that should be sought in the diagnostic material of the newly presenting child with AML. The response to treatment can be determined by microscopy and immunophenotypic or molecular assessments of minimal residual disease (MRD).

4. Remission induction is with chemotherapy containing an anthracycline and cytarabine. Treatment is intensive, and supportive care of infection and nutrition is important. Effective supportive care of this type improves AML prognosis.

5. HSCT is an effective therapy in AML and is employed when the risk is adverse and in relapsed or refractory cases. HSCT is not applied in all cases because of the risk associated with such therapy, including the long-term risks.

6. Special consideration is given to relapsed AML, to acute promyelocytic leukemia, and to HSCT in AML.

7. There are some late effects of AML treatment, and these are discussed specifically.

Introduction

AML is a rare disease with an incidence of about 7 per 1 million children. It is a heterogeneous disease clinically and biologically. In high-income countries, intensive treatment (including HSCT) with effective supportive care has seen the survival for this disease rise to about 70 percent.

There are several key advances in our understanding of the biology of AML that might be expected to translate into furthering our treatment outcomes that have somewhat reached a plateau:

- There are cancer stem cells in AML – leukemia stem cells (LSCs) – that, like normal hematopoietic stem cells (HSCs), are capable of unlimited self-renewal. Such LSCs are rare but are capable of recapitulating the leukemia in an immunodeficient mouse. Such *in vivo* repopulating ability defines LSCs, just as the ability to repopulate normal hematopoiesis in such a model defines a normal, nonmalignant HSC. (Interestingly, the biology of ALL is different, and this disease does not appear to have such an LSC population). This is illustrated in Figure 37.1.

- Genomic sequencing of individual AML cells demonstrates that all cells in AML are clonal, but there may be several clones that are related to each other. Evolved clones will hold the genetic lesions of the parent clone but have additional new lesions. Relapse of AML after therapy may proceed from one of these evolved clones. This is illustrated in Figure 37.2.

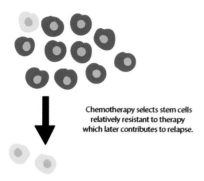

Figure 37.1 The hierarchy of AML recapitulates that of normal hematopoiesis. There is a stem cell fraction and there are more mature cells. The stem cells can give rise to the leukemia when injected into an immunodeficient mouse, while the more mature cells do not have such clonogenicity. They also may be more resistant to chemotherapy, and such resistance might contribute to disease relapse.

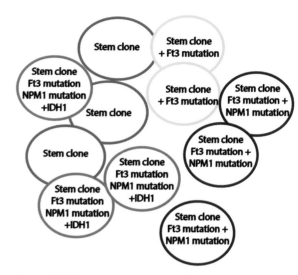

Figure 37.2 There are several genetically related clones in AML. These clones are defined by molecular evolution – here subsequent clones gain mutations in *FLT3*, *NPM1*, and *IDH1*. These additional molecular events in the different clones mean that they may have different treatment sensitivities and contribute differently to relapsed disease than in the presenting disease.

- Such genome-wide analyses define the total genetic, molecular lesions that are present in AML. AML in general and pediatric AML in particular contain relatively few such lesions compared to solid tumors. These analyses have yielded gene mutations that have prognostic relevance, including mutations in *FLT3* and *NPM1*, that are discussed in more detail later.

Some myeloid malignancy in pediatrics is associated with genetic illness or with previous therapy. Predisposing illnesses include the bone marrow failure syndromes, especially Fanconi Anemia, severe congenital neutropenia, and familial leukemia syndromes such as Li Fraumeni and MonoMAC (*GATA2* mutation) syndromes. Therapy-associated AML may follow alkyator agent therapy or radiotherapy, in which the cytogenetics are complex, or etoposide therapy, in which the interval between treatment and leukemia is short and there is translocation of the *MLL* gene on 11q23. Secondary leukemia will need HSCT for cure – chemotherapy alone is not considered sufficient, although outcomes after HSCT are better if the leukemia is in remission.

Diagnosis of AML

The essential diagnostic procedures in AML include

- *Blood film.* The blasts cells of AML are very different from those of ALL, which is the principal differential diagnosis. They are bigger, with prominent nucleoli, and they may have granulated cytoplasm. Auer rods will be diagnostic.
- *A bone marrow aspirate for morphology, immunophenotyping (for standard antibody panel, see later), cytogenetics, and molecular genetics.* Cytochemistry should be done to identify myeloblasts (myeloperoxidase positive) and monoblasts (nonspecific esterase positive). Interpretation of cytochemistry requires experience and should be performed routinely in all leukemia marrows and not just when the diagnosis is difficult so that experience can be gained.
- *A bone marrow trephine.* This procedure might not be diagnostically important in all cases, but it will always be there – archived in the laboratory – so that the diagnosis can always be reviewed if the clinical course, for example, is not as expected.
- *A lumbar puncture.* This can be deferred if there is a coagulopathy at diagnosis. Leukemic involvement is defined as more than 5×10^6 cells/liter, demonstrated on cytospin to be leukemic blast cells. CNS involvement is more common in infants and in monoblastic leukemia.

This assessment should allow a diagnosis of AML according to the FAB classification (Table 37.1). This has no prognostic importance except in its

Table 37.1 FAB Classification of AML

FAB AML type	Description
M0	Morphology and cytochemistry do not allow an AML diagnosis in AML M0, and only immunophenotypic evidence of myeloid differentiation distinguishes AML from other acute leukemias.
M1	Acute myeloid leukemia without differentiation
M2	Acute myeloid leukemia with differentiation
M3	Acute promyelocytic leukemia
M4	Acute myelomonocytic leukemia
M5	Acute monoblastic leukemia
M6	Actyre erythroid leukemia
M7	As in AML M1, only immunophenotyping allows a diagnosis of M7, acute megakaryoblastic leukemia, following the demonstration of platelet markers, CD41, and CD61

diagnosis of acute promyelocytic leukemia (APML). FAB classification is part of routine laboratory hematology and remains a key part of AML diagnosis.

Immunophenotyping in AML

Immunophenotyping of childhood acute leukemia to make a diagnosis of AML can be considered in four separate stages, although frequently in the laboratory these stages will be performed concurrently:

1. A CD45 antibody is used to define the blast cell population better – usually CD45 expression is reduced compared to normal lymphocytes. Once identified, blast cell further analyses are undertaken on this gated population.
2. The core myeloid markers are MPO, CD13 and CD33, and they are expected to be positive
3. A subclassifcation can be undertaken to discriminate different lineage commitments in the different types of AML. More primitive AML (M0 and M1) expresses CD34 and CD117. Monocytic leukemia will express CD64 and cytoplasmic lysozyme. Erythroid leukemia will mark with CD235a, and the markers of megakaryocytic lineage commitment are CD41

and CD61. Note the promyelocytic leukemia is HLA-DR negative in contrast to other AMLs.
4. There should be absence of markers suggesting B- or T-lymphoid commitment.

Cytogenetics and Molecular Genetics in AML

There are recurrent cytogenetic and molecular abnormalities in AML. They are listed in Table 37.2, but the following points should be noted:

- They contribute to the WHO classification of AML. One classification is AML with recurrent genetic abnormalities and includes AML with t(8;21), inversion 16, t(16;16), t(15;17), t(9;11), t(6;9) inv(3) and t(1;22).
- Cytogenetic changes in AML are key determinants of disease prognosis and risk assessment, as discussed in the next section.
- Where there is no cytogenetic change in AML, there is likely associated molecular genetic change. This is a changing field with advent of the ability to sequence the genome of even single leukemia cells. There may be different clones within a leukemia that carry different mutations, and such clonal diversity may underpin disease relapse. AML with mutated *NPM1* and *CEBPA* also forms part of the WHO classification. Some of these mutations, including in genes *IDH1* and *IDH2*, are more common in adult than pediatric AML. Such molecular analysis contributes to disease risk assessment, especially in leukemia in which there is no cytogenetic abnormality.
- There is enormous genetic diversity between the AML of one child and that of the next. Routine evaluation should include evaluation of the relevant selected set of molecular genetic markers after routine cytogenetic evaluation.

Risk Assessment in AML

Treatment intensity is adjusted against disease risk in *de novo* AML. AML that arises after treatment or as part of another condition such as a constitutional bone marrow failure syndrome is always considered as adverse risk. Poor-risk disease is not undertreated, and good-risk disease is not overtreated. Risk assessment is made after consideration of three factors:

263

Table 37.2 Cytogenetic and Molecular Abnormalities Associated with AML in Children

Karyotype	Affected genes	Frequency (%)	Clinical significance
t(8;21)(q22;q22)	RUNX1-RUNX1T1	15	Favorable Not for HSCT in CR1
inv(16)(p13.1;q22) t(16;16)(p13.1;q32)	CBFB-MYH11	10	Favorable Not for HSCT in CR1
-7	N/A	1	Poor prognosis
11q23 • t(1;11)(q21;q23) • t(9;11)(p12;q23) • t(6;11)(q27;q23) • t(10;11)(p12; q23) • Unknown partner	MLL • MLL-MLLT11 • MLL-MLLT3 • MLL-MLLT4 • MLL-MLLT10 • Unknown	20 1 8 1 3 9	Variable, depends on partner • Favorable • Intermediate • Adverse • Adverse • Intermediate
t(1;22)(p13;q13)	RBM15-MKL1	1	Megakaryoblastic leukemia Infants Intermediate prognosis
inv(3)(q21;q26.2) t(3;3)(q21;q26.2)	RPN1-EVI1	1	Adverse
t(6;9)(p23;q34)	DEK-NUP214	1	Adverse
t(8;16)(p11;p13)	KAT6A-CREBBP	1	Adverse
t(16;21)(q24;q22)	RUNX1-CBFA2T3	1	Adverse
t(15;17)(q22;q12)	PML-RARA	8	Diagnostic of APML and not seen in other AMLs Favorable prognosis Not for HSCT in CR1
Normal	Mutated NPM1	8	Favorable except where FLT3 mutation as well
Normal	Mutated FLT3	12	Poor prognosis if high ratio of mutant to wild-type allele
Normal	Mutated CEBPA	5	Favorable prognosis except where FLT3 mutation as well

1. *Cytogenetics.* Certain karyotypes in AML are associated with a good prognosis and some with a poor prognosis. The good prognostic ones include notably t(8;21) and inversion 16 or t(16;16) AML, and these are collectively known as the *core binding factor* (CBF) *leukemias*. The t(15;17) that is found in acute promyelocytic leukemia (APML) is also associated with a good prognosis. The t (1;11) translocation involving *MLL* gene rearrangement is associated with a good prognosis. Cytogenetic alterations associated with an adverse prognosis include monosomy 7, t(6;11), t(10;11) (note the different prognosis with different *MLL* gene rearrangements),and t(6;9).

2. *Molecular genetics.* In cytogenetically normal patients, single-gene mutations of are greater importance. Several genes are of prognostic importance, including *NPM1* (imparts a favorable prognosis), balletic *CEBPA* mutations (good), and *FLT3-ITD* (adverse).

3. *Response to treatment.* The response to a first chemotherapy course is of prognostic significance, not surprisingly. This first course should include an anthracycline and cytarabine, and the response is assessed in three possible ways:

   a. *Morphology.* The clearance of disease blasts after 15 days and disease response and achievement of remission (normal marrow elements, normal cellularity, restoration of normal blood counts) after the first two course of treatment are strongly predictive of outcome.

b. The immunophenotype of the presenting leukemic blasts is significantly different from that of the normal primitive myeloid cells of the bone marrow, and this phenotypic leukemia signature – learned at diagnosis – can be used to detect residual leukemia cells in an apparently normal marrow. This is technically challenging laboratory science, and standardization and quality control are essential. However, it is possible in principle to use such techniques to detect residual leukemia in most pediatric AML.

c. Some AML has fusion genes – t(8;21), t(15;17) – and therefore there are DNA sequences specific to the leukemic clone that can be tracked using polymerase chain reaction (PCR) in the same way immunoglobulin gene rearrangements are used to quantify residual leukemia in ALL. However, such techniques are not applicable in AML patients who lack such rearrangements, and it is well recognized that some leukemia that remains in long-term remission will be PCR positive even after treatment has ended.

Management of AML

There are unanswered questions in AML management. All children should be entered into clinical trials so that they receive evidence-based, best-available treatment and so that these questions can continue to be addressed. AML therapy is both supportive and specific. Many of the advances in AML outcomes have come from advances in supportive care. Children should be cared for in units that have experience in this area. There should be institutional protocols for infection prophylaxis and management (including fungal prophylaxis because neutropenia is deep and prolonged) and for nutritional support. Intensive care should be available. Usually children remain inpatients for many months, and their education must be catered to and attention given to the effects such treatment has on the child and family.

Specific treatment of AML includes remission-induction chemotherapy (one or two courses) and postremission consolidation with either further chemotherapy or HSCT. CNS-directed therapy is important and is with intrathecal treatment. More courses of treatment are given to children with cerebrospinal fluid (CSF) blasts, and usually three drugs (methotrexate, cytarabine, and hydrocortisone) are given at each administration.

AML treatment begins with one or two courses of induction chemotherapy that includes an anthracycline drug (such as daunorubicin 60 mg/m^2 for 3 days) and cytarabine (100 to 200 mg/m^2 continuously or twice daily by intravenous injection). The role of additional drugs such as etoposide and gemtuzumab has not been demonstrated clearly to be beneficial. After such a treatment course, children will be transfusion dependent with no neutrophils for at least 2 weeks.

A risk assessment should be made after the first course of treatment based on the response to that first course and the cytogenetics and molecular genetics of the AML.

- Children in remission with good-risk cytogenetics should be treated with chemotherapy alone. In most studies, two such courses are given after two induction courses. Often high-dose cytarabine (3 g/m^2 given twice a day on days 1, 3, and 5) forms the basis of such treatment. Such courses are better tolerated than induction treatment, but there is still at least several weeks of severe neutropenia and transfusion dependence.

- Children who achieve remission and have adverse cytogenetics [e.g. t(10;11) or t(6;9)] should have allogeneic HSCT during that first remission. Most such transplants in children have been performed using myeloablative chemotherapy (such as busulfan and cyclophosphamide). Radiation has not been shown to be necessary in AML and is generally not employed because there are more significant late effects of treatment.

- Children who have refractory disease should have further chemotherapy and then HSCT. Some patients who continue to be refractory after a second course of therapy proceed directly to HSCT because this therapy can eradicate AML through intensified chemotherapy and a *graft-versus-leukemia* effect.

265

Many patients are in the intermediate group. They are in remission and have neither good- nor poor-risk cytogenetics. HSCT will reduce the relapse risk, but this has not been shown to translate into improved survival in many trials because of the treatment-related risk. This risk has declined with improvement in HSCT technology and donor matching, and its role in AML will be better defined in continuing clinical trials.

Specific Situations in AML Management

Relapsed AML

About 30 percent of children with AML will relapse. The highest-risk time for relapse in AML is in the first year after treatment. For children who suffer AML relapse, the prognosis is related to the duration of first remission (the longer the better) and to the response to reinduction treatment. Usually reinduction treatment is with fludarabine/cytarabine G-CSF (FLAG) treatment to which an anthracycline might be added, including liposomal daunorubicin (less cardiotoxic). For children who achieve remission, transplantation is usual using the best-available donor and with myeloablative conditioning. This conditioning intensity might be reduced for children who have had a previous transplant. For children who do not enter remission, prognosis is poor indeed. Experimental therapeutic approaches may be indicated.

Myeloid Sarcoma

This is a localized deposit of AML in the absence of disease in the marrow. Myeloid sarcoma might be found in the skin, orbits, or testes, and it should be managed as AML is managed with a sequential intensive course of systemic chemotherapy. There is no role for local therapy alone such as radiotherapy, and systemic therapy is always required.

Acute Promyelocytic Leukemia (APML)

APML is morphologically, immunophenotypically, cytogenetically, and molecularly distinct.

- There are classic malignant promyelocytes in the blood and marrow, often with abundant Auer rods.
- These cells are HLA-DR negative on immunophenotyping.
- There is t(15;17)(q22;q21), which is diagnostic of this leukemia.
- There is a novel fusion gene *PML-RARA*. In a small number of APML cases, *PML* is fused to a gene other than *RARA*, and there is variable sensitivity to all-*trans*-retinoic acid (ATRA).
- APML has a dramatic presentation with disseminated intravascular coagulation and bleeding. ATRA administration (25 mg/m^2 per day) corrects this coagulopathy, but in children with a high WBC count it is associated with the APML differentiation syndrome with fever, weight gain, pulmonary infiltrates, and pleural/pericardial effusions. Concomitant chemotherapy will reduce the syndrome incidence. Adult APML is managed with anthracycline, but in children, cytarabine is used with more modest anthracycline doses in order to reduce the cardiac toxicity of a big cumulative dose of such drugs. ATRA is continued. There is an international collaborative protocol for the management of APML in children.

AML of Down Syndrome

This is considered separately in Chapter 6.

Late Effects of AML Treatment

The late effects will depend on the intensity of the treatment applied. For those who have had a myeloablative HSCT, there will be more effects than for those who have been treated with chemotherapy alone. Each treated child should have a long-term follow-up plan for late effects as well as disease surveillance on completion of their treatment.

Cardiac toxicity is related to the cumulative dose of anthracycline received. Routine echocardiography – at completion of therapy and regularly thereafter – should be part of follow-up. Patients with an abnormal echocardiogram should be seen by the cardiology team.

Chapter 38

Juvenile Myelomonocytic Leukemia (JMML) and Myelodysplastic Syndromes (MDS)

1. JMML is a rare myeloproliferative disorder of early childhood with an incidence of about 1 per 1 million children. Few centers will see many cases in a year.

2. JMML is seen at increased frequency in children with certain inherited disorders, such as Noonan syndrome and neurofibromatosis (NF1).

3. Our understanding of the molecular pathogenesis of this condition has increased greatly in recent years, so molecular investigation of newly diagnosed or suspected JMML and screening for mutations in candidate genes have become routine and have increased the sensitivity of diagnosis in this illness.

4. The diagnostic criteria for the diagnosis of JMML have evolved from the previous clinical criteria to include the now-known molecular criteria.

5. Usually, hematopoietic stem cell transplantation (HSCT) is required for cure, although occasionally an indolent and self-limiting course is described, especially in combination with Noonan syndrome. During HSCT, a clear graft-versus-leukemia phenomenon is recognized in JMML. There is little consensus in terms of therapies other than HSCT, but children have received chemotherapy regimens of differing intensities to control the disease, and splenectomy has been performed not infrequently in these patients.

6. MDS is unusual in children and is seen in association with the bone marrow failure syndromes and in children with Down syndrome.

Making the Diagnosis of JMML

JMML is an uncommon malignancy – an incidence of 1 in 1 million – and the diagnosis therefore should be borne in mind when consulting on a child with splenomegaly and a raised white blood cell (WBC) count so that the diagnostic features of the condition can be specifically sought. The condition is more common in children with Noonan syndrome and NF1. Diagnostic criteria have been established and are given in Table 38.1.

JMML can be diagnosed if all criteria of category 1 are met with *either* one of category 2 *or* two of category 3. For the practicing clinician who is considering a diagnosis of JMML, the following should be considered:

Table 38.1 Diagnostic Criteria of JMML

Category 1	Category 2	Category 3
All of the following:	At least one of the following:	At least two of the following:
1. Splenomegaly	1. Somatic mutation in *PTPN11* or *NF1*	1. Absolute WBC $> 10 \times 10^9$/liter
2. Blasts in blood and marrow < 20 percent	2. Clinical diagnosis of NF1 or *NF1* gene mutation	2. Clonal cytogenetics other than monosomy 7
3. Absolute monocyte count $> 1 \times 10^9$/liter	3. Homozygous mutation in *CBL*	3. Hypersensitivity to GM-CSF
4. Absence of Philadelphia chromosome	4. Monosomy 7	4. Myeloid precursors in blood smear
		5. Raised fetal hemoglobin (Hb F)

- Physical examination confirming the enlarged spleen. Many other clinical features may be present, including fever, rash, and lymphadenopathy, but these do not form part of the diagnostic criteria.

- The clinical features of the associated genetic syndromes – Noonan and NF1 – should be sought. In practice, it is usual to refer all children with a suspected diagnosis of JMML to clinical genetics for their opinion.

- The blood smear blasts should be enumerated and the presence of immature precursors specifically sought. Peripheral blood should be sent for hemoglobin F quantification.

- A bone marrow examination should be performed and cytogenetic analysis should be done. The blast count again should be enumerated to exclude acute leukemia. Marrow can be sent for colony analysis to demonstrate hypersensitivity to GM-CSF. This analysis is not often performed, and few laboratories will perform it.

Molecular Etiology of JMML

This is a changing area in hematology. Recently there is more understanding about the molecular etiology of JMML. This is of diagnostic utility to the practicing clinician, and may allow risk stratification of disease to some extent. This is also likely to be an area for future development.

In summary, 85 to 90 percent of newly diagnosed cases of JMML can be shown to have mutations in genes that regulate the *Ras* pathway. When Ras is switched on by incoming signals, it activates 'downstream' proteins involved in cell growth, cell survival, and proliferation, so mutations in *Ras* that constitutively activate Ras are among the most common mutations in cancer.

- The *NF1* gene encodes neurofibrin that negatively regulates Ras. In NF1-associated JMML, the child has inherited one allelic loss of *NF1*, and there is a second loss of the other allele in the tumor (somatic loss of heterozygosity). *NF1* in this way is acting as a classic tumor suppressor gene. *NF1* mutation is implicated in 10 to 15 percent of JMML.

- The most common gene involved in JMML is *PTPN11*, and this mutation is found in 35 percent of JMML. This encodes a protein tyrosine phosphatase, SH2. Germ-line missense mutations in *PTPN11* are found in about 50 percent of

Noonan syndrome patients, in whom is seen a rather indolent JMML that may resolve spontaneously. The acquired *PTPN11* mutations that are seen in JMML are dissimilar and are thought to be 'more transforming,' which would not be tolerated as germ-line events.

- Mutations in *Ras* itself – *NRAS* or *KRAS* – are seen in 30 percent of JMML.

- About 10 percent of patients with JMML have homozygous mutations in *CBL*. In a similar way to *NF1*-mutated JMML, these mutations are thought to be heterozygous germ-line events and somatic loss of heterozygosity.

Clinical Management of JMML

It follows from the preceding that JMML is not a single disease but many different diseases of diverse molecular etiology. Some disease is indolent, particularly in the context of Noonan syndrome. Such disease is the exception, but there are reports of spontaneous resolution of non-Noonan JMML.

Most disease requires HSCT for cure. Registry studies do not make clear whether pre-HSCT chemotherapy regimens favorably affect HSCT outcomes. Such regimens include low-dose schedules such as with mercaptopurine or low-dose cytarabine or are similar to acute myeloid leukemia (AML) treatment blocks in duration and intensity. Similarly, splenectomy has not been shown to influence long-term disease outcomes, although it has been employed in this disease not infrequently historically. In general, chemotherapy and splenectomy might be considered only in individuals with accelerating or transforming disease.

Several statements can be made about HSCT in JMML:

- Usually myeloablative conditioning using busulfan has been employed, although intensive but reduced-toxicity regimens are also employed, and there is no clear evidence of superiority to either approach. Reduced-intensity regimens will be employed rarely in first allografts in this condition.

- There is likely a graft-versus-leukemia effect in this disease, so immune suppression after HSCT probably should be withdrawn early in the absence of graft-versus-host disease.

- Children with disease relapsing after a first transplant are curable with a second procedure, including from the same donor.

- Survival rates are still not great, with published registry survival rates of only just over 60 percent, so there is room for improvement in outcomes in the next years with consensus conditioning regimens, donor selection criteria, and post-HSCT immune suppression protocols.

Pediatric Myelodysplasia

The core features of myelodysplasia (MDS) are bone marrow single- or multilineage dysplasia with peripheral blood cytopenia. MDS is common in adult hematology, but it is a rare disease in children, perhaps affecting only 1 in 10^6 children. Furthermore, in comparison with adult MDS,

- The most common presentation of MDS in children is refractory cytopenia. This is known as *refractory cytopenia of childhood* (RCC). There is rarely isolated anemia, which is more typical of adult MDS, and more commonly bilineage cytopenia. Refractory thrombocytopenia is more common than refractory neutropenia. After RCC, in which there are fewer than 2 percent blood blasts and fewer than 5 percent marrow blasts, there are 'adult-type' refractory anemia with excess blasts (REB) where there are blasts in marrow and blood but insufficient to diagnose AML (i.e. <20 percent) and REB-t (in transformation) (<30 percent blasts in marrow and blood). RCC, REB, and REB-t constitute the World Health Organization (WHO) classification of pediatric MDS and allow classification of most cases.

- The bone marrow is frequently hypocellular, while in adult MDS it is more typically hypercellular. A bone marrow biopsy may better determine the cellularity in suspected MDS.

- The cytogenetic abnormality is most commonly monosomy 7 or deletion of 7q, and trisomy 8 and the loss of part of chromosome 20 (e.g. 20q-) occur next. Adult 5q- is almost unheard of in pediatric MDS.

In considering a possible diagnosis of pediatric MDS, it is imperative to consider that MDS is frequently secondary to a primary condition that may be undiagnosed. The followed should be specifically considered:

- Pediatric MDS is strongly associated with the inherited bone marrow failure syndromes, including Fanconi anemia, Scwachman-Diamond syndrome, amegakaryocytic thrombocytopenia, dyskeratosis congenita, and severe congenital neutropenia (Kostmann syndrome). These conditions and their diagnosis are considered more completely elsewhere.

- The AML associated with Down syndrome (ML-DS) is not infrequently preceded by a myelodysplastic prephase with blood thrombocytopenia.

- It may be difficult to distinguish severe aplastic anemia from hypoplastic MDS.

- There is a heterozygous germ-line mutation in the transcription factor GATA2 in the monoMAC syndrome and Emberger syndromes. In the former, there is monocytopenia, B- and NK-cell lymphocytopenia, increased susceptibility to mycobacterial and papilloma virus infections, pulmonary alveolar proteinosis, and a predisposition to MDS/AML. In Emberger syndrome, the same predisposition to MDS/AML is associated with lymphopenia.

- Nonsyndromic familial MDS/AML conditions are described. These might include mutations in *RUNX1* (*AML1*), *CEBPA*, and *GATA2*. These are rare disorders, and only a handful of such families are described.

Management of MDS is both supportive and definitive. Definitive therapy is with HSCT. The inclination to proceed to HSCT will depend on the severity of the disease and the availability of a matched donor. Thus, the child with asymptomatic cytopenia may not be transplanted, but in progressive disease in symptomatic children, unrelated or even mismatched donor HSCT may be considered.

Chapter 39

Principles of Blood and Bone Marrow Transplantation (BMT) in Pediatric Medicine

Key Messages

1. For any transplant patient, there are five essential considerations: (a) What is the indication? (b) Who is the donor? (c) What is the donor cell source? (d) What conditioning regimen is to be given? And (e) what supportive care after hematopoietic stem cell transplantation (HSCT) is being applied?

2. BMT is used to correct malignant diseases (including leukemia), nonmalignant hematologic disorders (such as hemoglobinopathy), and nonmalignant, nonhematologic disorders (such as metabolic disorders).

3. Each BMT can be understood as four phases: indication, conditioning, donor selection and cell administration, and supportive care after transplantation.

4. BMT is explicitly about risk. The risk of the disease is balanced against the risk of the transplant.

5. There are donor selection criteria. Tissue typing is the first consideration. Tissue type is inherited as a haplotype, and each individual has two haplotypes. The usual typing is at class I (HLA-A, -B, and -C) and class II (HLA-DR and -DQ). Matching is therefore at 10 points.

6. The risk of BMT is reduced in children without major comorbidities and whose donor is closely matched. In general, risk to the patient in BMT comes from conditioning-related toxicity, infection, and graft-versus-host disease. Trying to reduce each of these risks in individual patients makes transplants safer.

7. There are long-term toxicities of BMT, including effects on growth and fertility. These should be taken into account when planning or considering BMT for any patient.

Introduction

The principles that underpin blood and marrow transplantation, more properly known as *hematopoietic stem cell transplantation* (HSCT), in children are straightforward but are sometimes lost in the apparent technical complexity. Transplantation in clinical practice is about balancing the risks of the process against the risks of the disease. The former risks are reduced in advance by correct donor selection, correct and appropriate conditioning therapy, and optimization of patient well-being and performance.

HSCT can be considered as four phases, which are summarized in Figure 39.1:

- *Pretransplant planning*, including consideration of type of transplant planned, indication, and risk balance
- *Conditioning therapy*, including consideration of drugs or radiotherapy, myeloablative conditioning (MAC) or reduced-intensity conditioning (RIC), and use of T-cell-depleting antibodies
- *Stem cell infusion* – donor selection, donor cell source, stem cell product manipulation (e.g. red blood cell depletion), and T-cell depletion
- *Supportive care* – strategies to prevent regimen-related toxicity, infection, and graft-versus-host disease

In more detail, each transplant can be considered in terms of

- The type of transplant
- The indication for HSCT (and the risks of the underlying disease)
- The conditioning process (which enables engraftment of donor hematopoietic stem cells and the types of conditioning used in different diseases)
- Donor selection
- The source of donor hematopoietic stem cells (related or unrelated donors; bone marrow,

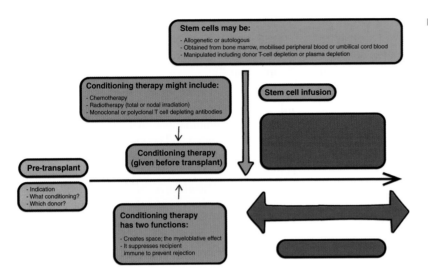

Figure 39.1 BMT process.

umbilical cord blood, or mobilized peripheral blood)

- Graft manipulation
- The short-term risks associated with HSCT
- The long-term risks associated with HSCT

Types of Transplants

HSCT may be *autologous*, in which the patient receives his or her own HSCs – which have been cryopreserved outside the body following a prior harvest procedure – after receiving high-dose chemotherapy/radiotherapy. This is usually part of a treatment protocol for a solid tumor. In *allogeneic* transplantation, the HSCs come from a donor who maybe be related or unrelated, and may be from marrow, mobilized blood, or umbilical cord blood. It will be tissue type matched to the recipient. In *syngeneic* transplant, an identical twin is the donor.

Indications for HSCT

The indications for transplantation fall into three groups:

1. *Disorders of number or function of the recipient HSCs or their mature progeny.* If there are too few recipient HSCs (constitutional or acquired aplastic anemia) or there is a deficient number or function of mature red blood cells (RBCs) (thalassemias, sickle cell anemia), neutrophils (Kostmann syndrome, chronic granulomatous diseases), lymphocytes (severe combined immune deficiency [SCID], hemophagocytic lymphohistiocytosis [HLH] illnesses), or platelets (amegakaryocytic thrombocytopenia, Glanzmann syndrome), then engraftment of normal donor HSCs will correct the underlying condition.

2. *Malignant hematologic disorders.* Most hematologic malignancy is cured with chemotherapy and without transplantation in this era. Transplantation is reserved for patients in whom such a chemotherapy approach has already failed or in whom factors associated with the disease in an individual patient predict for such failure. HSCT may succeed for two reasons:

   a. Conventional chemotherapy dose is limited by bone marrow suppression. During HSCT, the dose of chemotherapy can be escalated because recipient marrow suppression is irrelevant or even desired given that either autologous, stored marrow or fresh, donor marrow is given to restore marrow function after chemotherapy is complete.

   b. The engrafted donor immune system will reject the recipient hematologic tissue, including residual malignant hematologic disease in a process known as *graft versus leukemia*. There is therefore reduced disease relapse following HSCT, where there is graft-versus-host disease (GvHD) and there is greater immunologic disparity between donor and recipient such as following unrelated donor transplant compared with family donor transplant.

271

3. *Inborn errors of metabolism (IEMs).* In certain IEMs in which there is a deficiency of a catalytic enzyme, the transplanted and engrafted donor leukocytes are able to make that deficient enzyme and donate it to the host cells. The most common indication is Hurler syndrome, and the enzyme is the lysosomal enzyme α-iduronidase, which should catalyze the breakdown of heparin sulfate, which otherwise accumulates in the affected child to cause multisystem illness and premature death.

The Conditioning Process

The child receives pretransplant conditioning therapy – known as a *conditioning regimen*. This is usually chemotherapy drugs, but radiotherapy is still sometimes employed, especially in HSCT for acute lymphoblastic leukemia (ALL). Polyclonal or monoclonal T-cell-depleting antibodies may be included in the conditioning regimen.

The conditioning regimen has two functions:

- To *make space in the recipient marrow* into which the subsequently infused donor HSCs can engraft. HSCs are resident within a specialized, physical space (known as a *niche*) in the marrow. This is the *myeloablative* component of conditioning. Without this effect, the niche space remains occupied, and donor HSC engraftment cannot occur. Total-body irradiation and busulfan will each have a myeloablative effect.

- To *immune suppress* the recipient so that the subsequently infused donor HSCs are not rejected. Drugs that are included in a conditioning regimen and that are immunosuppressive include cyclophosphamide or fludarabine. These drugs are not myeloablative. Often antibodies that deplete recipient T cells are given in conditioning too. Such serotherapy includes the monoclonal antibody alemtuzumab and the polyclonal antibody product anti-thymocyte globulin (ATG). Because the half-life of such serotherapy may be considerable, they are likely still present in the recipient circulation after conditioning is complete. Circulating T-cell-depleting serotherapy present in the circulation on the day of transplant will deplete donor T cells and reduce the risk of GvHD that is mediated by those donor T cells. The closer in time to the transplant this serotherapy is given, the greater will be this donor T-cell-depleting action because there will be more circulating antibody. Donor T-cell depletion will both reduce GvHD and delay donor immune reconstitution, increasing the risk of viral infection.

Usually a conditioning regimen that is given pre-HSCT will contain both myeloablative and immunosuppressive agents. Combinations that are commonly used will include busulfan and cyclophosphamide, busulfan and fludarabine, or total body irradiation (TBI) and etoposide or cyclophosphamide. Such combinations are known as *myeloablative* (MAC) *regimens.*

In certain circumstances, MAC regimens are not employed:

1. Where the recipient is HSC deficient, such as in acquired or constitutional aplastic anemia, there is no need for the myeloablative component because the recipient marrow niche space is already empty. In these aplastic anemias, the conditioning regimen contains only immune-suppressant agents.

2. High-dose myeloablative agents have increased toxicities – including long-term toxicities such as infertility – and may not be tolerated. In reduced-intensity conditioning (RIC) transplantation, the dose of the myeloablative agent is reduced to a dose that the patient can tolerate, and engraftment of donor cells is achieved by the immune action of engrafting donor cells that clear the niche space. This is a graft-versus-marrow effect. RIC transplantation is common in adult practice and in children with significant comorbidity – with organ dysfunction or active infection – or those who have been heavily pretreated before transplantation.

Donor Selection

The HSC donor should be closely tissue type matched to the recipient. Usually high-resolution typing is performed at human leukocyte antigen (HLA) class I antigens (HLA-A, HLA-B, and HLA-C) and HLA class II antigens (HLA-DR and sometimes HLA-DQ). At each antigen, the recipient will have inherited two alleles, so matching can be at 10 points. Thus, a well-matched donor will often be referred to as a 10/10 match or 8/8 match (if HLA-DQ is not considered, as it often isn't).

HLA antigens are inherited as a haplotype because all antigen genes of class I and class II are colocated on chromosome 6. Two children with the same parents will therefore have a one in four chance of inheriting the same haplotype from each parent and being tissue type 'matched' to each other. An HLA-identical sibling is the donor of choice in most circumstances, but the following should be borne in mind when considering sibling donors:

- Most patients do not have an HLA-identical sibling because family size is small, and unrelated donors that are well matched have nearly comparable outcome data to the sibling outcome.
- The sibling will have to undergo a bone marrow harvest under general anesthetic and should be carefully assessed medically because this operation, although of very low risk, is in the strictest medical sense not to their benefit.
- Much pediatric transplantation is for genetic disease, and the donor must be clearly shown not to have the same genetic disease. Sometimes such a demonstration may be difficult because the sibling may be younger or the disease manifestations heterogeneous and the gene responsible not known.
- In metabolic disease in which the beneficial effect is from enzyme donated by engrafted donor WBCs, the sibling, if a carrier, may donate less enzyme than a completely unaffected unrelated donor. Patients engrafted from donors with higher enzyme levels have superior outcomes following transplantation.

Unrelated donors are identified through an unrelated donor registry such as the National Marrow Donor Program (NMDP). The closeness of the tissue type match is the most important factor in determining the suitability of a particular donor for a particular patient.

Where several matched donors are available, a younger male donor with the same blood group and the correct cytomegalovirus (CMV) exposure is preferred. For a CMV-seropositive recipient, in whom CMV may reactivate during the immune suppression of transplant, a CMV-seropositive donor is preferred because the engrafted donor immune system will bring immunologic anti-CMV 'memory' to better deal with this reactivated CMV. Similarly, in a CMV-seronegative recipient, a CMV-seronegative donor is preferred so as not to infect the patient with CMV through infused donor leukocytes. Such considerations are always secondary to the tissue type match.

In haploidentical HSCT, a parent donates to the child. There is a match only of the tissue type haplotype that the recipient has inherited from the donor. There is

usually complete mismatch of the haplotype inherited from the other parent. There is an increased risk of graft rejection and of GvHD because of this tissue type disparity. Considering haploidentical HSCT:

- Almost all patients have a donor; – there is no need for a matched family donor, and the expense of unrelated donor identification is also spared.
- The risk of rejection is overcome by using a large cell dose of donor HSCs, usually obtained by peripheral blood mobilization of donor HSCs.
- The risk of GvHD is reduced usually by T-cell depletion of the donor product. This can be done in several ways:
  - Positive selection of donor HSCs from the donor cell product. This is commonly performed as CD34 cell selection. CD34 is an antigen expressed on HSCs. The process is depicted in Figure 39.2.
  - Negative selection of the cells that cause GvHD from the product. CD3 T cells can be depleted or, more recently, alpha and beta CD3 cells can be depleted. This has the advantage of leaving in the graft both HSCs and other cells that might contribute to infection prevention but that do not cause GvHD, such as monocytes, NK cells, and gamma-delta T cells.
- GvHD may also may prevented by administration of post-transplant cyclophosphamide (PTC). This is used increasingly and is attractive partly because it is far cheaper than graft cell selection strategies. PTC is given on days 3 and 4 after the donor cell infusion, and the PTC selectively destroys the alloreactive T cells in the donation that have begun to proliferate in response to the recipient tissue type difference. Antiviral T cells will not be proliferating yet and will not therefore be affected by cyclophosphamide, which destroys proliferating cells.

Stem Cell Source

Donors may donate bone marrow, mobilized blood, or umbilical cord blood (UCB). The advantages of each are discussed next. The cell dose from any source is important. It can be expressed as the number of mononuclear or nucleated donor cells in the product, or the CD34 cell content of the donor product is often given. CD34 is a surface antigen that is expressed on more

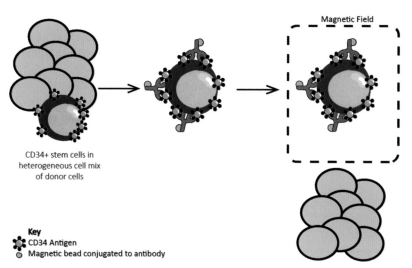

CD34+ stem cells in
heterogeneous cell mix
of donor cells

Magnetic Field

Key
CD34 Antigen
Magnetic bead conjugated to antibody

Figure 39.2 Positive selection of CD34⁺ HSCs from the mobilized donor peripheral blood. The harvest product is a heterogeneous mix of different cell types. CD34 cells are identified and bound by monoclonal antibodies that have attached a magnetic bead. The now-magnetic bound cells are held up and separated in a column within a magnetic field. Nonmagnetic cells including donor CD3⁺ T cells that mediate GvHD pass through the column and can be discarded. The CD34⁺ fraction is eluted as a final stage in the process after the magnetic field has been removed.

primitive blood cells including HSCs. Its expression is determined by flow cytometry. The dose of donor HSCs available for HSCT is different for different donor cell sources (Table 39.1).

Umbilical Cord Blood

The first UCB transplant was performed in 1988 in Paris, and an older sibling had Fanconi anemia. There is increasing use of UCB, which is usually unrelated and cryopreserved in dedicated banks following altruistic and anonymous donation by mothers at the time of delivery. Where a family has a child who requires HSCT and they are expecting a second child, the cord of that child may be harvested specifically for use within the family. This is known as *directed cord*. Where that directed cord blood has come from an embryo selected to both be a tissue type match and to lack the genetic, transplantable disease of the index case, this is known as a *savior sibling HSCT*.

The advantages of umbilical cord blood as a cell source include the following:

- UCB is tissue typed and cryopreserved and so is rapidly available for use in a transplant procedure.
- UCB is taken from all women delivering in certain institutions. It therefore better reflects the current ethnic diversity and tissue-type spectrum of the population than unrelated adult donor registries using volunteer adult donors, where certain ethnic communities remain unrepresented.
- The tissue type match for UCB is less exacting than where an adult unrelated donor is used,

although the better the cord blood match is, the higher is the success rate and the lower is the complication rate. Where adult donors are required to match at high resolution, usually at 9 or all 10 of class I and class II HLA antigens (see earlier), the cord is often selected on less stringent criteria – low-resolution match at class I (and only HLA-A and HLA-B) and high resolution at class II (and only HLA-DR). Thus, tissue type matching for an UCB is often scored as out of 6 tested points rather than the 8 or 10 of an unrelated marrow donor. This permissiveness of mismatch increases the likelihood of finding an UCB donor for a child within an unusual tissue type.

- The cell dose available in the cryopreserved cord blood unit becomes critical. The dose required is related to the match. A threshold of 3×10^7 nucleated cells per kilogram of recipient is usually the minimum for a 6/6 cord and 4 and 5 $\times 10^7$/kg for 5/6 and 4/6 matching cord blood units, respectively. This means that for older and heavier patients, finding large enough matched units may be difficult. Sometimes, in order to overcome this difficulty, 2 units are selected for infusion that are matched to each other and to the patient and that together have a cumulative adequate cell dose.
- Engraftment of donor material is known as *chimerism*. A fully chimeric recipient has 100 percent donor blood DNA in the circulation, whereas in mixed chimerism there is some residual recipient DNA. In graft rejection, there

Table 39.1 Donor Stem Cell Sources

	Bone marrow donation	Mobilized peripheral blood	Umbilical cord blood
Advantages	• Reduced donor T cells in the graft, and less GvHD • Can take from pediatric donor	• No operation required for donor • Large donor CD34 stem cell dose	• Ubiquitously available • Reduced matching; easier to transplant across HLA barriers • Higher rates of donor chimerism in some diseases • Rapid immune reconstitution where no serotherapy • Possible augmented anti-leukemia action
Drawbacks	• General anesthetic and operation for donor • Reduced donor T-cell contamination of graft (less anti-leukemia action) • Limited cell dose (limit to volume of donor marrow) • Contaminating RBCs may need to be depleted when donor and recipient are ABO incompatibilty	• Significant T-cell dose contaminates harvest and increased GGvHD • Difficult to take from pediatric donor – ethics of G-CSF and venous access	• Cell dose is limited especially for larger subjects (can use double cord) • Expensive (especially if using double cord) • Engraftment might be slow
Cell dose	3×10^8 mononuclear cells per kilogram	3×10^6 CD34$^+$ cells per kilogram of recipient	• If 6 of 6 match, then 3×10^7 nucleated cells per kilogram of recipient (increased dose where mismatch)

Note: This table summarizes the advantages of the various cell sources, and these are discussed in more detail in the text.

is loss of donor DNA in the blood and return of recipient material. Chimerism is often higher in UCB recipients than in marrow recipients, and there is increasing interest in the use of UCB in children with difficult or refractory leukemia for this reason because the high chimerism rates reflect the ability of the UCB cells to displace host HSCs, including host malignant cells.

Bone Marrow Donation

HSCs were first harvested from the bone marrow. It remains the only cell source where the donor is a child and an HLA-matched sibling donor (MSD) because it is considered unethical in MSDs who are children to give G-CSF or other cytokines to mobilize HSCs into the blood or to place a central venous line that is usually necessary to support a leukapheresis in small children without good peripheral venous access.

• Bone marrow harvesting requires a general anesthetic, although the procedure is low risk. The volume that can be aspirated is limited – to about 15 ml/kg of donor weight – because healthy donors should not be given allogeneic blood owing to the fact that it is not in their interest to be exposed to any risk associated with such a transfusion.
• Compared with a peripheral blood donation, there are fewer T cells in a bone marrow HSC donation. For this reason, bone marrow is usually the preferred donor source in nonmalignant conditions where GvHD after the transplant confers no benefit to the subject at all.
• A bone marrow will be significantly contaminated with donor RBCs. Where these RBCs are incompatible with the recipient (e.g. a group A donor and a group O recipient), they must be depleted in the stem cell laboratory before the product is issued to the recipient. The RBC depletion procedure is technically quite

challenging and will be associated with some loss of the WBC fraction and the stem cell dose available to the recipient.

Peripheral Blood Stem Cells

In a normal subject, the HSCs reside in the marrow niche, and very few circulate in the blood. Following growth factor administration (usually granulocyte colony-stimulating factor [G-CSF] for 4 days), these resident HSCs are mobilized from that niche space into the blood, from which they can be harvested using a leukapheresis procedure.

- The harvest is more tolerable to the donor than a bone marrow harvest procedure. There is no operation, and there is no discomfort. The growth factor mobilization is considered safe, and adult donors can consent to it. For donating children, blood is rarely used as a donor source because the long-term effects of the growth factor are unknown and therefore not something to which children should be subjected and to which they cannot consent. Furthermore, good peripheral venous access is required. When mobilized HSCs are obtained in children, such as in oncology children, in whom mobilized autologous cells are used to support an autologous high-dose chemotherapy procedure, a central venous catheter is usually placed for this purpose. This is not possible in a healthy pediatric donor.
- The possible dose of stem cells is higher in a peripheral blood procedure. The dose can be expressed as either nucleated cells per kilogram of recipient or as stem cells (HSCs express the antigen CD34 on their cell surfaces). Usually in allogeneic transplantation the nucleated cell dose is 3×10^8/kg of recipient, and the CD34 dose is 3×10^6 cells/kg. For large subjects, this is more readily achieved using mobilized peripheral blood than marrow because a second days' donation could easily be managed and more cells collected.
- There are more T cells in the peripheral blood than in a marrow HSC donation. These may help to drive engraftment in a RIC procedure and may aid leukemic remission via their action in graft versus leukemia and GvHD. For these reasons, blood is often the preferred donor source in certain HSCT procedures.
- There are far fewer contaminating RBCs in a peripheral blood HSC product than in bone

marrow, and RBC depletion is not necessary. Plasma from the product is easily removed when that plasma is incompatible with recipient RBCs (e.g. a donor of group O and a recipient of group A).

Graft Manipulation

The donor cell product may need to be manipulated prior to infusion into the recipient.

- A cryopreserved product may need to be washed of the dimethyl sulfoxide (DMSO) – the agent used to protect cells during freezing. There is a DMSO dose limit for the recipient weight. Washing will remove some donor cells.
- A bone marrow donation might contain RBCs against which the recipient has antibodies. For example, a recipient of blood group O is ABO incompatible with a donor of blood group A. The bone marrow donation will need to be RBC depleted. Some stem cells may be lost in this process, and it requires stem cell laboratory expertise. Peripheral blood donations do not contain sufficient contaminating RBCs. RBCs are lysed during cord blood freezing, and if significant numbers are present, they should be washed before administration to prevent renal injury from hemoglobinuria
- The product may be T-cell depleted or CD34 selected, as discussed earlier, with haploidentical transplant (Figure 39.2).

Risks of HSCT

Complications of BMT are related in general to the conditioning regimen, infection, and GvHD. Different complications are seen at different times after the transplant, and the focus of clinical follow-up of these patients depends on the time from transplantation. The total risk of transplantation is minimized during the BMT planning process and is set against the risk of the underlying disease.

There are risks associated with HSCT, including a risk of recipient mortality. Mortality following transplantation may be due to the original disease or to the transplant itself. For leukemic transplantation, death after HSCT is often considered as either due to disease relapse or to nonrelapse causes.

These risks are explicitly shared with the family and are accepted if they are less than the risks that are posed by the underlying disease. The risk of a transplant procedure is not constant and is reduced when the donor is well matched and the recipient is well (e.g. with good organ function, without active infection, and in remission from the malignancy). Transplants from mismatched donors and into sick children are associated with higher risk and will be performed only when the indication for that transplantation is also associated with higher risk.

Risk from transplantation is generated in three ways – risks from the conditioning therapy, risks from infection, and risks from GvHD. The transplant team will reduce these risks as far as possible.

Conditioning Therapy Risks and Noninfectious Early Complications

Intensive conditioning that is given to damage recipient marrow may damage other organs, including liver, lung, brain, and kidney. Where such organs are already

dysfunctional, the risks of transplant-associated organ damage are significantly greater. In such instances, the intensity of conditioning may be reduced and a RIC procedure offered. The conditioning might be individualized. Busulfan has highly variable pharmacokinetics between children, especially small children. After a given dose, those with high exposure are more likely to experience toxicity, and those with low exposure are more likely to experience graft failure. If the drug pharmacokinetics is measured during the transplant, the dose for that child can then be targeted into the therapeutic window.

A specific hepatic toxicity associated with HSCT is veno-occlusive disease (VOD). In VOD, there is hepatic sinusoidal obstruction, and it is clinically diagnosed by jaundice, tender hepatomegaly, and weight gain with fluid retention as edema and ascites. It is more common with certain conditioning regimens (busulfan with melphalan), when the liver is already damaged, and with certain diseases (osteopetrosis or

Table 39.2 Complications of BMT

	Early complications, weeks	Later complications, months	Long-term complications, years
Conditioning and drugs	• Mucositis (first weeks after MAC transplant) • Veno-occlusive disease, especially with preexisting liver disease and/or MAC transplant • Noninfectious pneumonitis • Graft rejection	• Organ toxicity related to drugs (e.g., renal impairment with tacrolimus) • Transplant-associated microangiopathy • Late graft rejection with autologous recipient blood cell reconstitution (including leukemic relapse)	• Growth • Cataracts • Second malignancy • Puberty • Fertility • Reduced bone mineral density
Infection	• Bacterial infection during early neutropenia • Fungal infection risk related to duration and depth of neutropenia, use of antibiotics, T-cell immune deficiency (including from GvHD and its treatment), and use of steroids	• Virus infection – reactivation (CMV, EBV, adenovirus) during T-cell lymphocytopenia • Fungal infection risk related to duration and depth of neutropenia, use of antibiotics, T-cell immune deficiency (including from GvHD and its treatment), and use of steroids	
Graft-versus-host disease	• Acute GvHD • Skin, gut, liver • For grade/stage, see text	• Chronic GvHD • Other organs including lung • Scleroderma of skin	• Chronic GvHD • Other organs including lung • Scleroderma of skin

HLH). If VOD is expected to be a problem, the conditioning may be changed (away from busulfan/melphalan and toward a RIC) or a prophylactic agent such a defibrotide given.

Risks from Infection

The recipient is immune suppressed so that the donor HSC is not rejected, and there is a period of time before the engrafted donor immune system is fully reconstituted. The time to immune reconstitution will be increased when there is donor-recipient mismatch and when donor T-cell-depleting serotherapy has been given or the graft has been *ex vivo* T-cell depleted. Early after transplant while there is neutropenia, the risk of bacterial infection is highest, and the risk of virus infection is more prolonged because donor T-cell recovery is more protracted and measured in months where donor neutrophil recovery has occurred within the first weeks. The infection risk is managed

- By using prophylactic drugs to prevent herpes simplex virus (HSV) infection, fungal infection, bacterial infection, and *Pneumocystis* infection associated with immune suppression
- By nursing children in HSCT facilities where they are isolated from each other and from many visitors, where rigorous attention is given to cleanliness and to hand washing, and where the air is filtered of fungal spores
- By screening blood, urine, and stool for virus infection (Many virus infections, including CMV, EBV, and adenovirus, are reactivated infections that were previously controlled by a competent recipient immune system. Once that immune system is impaired, the virus returns. There is usually a period of asymptomatic and rising viral load that is quantifiable by PCR before children become sick from the virus. The principle of screening is to identify infection early and treat it before children are ill.)
- Epstein-Barr virus (EBV) infection after HSCT may be associated with B-cell lymphoproliferation. This is known as *post-transplant lymphoproliferative disease* (PTLD). PTLD is more common when T-cell depletion of the donor has been employed. It might present as lymph node or extranodal disease. Since the advent of EBV screening and the early use of B-cell-depleting antibodies such as rituximab when EBV is detected, the incidence of PTLD has declined.

- Effective therapy is given for infection. There are antibiotics for neutropenic fever, antifungal drugs, and cidofovir for adenovirus, rituximab for EBV, and ganciclovir for CMV.
- In the end, infection is only controlled by restoration of the immune system. That immune system restoration may be accelerated when there is infection by reduction of immune suppression or administration of additional donor lymphocytes. There is a balance between accelerated immune recovery that reduces virus and accelerated immune recovery that causes GvHD. At any time and in any patient, that balance may be altered in favor of reducing immune suppression when there is infection or increasing it when there is GvHD.

Graft-versus-Host Disease (GvHD)

Recipient immunity is removed so that the recipient does not reject the donor cells, but engrafted donor T cells can reject the recipient with GvHD. In most HSCT in children, engrafted donor T cells become tolerized within months to the recipient so that all pharmacologic immune suppression can be withdrawn. GvHD may reduce the risks of graft rejection and disease relapse. Acute GvHD occurs in the first months after HSCT and manifests as a skin rash or diarrhea and is graded according to its severity from grade 1 (the mildest) to grade 4 (where it might be life threatening) depending on the number of organs involved and the extent of involvement.

The risk of GvHD is reduced by matching so that the risk is reduced when the donor and recipient are tissue typed matched. T-cell-depleting serotherapy will reduce the number of T cells in the donor HSC donation and reduce acute GvHD, but such serotherapy will slow donor T-cell immune reconstitution and increase the risk of virus infection. Drugs such as ciclosporin and methotrexate are given in the early post-transplant period to suppress T-cell proliferation in GvHD as recipient is recognized as foreign. Such drugs are required until tolerance has occurred.

Acute GvHD is usually treated with intensified immune suppression, including with steroid drugs. In severe disease, monoclonal antibodies directed at cytokines or their receptors may be employed. In a small number of children, the GvHD does not resolve and is chronic. This can affect all organs of the body (extensive) and can be difficult to treat and be associated with a poor quality of life. It is a devastating but fortunately rare complication of HSCT.

Graft Rejection

The engraftment of donor cells is closely monitored. This is usually performed by molecular discrimination of donor-derived versus recipient-derived cells. Highly polymorphic and individual-specific sequences known as short tandem repeats (STRs) are amplified by PCR in this process. Following HSCT, this STR pattern may be fully donor (transplant success), fully recipient (graft rejection), or mixed.

The mixture of donor and recipient cells is known as *chimerism*. Mixed chimerism may be acceptable in nonmalignant disease as long as the donor cell fraction is sufficient to correct the underlying disease (e.g. to achieve transfusion independence in thalassemia). In malignant disease, mixed chimerism will predict disease relapse or recurrence. In some leukemic transplants with mixed chimerism escalating doses of additional donor lymphocytes are given to the recipient after transplant in order to establish full donor chimerism (donor lymphocyte infusion, DLI) and reduce leukemic relapse risk. Graft loss may be more likely following RIC conditioning or when the donor cell dose is small or the donor material has been T-cell depleted, especially *ex-vivo* T-cell depleted.

Long-Term Toxicities of BMT

Post-transplant follow-up has three components:

1. *The early period during which organ complications, infectious complications, and GvHD are identified and managed.* This phase continues until the immune system is fully reconstituted and prophylactic drugs withdrawn. In most patients, all drug therapy except lifelong prophylactic penicillin is withdrawn by 6 months.

2. *Disease-related follow-up.* If the transplant was indicated for malignant disease, the risk of relapse persists for at least a few years after the transplant, and follow-up will include relapse surveillance. If the transplant was for nonmalignant disease, then the engraftment of donor cells will be monitored by donor chimerism to ensure that it is adequate to correct the condition.

3. *Generic late effects associated with HSCT itself.* The conditioning agents, especially in MAC conditioning, may have long-term effects, and the patient should be referred to a specialist so that long-term late effects can be monitored and managed. This clinic is separate from the clinics that will have monitored the first two components. These complications include the effects of HSCT

   a. On growth. This is particularly true when radiation was part of conditioning because there was irradiation of the growth plate. Radiation is much less commonly used in conditioning now.

   b. On bone health, including bone mineral density.

   c. On endocrine function. The use of MAC conditioning will frequently affect gonadal function and pubertal development, especially in girls. Hypothyroidism is increasingly common with time after radiation conditioning.

   d. On fertility. This is likely more pronounced in males than in females.

   e. Second malignancy. This is only ever at all likely after radiation conditioning and is often a malignant brain tumor.

Index